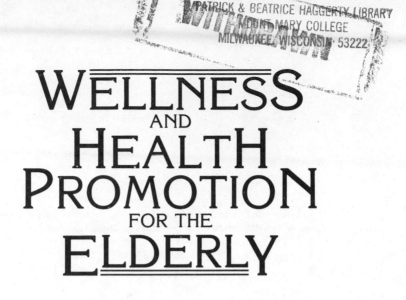

WELLNESS
AND
HEALTH
PROMOTION
FOR THE
ELDERLY

Edited by

Ken Dychtwald, Ph.D.
Dychtwald & Associates
Berkeley, California

Judy MacLean
Consulting Editor

AN ASPEN PUBLICATION®
Aspen Systems Corporation

1986

Rockville, Maryland
Royal Tunbridge Wells

Library of Congress Cataloging in Publication Data

Main entry under title:

Wellness and health promotion for the elderly.

"An Aspen publication."
Bibliography: p.
Includes index.
1. Aged—Care and hygiene. 2. Health promotion. 3. Aged—Care and hygiene—United
States. 4. Health promotion—United States. I. Dychtwald, Ken, 1950-   . II. Aspen
Publishers, Inc.
RA564.8.W45   1985   362.1'9897   85-20150
Hard Cover ISBN: 0-87189-238-3
Paper Cover ISBN: 0-87189-385-1

Editorial Services: Carolyn Ormes

Library of Congress Catalog Card Number: 85-20150
Hard Cover ISBN: 0-87189-238-3
Paper Cover ISBN: 0-87189-385-1

Printed in the United States of America

2   3   4   5

To Seymour Dychtwald

with my deepest love and appreciation for a
lifetime of support and encouragement

Contributors

Sharon Arnold, MSPH
Researcher and Graduate Fellow
The Rand Corporation
UCLA Center for Health Policy
  Studies
Santa Monica, California

Robert N. Butler, MD
Brookdale Professor of Geriatrics and
  Adult Development
Chairman, Gerald and May Ellen
  Ritter Department of Geriatrics and
  Adult Development
Mount Sinai School of Medicine
New York, New York

Nan W. Cisney
Consultant for Pritikin Research
  Foundation
Santa Monica, California

Lawrence M. Crapo, MD, PhD
Associate Professor of Medicine
  (Endocrinology)
Stanford University
Chief, Endocrinology
Santa Clara Valley Medical Center
San Jose, California

James A. Davis, EdD
Research Faculty, Center on Aging
Assistant Director of Experiential
  Learning Programs
University of Maryland
College Park, Maryland

Dr. Ken Dychtwald
President
Dychtwald and Associates
Berkeley, California

Carroll L. Estes, PhD
Director, Institute for Health and
  Aging
University of California
San Francisco, California

Stephanie J. FallCreek, MSW, DSW
The Institute for Gerontological
  Research and Education
New Mexico State University
Las Cruces, New Mexico

Mary Farrar
formerly American Red Cross
New York, New York

Sherry Fox, RN, MA
Associate Professor of Nursing
California State University
Chico, California

James F. Fries, MD
Associate Professor of Medicine
Stanford University Medical Center
Stanford, California

P. Allen Frisk, RPh, MS
St. Alphonsus Regional Medical
  Center
Boise, Idaho

Willis Goldbeck
President
Washington Business Group on
  Health
Washington, DC

Martha Holstein, MA
Deputy Director
Western Gerontological Society
San Francisco, California

Robert L. Kane, MD
Dean
School of Public Health
University of Minnesota
Minneapolis, Minnesota

Rosalie A. Kane, DSW
Professor
Center for Health Services Research,
    School of Public Health
School of Social Work
University of Minnesota
Minneapolis, Minnesota

Donald W. Kemper, MPH, MSIE
Healthwise, Inc.
Boise, Idaho

Anne K. Kiefhaber, BSN, RN
Office of Disease Prevention and
    Health Promotion
Public Health Service
Department of Health and Human
    Services
Washington, DC

Theodore H. Koff, EdD
Director, Arizona Long Term Care
    Gerontology Center
Professor of Management and Policy
University of Arizona
Tucson, Arizona

Joyce Leanse, MPH
Associate Director
National Council on the Aging, Inc.
Washington, DC

Stephanie Lederman, MA
formerly National Center for Health
    Education
New York, New York

Mary E. Longe, MA
Manager, Community Health
    Promotion
Center for Health Promotion
American Hospital Association
Chicago, Illinois

Constance W. Mahoney, MA, MPH
Pew Health Policy Doctoral Fellow
Institute for Health and Aging
Institute for Health Policy Studies
University of California
San Francisco, California

Molly K. Mettler, MSW
Consultant
Healthwise, Inc.
Boise, Idaho

Meredith Minkler, DrPH
Associate Professor
Department of Social and
    Administrative Health Sciences
School of Public Health
University of California
Berkeley, California

Eugene C. Nelson, DSc, MPH
Associate Professor
Department of Community and
    Family Medicine
Dartmouth Medical School
Hanover, New Hampshire

Rena J. Pasick, DrPH
Public Health Consultant and Lecturer
School of Public Health
University of California
Berkeley, California

Kenneth R. Pelletier, PhD
Assistant Clinical Professor
Departments of Medicine and
  Psychiatry
School of Medicine
University of California
San Francisco, California

Nathan Pritikin, DSc
former Director
Pritikin Centers
Los Angeles, California

William Rakowski, PhD
Health Gerontology Program
School of Public Health
University of Michigan
Ann Arbor, Michigan

Ellen Roberts, MPH
Instructor
Department of Community and
  Family Medicine
Dartmouth Medical School
Hanover, New Hampshire

John H. Rutledge, MD, JD, MPH
Deputy Commissioner of Health
New Jersey Department of Health
Trenton, New Jersey

Jeanette J. Simmons, DSc
Clinical Professor
Department of Community and
  Family Medicine
Dartmouth Medical School
Hanover, New Hampshire

Gregory S. Thomas, MD, MPH
Preventive Cardiology Fellow
Harvard Medical School
Massachusetts General Hospital
Boston, Massachusetts

Anne Warner-Reitz, PhD
formerly Director, Healthy Lifestyle
  for Seniors
Health Promotion and Retirement
  Planning Consultant
San Francisco, California

Robin R. Wechsler, MPH
Project Administrator
Tenderloin Senior Outreach Project
San Francisco, California

Philip G. Weiler, MD, MPH
Department of Community Health
School of Medicine
University of California
Davis, California

Table of Contents

            Theodore H. Koff

            Long-Term Care Defined 119
            The Continuum of Care 120
            The Community and Public Policy 129

Chapter 9—Growing Old Healthy: Meeting the Emotional
            Challenges of the Senior Years 133
            James A. Davis

            Senior Life Adjustments 133
            Dealing with Emotional Turmoil 136
            The Truth about "Senility" 137
            Self-Help as a Treatment 138
            The Elderly and the Mental Health System 139
            Conclusion 145

Chapter 10—Worksite Wellness 147
            Anne K. Kiefhaber and *Willis B. Goldbeck*

            Program Initiation 148
            Eligibility 148
            Staff and Facilities 149
            Components of a Wellness Strategy 149
            Evidence of Effectiveness 158
            Worksite Wellness and Older Workers 161
            Conclusion 162

Chapter 11—Fitness and Exercise for the Elderly 165
            Gregory S. Thomas and *John H. Rutledge*

            Aerobic and Low-Intensity Exercise 165
            The Effects of Exercise on the Elderly 167
            Medical Evaluation Prior to Exercise 170
            The Exercise Program 172
            Conclusion 174

Chapter 12—Dietary Recommendations for Older Americans 179
            Nathan Pritikin and *Nan Cisney*

            Nutritional Requirements 179
            Diet-Related Diseases 184
            Food, Nutrient, and Drug Interactions 191

Wellness and Health Promotion for the Elderly: An Overview

Robert N. Butler, M.D.

Our broad conclusion may be stated as follows: As a consequence of a careful multidisciplinary pilot study, we have found evidence to suggest that many manifestations hereto associated with aging per se reflect instead medical illness, personality variables, and social-cultural effects. It is hoped that future research may further disentangle the contributions of disease, social losses, pre-existent personality, so that we may know more clearly what changes should be regarded as age-specific.

If we can get behind the facade of chronological aging we open up the possibility of modification through both prevention and treatment. In our lifetime (if at all) it is not likely that the inexorable processes of aging will be amenable to human intervention but it cannot be too greatly emphasized that it is necessary to be able to recognize those factors which are open to change.[1]

Many years ago, from 1955 to 1966, I had the good fortune to participate in a remarkable study of human aging. During the first phase of this work, I wrote an article that I entitled "The Facade of Chronological Aging" in which I emphasized the possibility of modifying the aging process. I envisioned the facade of aging as rather like an onion; one had to peel back layer by layer those features of the facade that were really accounted for by disease, disability, socioeconomic events, and personality. This approach provided us with an important conceptual and strategic approach to studying human aging and a principle, even a tool, for future altering of the facade of aging. It certainly made very clear that the calendar alone cannot account for what we see in human aging.

As a public health physician—my core identity—it seems so obvious that human behavior can be modified not only through the individiual doctor-patient relationship but perhaps even more effectively through broad social and economic policies. In that sense, politics and medicine intersect.

Organized medicine and individual physicians cannot continue to neglect public health, which perhaps we can label in its modern form as health promotion and disease prevention. The word "doctor" derives from the Latin for teacher. Therefore, I believe that physicians must join with psychologists, nurses, social workers, and other health providers in advancing improvements in health from both the public and individual perspectives.

To accomplish such a goal, of course, requires a continuing growth of the base of scientific knowledge. Our society through its institutions—the executive and legislative branches of federal and local government, as well as the private sector—has devoted very little money to fundamental research and to the prevention of disease. How dollar foolish! The ultimate service and cost-containment strategy is basic research and its applications, which prevent diseases and disabilities from ever developing.

Health promotion for older people comes as a surprise to some people who unfortunately link efforts at health promotion and disease prevention with the earlier years of life. How wrong they are! Indeed, there is much that we can do at this time to encourage three forms of fitness: social, personal, and physical fitness.

By social fitness, I mean the great importance of social networks and support systems in maintaining both the quality of life and even survival. We know from studies of individuals who have lost a loved one that men do not do as well as women, perhaps because of the greater availability of support systems for women. Women may also have greater capacities or have at least exercised greater capacities for human intimacy than men have. Women share grief and admit their concerns, in contrast to the socialized male's "stiff upper lip."

By personal fitness, I mean having a role and a life of substance. We found in our same human aging studies an unequivocal statistical relationship between survival and the presence of definitive goals and an organized daily life.

Finally, there is a physical fitness of which we have all heard a great deal—from good physical conditioning to nonsmoking to proper diet to avoiding the sun. Acquiring and maintaining the habits of physical fitness require the active participation of persons. The use of self-care and self-support groups can be helpful.

We certainly must move more rapidly in expanding both research and health promotion than we have been; we cannot wait until the baby boomers reach "Golden Pond."

NOTE

1. Robert Butler, "The Facade of Chronological Aging," *American Journal of Psychiatry*, 119 (1963): 235–242.

Preface

As America ages, we can look forward to continued advances in life expectancy. However, we are still far from successful in promoting health among our older citizens. Medical advances during the past century have allowed increasing percentages of us to live many more years than our grandparents and parents, but relatively little has been done to ensure that we live out this increased life expectancy with full mental and physical health and vigor.

In fact, almost 85 percent of American's 25.5 million elders suffer from at least one chronic degenerative disease. These diseases, although not necessarily crippling in nature, diminish personal independence and vitality and are a considerable drain on our nation's health care resources. America's elderly are by far the biggest consumers of health care, with spending most pronounced in the older age categories. Although people over 65 comprise less than 12 percent of the population, they account for more than 25 percent of all prescriptions written, 33 percent of all hospital beds occupied, and 30 percent of all health bills paid. If these trends continue, by the year 2000, 50 percent of all health care expenses will be related to the care and treatment of our over-65 population. Although this situation may be perceived as a boon to some health care providers, few responsible professionals would view the overall effect of an ailing aging population as anything but negative.

This dilemma is compounded by the fact that most medical, educational, and recreational services and programs for adults and elders are *not* presently focused on encouraging health, vitality, and self-responsibility. Instead, the typical focus is usually on symptom-oriented treatment, on dependency-producing drug prescription, and on often meaningless, pass-the-time activities. Most important, despite the nation-wide proliferation of health promotion programs, these efforts have largely bypassed the elderly, focusing instead primarily on young persons and those in the work force.

Whereas the nation could benefit profoundly from increased numbers of healthy, long-lived citizens, it could suffer a loss of profound magnitude if its growing older population is ill, functionally dependent, and socially impotent. Whether the trend toward an older America will ultimately be a boon or a drain on the nation is a question that the expanding field of health promotion is becoming increasingly equipped to address. As our understanding of the mind, body, and human aging expands, a growing body of evidence clearly suggests that a great deal of the physical and mental decline so prevalent among older citizens is due not to aging *per se,* but rather to an absence of comprehensive disease prevention and health maintenance strategies.

We are learning that, as the body ages, it requires even more attention to health-promoting behaviors and activities than it did in earlier years. Yet, relatively little effort is made to educate or motivate older persons to achieve the high level of wellness so crucial to independence and an active life style. The assumption is made that older persons are unwilling or unable either to prevent illness or to minimize its effects, let alone to reverse its progression through health-promoting activities. Instead of being offered information, resources, and programs for preventive health care and self-reliance, all too often the older person is only encouraged at most to maintain his or her present status. Yet, the maintenance of health with such limited support is difficult at best.

In recent years, however, in response to several demographic and social trends, such as the age shifts in our population, the change in health focus from acute infectious diseases to chronic degenerative diseases, the recognition of life style and individual behavior as significant factors in the health/disease process, the increasing shortcomings of traditional medicine, and the unbearable economic prospect of maintaining an ailing elder population, there has been a growing national trend toward wellness-oriented health care, disease prevention, and health promotion that has begun to find its way into the world of our over-65 population.

Experiments already underway by hospitals, community and senior centers, YMCAs, American Association of Retired Persons' chapters, Red Cross centers, health clubs, colleges and universities, and at worksites throughout the United States suggest that many of the basic tools and methods of health promotion for younger persons—for example, exercise, proper diet and nutrition, stress management, hypertension control, back care, proper use of medications, wise health consumerism, personal safety practices, and effective health advocacy—can readily be modified to meet the particular problems and potentials of those in older age groups. Preliminary research findings suggest that the elderly not only enjoy the opportunity to take part in such activities but also respond quickly and positively to them.

As we approach the 21st century, the aging of our nation will challenge and shake every aspect of our social, political, economic, and global dynamics. Will we be able to reshape our ailing health care system into a more humane and health-promoting institution? And, most important, can we create a healthy aging America? This will be an issue of mounting concern in the coming years. Indeed it may well prove to be the single most controversial issue in the twilight of this century.

History may even show that, as the primary focus of health care shifts from the diagnosis, treatment, and reimbursement of acute infectious disease to the promotion and maintenance of high levels of mental and physical health, a long, healthy, vibrant life may become the norm of the 21st century. Further, a broadened field of health promotion, including primary, secondary, and tertiary preventive measures, may very well serve as the cornerstone for this development.

In this book, leading researchers, seminal thinkers, pioneering program designers, and key policy analysts have contributed their thoughts, visions, concerns, and assessments of the emerging fields of wellness and health promotion for the elderly. It is hoped that this volume may serve as a timely supportive base from which further ideas and applications might be developed, funded, and put in place to promote further the health and well-being of our growing elder population.

Ken Dychtwald
August 1985

Acknowledgments

I would like to extend a very special thank-you to the following people for their support and assistance in bringing this book to life:

- Judy MacLean, for her sensitivity, intelligence, and masterful editing skills;
- Gloria Cavanaugh and Martha Holstein, my dear friends at the American Society for Aging, who have consistently given me the opportunity to grow and expand my limits in the aging field;
- Gay Luce, for introducing me to the world of aging and for creating the vision for the SAGE project, the first of a generation of wellness programs for older people;
- Maggie Kuhn and Robert Butler, for setting such inspirational personal examples, and for helping to diminish cultural gerontophobia;
- Willis Goldbeck and Rick Carlson, for inspiring me with their integrity and commitment to wellness and social transformation, and for their wonderful friendship;
- Barbara Phipps and Andal Tomas, for their tireless administrative assistance and patience;
- Laurie Bagley, for her brilliant research assistance;
- Darlene Como, Carolyn Ormes, and Betty J. Bruner, my editors at Aspen Systems, for giving this book a home and for their exceptional level of professionalism and publishing vision;
- My terrific friends and family who, incredibly, put up with all of my theatrics and whose support and encouragement nurture me and give me the confidence to move forward: Pearl, Seymour, and Alan Dychtwald, Cayenne Dychtwald, Stan and Sally Kent, Richard and Linda Kent, Frieda Gordet, Anea Neuss, Bill Newman, Jaymie and Barbara Canton, Marc Michaelson and Diane Zinky, Jeremy Tarcher, Frank and Claire Wuest, Don Mankin,

xx   Wellness and Health Promotion for the Elderly

Kenny and Sandy Dorman, Alberto Villoldo, Jesper Juul, Anne Kiefhaber, Phil Polakoff and Nancy Pfund, Mark Goldstein, Marck Rocchio, and Marla Kaye.

- My wonderful wife Maddy, who with her bursting love and enthusiasm has introduced me to the context in which this project and, for that matter, all of my work has fresh meaning and purpose.

Chapter 1

The Aging of America: Overview

Ken Dychtwald, Ph.D.*

Throughout history, the major causes of illness and death have been natural disasters, infant mortality, and a host of infectious diseases such as pneumonia, influenza, tuberculosis, diphtheria, cholera, and smallpox. However, during the past century, as our understanding of health and disease has increased, a series of profound improvements in sanitation and public health has been accompanied by remarkable breakthroughs in diagnostic medicine, antibiotic therapy, and immunization. Together, these advances have nearly eliminated acute infectious diseases as causes of suffering and premature death.

These once-dreamed-of advances have brought about a radical decline in the death rate and a corresponding elevation in average life expectancy. After having risen only slightly during the past seven centuries from approximately 30 years in 1200 A.D. to 45 years in 1880, average life expectancy has vaulted in the past century to a high of 75—69.9 for men and 77.6 for women—and is still climbing (Figure 1–1).

In place of infectious illnesses, there has been a dramatic rise in the incidence of stress- and life-style-related chronic degenerative diseases in the twentieth century. The primary killers are now heart disease, cancer, stroke, accidents, cirrhosis of the liver, and diabetes. These noninfectious diseases, the high incidence of which is more reflective of unhealthy life styles than any other factors, have now become the primary obstacles to high levels of health and long life among our older population.

---

*Ken Dychtwald is a psychologist, gerontologist, author, public speaker, and consultant to government, industry, and media on issues relating to aging, health care, and health promotion. As a leading pioneer in these fields for the past fifteen years, he has played an influential role in creating the vision, the programs, and the motivation for several hundred wellness and health promotion programs for the elderly throughout North America and Europe.

His other publications include: *Bodymind, Millennium: Glimpses into the 21st Century, Stress-Management: Take Charge of Your Life,* and *The Aging of America* (forthcoming).

Figure 1–1 Life Expectancy at Birth: 1000–1980 A.D.

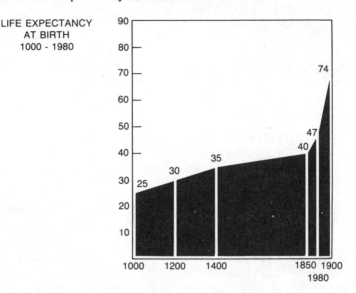

Source: From *Statistical Abstract of the U.S. 1985*, pp. 69, 838, U.S. Bureau of the Census; *Historical Statistics of the U.S., Colonial Times to 1970*, p. 55, U.S. Bureau of the Census; and *Length of Life*, by Louis Dublin et al., p. 42, Ronald Press Company, © 1949.

However, with continued advances in our understanding of the mind, body, and the human aging process, some demographers predict that average life expectancy at birth will continue to rise in the coming decades, approaching 80 or 85 years by the turn of the century. And, as we anticipate a broad variety of breakthroughs in such areas as preventive health care, genetic engineering, biopharmacology, bionics, organ transplantation, and reconstructive surgery, we can envision the time when much age-related physical degeneration and illness will become a thing of the past.

Already, as the war on disease continues to lower the death rate, a larger proportion of each successive generation of Americans is surviving into the later years of life. Until the nineteenth century, less than one in every ten persons ever lived past the age of 65, presently nearly 80 percent of our population can expect to live through most of their seventh decade of life. Moreover, once having reached that age, older people can expect to live considerably longer than their predecessors. For example, the average 65-year-old American man can presently expect to live another 11 years, whereas the average woman can expect to live to age 84.

Thus, as life expectancy continues to increase, the number and percentage of older Americans will continue to grow, especially in the upper age categories.

Whereas our grandparents might have felt themselves fortunate if they lived to age 60, increasing numbers of Americans will be expecting and, indeed, planning to live a long healthy life spanning nine, ten, or more decades.

DEMOGRAPHIC UPHEAVAL

These changes in health care and the resulting increases in life expectancy profoundly influence all aspects of life from the way we dress and how long we work to the way we promote and maintain our nation's health. This age-related population shift, the result of numerous interwoven trends and social undercurrents, is being fueled by three simultaneous demographic events. each one compounding the effects of the others.

Senior Boom

The first element contributing to the aging of America is a tremendous increase in the sheer numbers of older people, as the elderly currently make up the fastest growing segment of the American population.

In 1880, there were less than two million Americans over 65 years old, who represented approximately 3 percent of the population. However, by 1980, with approximately 25 million Americans age 65 or older of a population of 227 million (Figure 1–2)—more than 11.3 percent of the population (Figure 1–3)—the social presence of the elderly had increased significantly. In fact, in the past 100 years, during which the total United States population multiplied 5 times, the over-65 segment of our population multiplied an incredible 15 times. Every day, approximately 3,400 older Americans die and 5,000 Americans celebrate their 65th birthday, leaving a net increase of approximately 1,600 elders per day. Never before in the history of this country have older people made up such a large proportion of the population. And the numbers continue to swell. By 2020, every fourth American could be over 65 years old.

Another more recent characteristic of today's elderly population is that it is increasingly composed of women. As recently as 1930, the number of males and females over age 65 was approximately equal, but since then, female life expectancy has been increasing much faster than that of men, and the survival gap increases with increasing age.

According to the 1980 census, up to age 50, women and men are still approximately equal in number. However, between age 65 and 74, there are only 77 men for every 100 women; between ages 75 and 84, the ratio drops to 50 men per 100 women; and among those aged 85 and older, there are only 44 men per 100 women. Increasingly, then, the issues of old age are also principally issues of women.

Figure 1–2 The Aging of America: Population Growth Aged 65 and Over (in Millions) 1890–1980

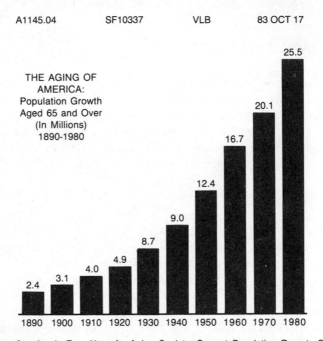

Source: From *America in Transition: An Aging Society,* Current Population Reports Series P–23, No. 128, p. 3, U.S. Bureau of the Census; and *Historical Statistics of the U.S., Colonial Times to 1970,* p. 15, U.S. Bureau of the Census.

The Baby Bust

The decline in the national death rate and the ensuing senior boom made up only one of three major factors contributing directly to the aging of America. It is the balance between the generations at the beginning and end of the life span that ultimately shapes the overall population size, social characteristics, and age distribution.

For example, if fertility rates were to increase, a rise in the number of older Americans, although influential, would nevertheless be counterbalanced by the continued growth in the number of births. With rising fertility and declining mortality, the overall population make-up and the corresponding social characteristics would remain essentially constant, except for a gradual increase in activities, services, and products for older people. In this context, youth would, in all likelihood, still dominate the culture.

However, the United States is presently undergoing an extraordinary change in the sensitive balance between fertility and mortality. Except for the post-World

Figure 1–3 The Rise of the Senior Boom: Percent of the Total
Population 65 and Over

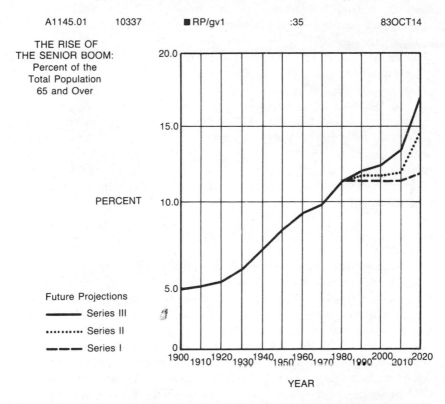

A1145.01   10337   ■RP/gv1   :35   83OCT14

THE RISE OF
THE SENIOR BOOM:
Percent of the
Total Population
65 and Over

PERCENT

Future Projections

———— Series III

·········· Series II

— — — Series I

Source: From *America in Transition: An Aging Society,* Current Population Reports Series P–23, No. 128, p. 3, U.S. Bureau of the Census; and *Population Profile of the United States: 1982,* Current Population Reports Series P–23, No. 130, p. 65, U.S. Bureau of the Census.

War II period from 1946 to 1964 when there was a volcanic boom in the birth rate and 76 million babies were born, the increase in the size and strength of the elder culture has been consistently paralleled by a steady decline in the rate of births. In the years since 1964, sweeping social and cultural changes have caused the birth rate to plummet, which by comparison to the dramatic postwar years of pro-creativity appears to be somewhat of a "baby bust." Whereas the fertility rate was at a high of 3.8 at the 1957 peak of the baby boom, it dropped to only half that figure—1.9—by 1980.

Some demographers and futurists predict that the number of births will swing sharply upward once again, now that so many women of the baby boom generation have entered their prime childbearing years. Thus far, however, this so-called echo effect has not come close to achieving the proportions of a second baby boom and instead appears to consist of a series of lesser baby "boomlets." Although the total number of births has been increasing slightly, due principally to the enormous mass of women of childbearing age, the birth rate and the proportion of young people to the population at large continue to drop consistently.

In fact, the women of the baby boom generation are marrying three years later than their mothers, and a high percentage are not marrying at all, as marriage is no longer considered a necessary ingredient of a normal, healthy life style. Demographers now estimate that as many as 25 percent of the baby boom generation will have no children at all, and another 25 percent will have only one per couple.

Reflecting this life-style shift, in 1980, the total number of Americans under the age of 25 actually shrunk by 650,000, and on July 1, 1983, for the first time in our nation's history, the number of people over age 65 actually surpassed the number of people under age 25. Indeed, the position of the demographic see-saw is reversing, and with it, the exalted position of youth will continue to give way to a new and rapidly emerging *American gerontocracy*.

The Baby Boom: Like a Pig in a Python

The tipping of the population see-saw away from youth toward old age is further compounded by the third force. The World War II baby boom, comprising more than one-third of our total population, is poised between youth and old age.

Even before the baby boom, America had been an increasingly youth-oriented society. When the number of births increased so dramatically in that unusual period from 1946 to 1964, all elements of American culture focused on this huge generation. Never before had the moods, styles, interests, and age-related activities of a single generation of children so completely dominated a nation.

Many social observers predicted that the national obsession with members of the baby boom generation was really a natural love for youth and that their aging would not detract from a long-term fascination with the early years of life. These observers were wrong. The object of interest turned out to be not youth itself, but rather this extraordinary generation. And so, inch by inch, day by day, as the more than 76 million baby boomers grew older, every institution of American culture sought a good position from which to support, service, or otherwise cash in on this energetic population mass.

Yet, the real excitement and the most radical changes are yet to come. In the second decade of the twenty-first century, when the first members of the baby boom generation celebrate their entrance into senior citizenry, there will be born a generation of elders larger and more commanding than any cohort that has ever come before or after. The continued decline in the birth rate, coupled with extended life for the baby boom generation, will swell the ranks of the elderly incredibly. In the coming decades, the planners, policymakers, and product developers of America will, in all likelihood, scramble to refurbish and reconfigure our nation to meet the problems and potentials of the approaching mass of senior boomers.

Similarly, a parallel shift will be taking place within our values and expectations for the future as we begin to conceptualize a full, healthy life span of 90 or 100 years. The opportunities to learn, teach, travel, rest, play, work, love, and be loved will grow more, rather than less, with each additional year of life.

Evidence of the aging of America is already visible and includes the heightened public interest in preventive health and life extension; a bevy of older models and stars in the media; growing concern for the future of Social Security, Medicare, and other age-dependent economic support systems; enhanced interest in leisure and recreational activities for the mature consumer; increasing interest in the older worker and retirement; and a rash of television shows, movies, and magazines focused on the needs, interests, and potentials of middle-aged and older people such as, "Over Easy," "Going in Style," *Prime Time* magazine, and "On Golden Pond."

In addition, scores of organizations and coalitions now exist to give voice to the wishes and preferences of a graying population. Certainly, the emergence of the Gray Panthers as an outspoken national coalition; the swelling of the ranks of the American Association of Retired Persons (AARP) to nearly 20 million members; and the proliferation of professional aging organizations and institutes such as the Administration on Aging, the National Institute on Aging, the Gerontological Society of America, and the National Council on the Aging mark the beginning of this irreversible trend toward the aging of America. Just as 40 years ago, pediatrics was the growing profession, now geriatrics is the field of the future.

TOWARD A NEW IMAGE OF AGING

At this time, our society's images of aging and growing older are still far from positive. These negative images of aging reveal a sad and twisted attitude toward the aging process, reflecting the youth focus and gerontophobia of most of our cultural values and life-style preferences. The profound task we have before us is to transform a youth-focused culture into a healthy nation of middle-aged and older people.

Currently, the impression persists that growing old is a sad and negative occurrence, fraught with loss, poverty, loneliness, sickness, and impotence. We are led to believe that, as we gradually approach our 65th birthday, our circumstances become increasingly desolate, hard to manage, and ultimately unpleasant. And we are certain that when we cross the marker of our 65th year, the road turns downhill, with an ever-increasing slope, racing us quickly toward death.

This point of view is projected by all the institutions and values of our culture. In magazines, popular books, newspapers, and on television, the experience of older people is distorted and discounted, if represented at all. In particular, advertisements seldom portray older people in a positive light, particularly if the product relates to health, beauty, romance, or sexuality. Even many of the magazines and television shows especially designed for the elderly actually use younger people in their advertisements and commercials. The powerful message that is being communicated to all of us each day is that the elderly are not worth writing about; neither are they interesting, beautiful, or sexy, nor do they deserve products created especially for them.

When older people take in this negative image of aging, they cannot help but feel left out and worthless. The message comes through clearly: "You have to be young to be okay."

Not only do negative attitudes toward aging and the elderly limit the opportunities inherent in the full life span but they also degrade and stifle the expectations of the young regarding their own aging process. The popular expression tells us, "You can't teach an old dog new tricks," so as we pass our 30th birthday, we assume that it is too late to start a new career or go back to college. We are told that with aging comes physical degeneration, so we tend to shy away from exercise and the kind of vigorous physical activities that we normally associate with youth. Disease is an inevitable part of aging, we are told, so when our joints stiffen and our muscles atrophy, we naturally interpret this condition as a sad symptom of aging, and not as a reflection of improper self-care. Sexual interest, desirability, and potency fade with the years, we are told, so we come to associate the teenage years with sexual excitation and intimacy and, at the same time, assume that the few older people who are sexually interested or active are "dirty old men and women." We are told that real love is the love of youth, so if we become widowed or divorced, we believe that our lives as lovers are over.

The low cultural priority placed on aging has more than a psychological effect on the elderly. These same ageist beliefs also affect the physical environment as they are reflected in the plans and visions of architects, designers, and city planners. Most environments are tailored to meet the needs and physical capabilities of a youthful body.

For instance, many older people cannot ride public buses because the entrance steps are too high. They cannot attend public events because the transportation is inappropriate, or walkways are too slippery, or the lettering on the exit signs is too small, or the bathrooms are hazardous, or there are no elevators, or there are too many steps, or the rooms are too dark.

The exclusion of the elderly continues across all the other areas of our personal and cultural life. It is remarkable that although there are more than 50 million Americans over the age of 50, there are still less than 100 fully trained geriatric physicians in this country. Even though the elderly are the principal consumers of prescription and over-the-counter drugs, very few pharmaceutical manufacturers test their products on people over 50 years old. Of course, our prejudicial and incorrect belief that older workers are less competent than young workers also serves to fuel this gerontophobic fire.

These factors, coupled with the rise in crime and violence, make it unpleasant and difficult for the older person trying to function as a vital member of the community. The saddest part of this predicament is that only a small, but growing, number of older people consciously realize that we have collectively created a world in which they are not meant to fit. Instead, they pick up and internalize these negative messages and signals, and therefore, where outrage might be an appropriate and reasonable response, too often we see resignation, low self-esteem, and anomie. In some instances, the response is outright self-destruction: The suicide rate for older men is four times higher than that of the overall population.

THE MYTHS AND REALITIES OF AGING

There are a host of erroneous myths and age-related stereotypes that pervade American culture. These myths obscure the truth about the later years of life and ultimately undermine our images and expectations of our potential for vigor and health as we grow older. For a healthy aged America to arise, it is essential that these myths be identified and disavowed.

Myth 1: Old Age Sets in at Age 65.

Absolutely no biological or psychological event occurs on or around the 65th year of life that would mark it as being very difficult from the 5 or 10 years before or after. Yet, if there is no scientific reason for choosing 65 as the year at which to mark a dramatic life transition, where does this number come from, and why must we continue to be so traumatized by it?

The age of 65 first emerged as the measure of the onset of old age in the 1880s when Chancellor von Bismarck of Germany was trying to decide at which age to retire some of his military personnel. In fact, von Bismarck knew nothing of gerontology or the human aging process. In an era when life expectancy hovered around 45 and nearly 90 percent of the world's population could expect to die before reaching their 65th birthday, von Bismarck, with good intentions, felt that 65 was indeed a very advanced point in life.

However, with today's elevated and continually increasing life expectancy, and with more than 80 percent of our population virtually assured of celebrating their 65th birthday, von Bismarck's choice of age has no place whatsoever in the contemporary life-span model. If we were to factor in the elevations in life expectancy that have occurred since the late nineteenth century, a corresponding contemporary marker of old age would be 108 years!

Myth 2: America Has Always Been a Youth-Focused Culture.

Remarkably, our nation was not founded on the premise of the superiority of youth over age. During the early years of our nation's history, it was the elderly who were exalted and given superior status.

In Colonial America, the aged were honored in all social rituals and on all public occasions. Young men and women were expected to treat the elderly with absolute veneration, an attitude of near-religious awe. In return, it was considered appropriate for the elderly to reciprocate with an attitude of condescension, which at that time meant treating one's social inferiors with sympathy, understanding, decency, and respect.

Why were old people so esteemed in Colonial America? One reason was that, according to the Puritan doctrine that was profoundly influential at that time, living to a great age was a sign of God's special favor. Because there were few ways to evaluate the relative value of a person's life and thereby judge his or her spiritual worth, longevity was used as a convenient scale along which to measure one's closeness to God.

Within this context, the elderly were thought to possess highly developed moral faculties. It was commonly assumed that they possessed divine wisdom regarding the secrets of health, happiness, spiritual perfection, and long life.

During this period, old people were expected to remain active in important leadership positions in the community. As long as they were capable of carrying out any of the tasks required to maintain a farm, a home, and a family, no matter how small or minimal those tasks were, the elderly continued working. With limited formal education available, experience usually counted as the best teacher; therefore, those who had been around the longest were the most knowledgeable about farming, home building, food preparation, and other practical matters.

Perhaps more than in any other aspect of early American society, it was in the family that the elderly held absolute authority. Because 90 percent of the businesses were family-owned and run, with farming accounting for the work of about 60 percent of all gainfully employed persons, being the family head was comparable to being the ruler of a small fiefdom. Therefore a fundamental dimension of social control lay in ownership of property, which was usually retained by elder parents until their death. In fact, it was quite common for children to be fully grown with families of their own before any part of their parents' (or even grandparents') property was turned over to them. Not surprisingly, the young people of that time associated aging with a gain in the so-called good things of life. In this agrarian culture, each year of life promised more, not fewer, rewards.

So highly valued was old age that people actually tried to appear older than they really were, the exact opposite of what we see today. Fashions were designed to flatter the old, as men and women hid their hair beneath wigs or powdered it to make it white as if with age. Men's clothing was even cut in a way that emphasized the posture and physique of the elderly; the hips and waists of coats were broadened, and the shoulders were made to appear narrow and somewhat rounded to mimic the posture of the elder.

For the same reasons, in the seventeenth and eighteenth centuries, women hid their bodies beneath their dresses. Only the upper breasts and shoulders, the areas of the body that a mature woman could usually reveal to her advantage, were revealed. Torsos and hips that may have shown the effect of childbearing were covered in large flowing skirts. Similarly, people actually tended to exaggerate their age when questioned by census takers, unlike today, when Americans usually subtract a few years.

Myth 3: Old Age Is a Disease.

As is explained in detail in subsequent chapters, aging and disease, although often intertwined, are *not* the same. Although, through lack of knowledge, many people think that most older people are severely limited by their ill-health, in fact, only four percent of those over 65 years of age currently reside in health care institutions, including hospitals, nursing homes, convalescent hospitals, and mental institutions. This figure is not much higher than the percentage of the institutionalized younger population.

Although vulnerability to disease does increase with aging, it is entirely possible to grow old and live one's entire life in the absence of physical disease and with traces of only the most subtle physical degeneration not appearing until the very latest years of life. Although we are led to believe that the elderly are mostly frail and disabled, in actuality, our nation is already populated by healthy and vibrant elderly individuals who are actively living out their lives with exceptional levels of health and vitality.

In 1982, Walt Stack, the San Franciscan septuagenarian athlete, competed successfully in the Hawaiian "Iron Man Competition." After 26 hours of nonstop output, including a 3-mile rugged ocean swim, followed by a 120-mile bicycle race and a 26-mile marathon run, he could be seen smiling and beer-drinking his way across the finish line with thousands of fans and well-wishers cheering him on!

In fact, some of the most exciting news in the world of sports these days is made by the master and senior athletes of the 1980s. Throughout our country, "Senior Olympiads" are proving that, with a good genetic start and the right frame of mind, proper diet and exercise can keep the body resilient, beautiful, and disease-free throughout the entire life span.

As the negative images of health and aging continue to be discarded, and as we learn about ways to prevent and better treat the illnesses of the aged, we can anticipate a future in which sickness has been significantly diminished, prevented, or postponed. In the coming decades, the current association of age and feebleness or disability may become outmoded.

Myth 4: Old Age Brings Feeblemindedness.

In the late 1800s, an American psychologist, George Beard, reported his controversial findings on how aging affected the mental faculties. Studying the age at which great creative works had been accomplished, he reported that "70 percent of creative works had been achieved by age forty-five, and 80 percent by age fifty."[1] Using vague and highly impressionistic data, Beard concluded that, as people grew older, their mental faculties deteriorated considerably. His conclusions were later totally discredited and shown to be invalid, and no further studies have ever been reported that prove there is any loss of judgment, knowledge, or intelligence that necessarily occurs with age. However, his work fanned the fire of the spreading gerontophobia of that era and began a tradition that has continued to this day. In fact, even now in America, many people assume—incorrectly—that intelligence declines with age. Beard and his followers had quite an important effect on the popular image of aging.

The idea that aging brings feeblemindedness is even further strengthened by the fear that senility looms in everyone's future. The word "senility" has the same origin as the word "Senate"; both come from the Latin "senex" meaning old. The root of the word connoted wisdom and experience, but in more recent years, it has come to be associated with mental degeneration and decline. Although people use the word "senile" to refer to any of a host of disorders such as, confusion, forgetfulness, dizziness, or lack of self-care, in reality, the term has no medical legitimacy whatsoever. In fact, there are more than 100 different conditions, all easily treatable, that can lead to such symptoms, as well as a few serious diseases that do produce the mental deterioration implied by the misnomer senility.

How many of us will actually lose our mental faculties as we grow older? In 1984, a group of young medical students were asked this question. After some discussion, they agreed that approximately 30 to 40 percent of the elderly population experiences signs of so-called senility.

These medical students were very wrong. Presently, of the 25 million Americans over the age of 65, only about 5 percent show serious mental impairment, and only 10 percent exhibit even mild to moderate loss of memory.[2] The odds of age-related brain impairment are slim, and with advances in medical research, they grow slimmer each day.

Recent research into the aging brain has begun to suggest a practical model of how the mind is affected by the aging process. According to Robin Marantz Henig, in *The Myth of Senility:*

The old mind is like an old muscle: It must be used and challenged in order to function well. If housed within four empty walls and left to wither, the mind will indeed atrophy, roaming back into the past when it was put to good use and unable to snap back to the dreary present even when called upon to do so. But if enclosed in an environment that challenges, that stimulates, the mind not only will survive, it will grow.[2]

How would Beard and his more contemporary ageists explain the fact that Goethe completed *Faust* when he was over 80, and Humboldt worked out his great contribution to science, the *Kosmos,* from ages 76 to 90? Michelangelo—sculptor, painter, architect, and poet of the Italian Renaissance—was 71 when he was appointed chief architect of Christendom's greatest architectural undertaking, the St. Peter's Cathedral in Rome. During the next 18 years, until his death at 89, he personally created the vast main body of the church while writing some of his finest poetry in his spare time.

Myth 5: All Old People Are Similar to Each Other.

Considering the elevated life expectancy, alterations in the life cycle, increases in early retirement, and the expanding number of older Americans, it makes no sense to talk about older people as though they were all the same. In fact, the older people are, the more varied in physical capabilities, family background, personal style, life-style preferences, and financial involvements they tend to be.

Our stereotyping of the elderly often leads us to believe that, as people grow older, they come to think and look alike, act similarly, feel the same, and have the same needs. Not only is this point of view incorrect, but it can actually make people uncomfortable about growing older for it suggests that the diversity and individualism we all cherish so much in our early years must come to an end, a thought that would frustrate many of us.

The diversity among America's elderly is great. Some older people are terribly sick and are waiting to die, whereas others are vigorous and are training to run marathons. Some are very poor and depend entirely on government support for food and shelter; others have vast fortunes and assets and travel the world first-class. Some serve on boards of directors of large multinational conglomerates, whereas others wait in breadlines for a warm meal.

Although it is correct that some elderly people have rigid and conservative life styles, others are extremely radical in their behaviors and, in many instances, live freer and more experimental lives than their children and grandchildren. Some of our elderly feel finished with work and thoroughly enjoy the experience of full retirement, whereas others love working and hope to continue at their jobs throughout their entire life span. Although some elderly individuals are lonely and live out their years in quiet desperation, many others belong to clubs and social groups and, in fact, are more socially active than at any earlier point in their lives.

In order to identify, understand, and serve more effectively the needs and problems of America's aging population, sociologists and demographers have recently begun to analyze the aged population in terms of three population segments.

The first of these new age categories, the "young old," corresponds to a new period of life that might be called "middlescence." In 1985, there were approximately 40 million Americans between ages 55 and 75, representing nearly 18 percent of the population. Members of this age group have very little in common with the stereotypical elderly.

The lower age limit of the young-old group is about age 55 because, in recent years, more and more men and women are choosing to retire at around this age, rather than after age 65. The upper age limit is about 75 years because, at present, this age more closely fits the cultural images of what an elderly person is than the current younger standard of age 65. In fact, if one were to take a poll and ask people to describe the average 65-year-old American, their description would probably more closely define the needs and characteristics of a typical 75-year-old person.

The next age grouping is the "old old," whose life experience and age correspond to the period of life we might call "late middlescence." Spanning the years between age 75 and 90, this age group is the fastest growing segment of the American population. With approximately 10 million members, representing roughly 4 percent of the total U.S. population, this age group is multiplying at nearly three times the rate of the overall population.

Finally, sociologists and demographers talk of a third period of life, "senescence," which is comprised of those people over the age of 90. There are already nearly 1 million "seniors," and this age group is expanding at nearly eight times the rate of the total population.

Even more than their younger counterparts, America's elders have a greater diversity in how they behave, what they look and feel like, what they do for a living, how they perceive retirement, and in how they wish to be treated.

Myth 6: All Old People Are Poor.

Although twice the percentage of the elderly are poor as compared to the general population, by far, the majority of older Americans are financially secure. In fact, the percentage of older persons living in poverty as compared to the percentage at poverty level in the general population has been dropping and stabilizing since the enactment of Social Security in 1935.

At present, more than one third of our nation's households—more than 30 million—are headed by a person age 55 or older. By any standard, the economics of the older population are impressive, even staggering. Young-old households headed by a person age 55 or over account for more than 30 percent of the annual income in America. Made up of long-time money savers, these households account for an amazing 80 percent of all the money in savings and loan institutions in the country. Even though most of the products and services in the marketplace have not been aimed at them, the young-old already spend an estimated 28 percent of all discretionary money in the marketplace; this amount is nearly double that available to households headed by persons age 34 and under.

Americans over the age of 65 have a great deal more money and assets than is generally assumed. Although the median income for families headed by persons over age 65 is approximately 60 percent of that for younger households, the per capita after-tax income of these households is actually more than that of the population as a whole.

Generally, as adults pass their child-raising years, they have fewer expenditures on clothing, school, children, and housing. Also, with inflation, the value of long-owned property and valuables rises. Therefore, it is estimated that older persons can maintain the same purchasing power as the young on an income of 65 to 80 percent of their preretirement earnings.

Myth 7: Old People Are Powerless.

In the past five decades, the power and clout of America's elderly have steadily increased so that they are now a population mass with which to be reckoned. According to Dr. Neal Cutler of the University of Southern California's Andrus Gerontology Center, "In 15 years, there won't be anybody as powerful as the organized elderly."

Probably the first major marker of the rising power of the elderly came in 1935 with the passage of the Social Security Act. Since then, the elders of America have played an increasingly active role in securing other aspects of their well-being and in encouraging political and human service groups to assist them in meeting their needs. Milestones have included:

- the first National Conference on Aging, which was sponsored by the Federal Security Agency (then the Social Security agency) in 1950
- the establishment of an Office of Aging and an interdepartmental committee that later became the federal Council on the Aging in 1973
- White House Conferences on Aging held in 1961, 1971, and 1981
- the passage of Medicare and Medicaid in 1965
- the 1965 Older Americans Act, which for the first time established a purpose, structure, and funding mechanism for a federal Administration on Aging to

coordinate efforts dealing with older people's income, housing, legal, health, and social needs

• legislation, passed in 1967, which eliminated discrimination in employment for people between the ages of 40 and 65

• indexing of Social Security benefits to inflation in the 1970s

• the 1972 Supplemental Security Program for the Aged, which provides minimal income

• federal legislation in 1978, which banned mandatory retirement for most workers under age 70

As elders have demanded better mental, physical, and social health care, the fields of research and clinical work with the aged have greatly expanded. Although slow to respond to the needs of an aging America, the medical specialty of geriatrics has now begun to provide medical care targeted at older Americans and their special medical problems. The American Geriatric Society, which had only 400 members when it was founded in 1942, grew to 5,000 members in 1984.[3]

The field of social gerontology has also grown with the aging of America. The Gerontological Society of America had 80 members when it was founded in 1945 and had multiplied to more than 5,600 active members in 1984.[4]

Myth 8: Tomorrow's Elderly Will Be Very Similar to Today's Older People.

With each passing day, the average older American grows healthier, better educated, more politically savvy, more accustomed to life-style change, more mobile, more youthful in appearance, more comfortable with technology, and more outspoken.

For example, today's elderly have less formal education than any younger group. Seventy percent have a seventh-grade education or less, one-fifth are functionally illiterate, and seven percent have had no formal education at all.

In contrast, the generation of Americans currently between the ages of 25 and 34, who will begin celebrating their 65th birthdays in around 30 years, are highly educated. Nearly one half of all 25- to 34-year-olds have been to college, and one-quarter have college degrees. In comparison, only one-fifth of that age group attended college 30 years ago. It is estimated that the percentage of high school graduates over age 65 will increase from 29 percent in 1970 to more than 70 percent in 2010.

Similarly, tomorrow's elderly will have traveled to more places, will have read more books and magazines, will have met more people, will have lived through more world changes, will have experienced more sexual and life-style experimentation, will have lived longer, and will be part of a more powerful "elderculture" than any previous cohort in the history of the world.

The world is changing so fast that each successive generation is, in some ways, light years different from the ones that came before. In the past 50 years, we have entered the atomic age, the space age, and the computer age; life expectancy has increased by more than 15 years; more than 80 new nations have appeared worldwide; and the global population has more than doubled. It is estimated that 75 percent of all the information ever known in the history of the world has been discovered in the past 25 years.

Although our present images of aging are a mixed bag of fears and curiosities, we will soon find that, as America ages, our internal images and expectations will also change and shift to reflect this cultural transformation. And underlying all the changes inherent in the aging of America is the absolute need for our people to grow older with the highest levels of health, vitality, and independence possible. The fields and strategies of wellness, health promotion, and disease prevention can make a significant contribution to this end.

NOTES

1. Tamara Hareven, "The Last Stage: Historical Adulthood and Old Age," in *Adulthood,* ed. Erik H. Erikson, (New York: W.W. Norton & Co., 1978), p. 201.
2. Robin Marantz Henig, *The Myth of Senility* (Garden City, NY: Anchor Press/Doubleday, 1981).
3. Denise S. Akey, ed., *Encyclopedia of Associations, 1985* (Detroit, MI: Gale Research Co., 1984), p. 972.
4. Ibid., 193.

Chapter 2

The Elimination of Premature Disease*

James F. Fries, M.D.
Lawrence M. Crapo, M.D.

Premature death in the United States has nearly been eliminated, and its passing has hardly been noted. Sometimes, progress occurs in such small steps and workers are so close to the problem that they do not realize the task is just about finished. The implications for how we live and die are momentous.

The mass media constantly emphasize the illnesses that remain. We hear of an ''epidemic'' of lung cancer in women. An outbreak of rabies in animals is reported in New Mexico. Gonorrhea is observed to be increasingly common and to appear at ever younger ages. Individuals are struck down by mysterious maladies and die, despite heroic efforts to save them. The adverse effects of our environment on our health are continually emphasized. Entirely new diseases, such as Legionnaire's disease or Lyme disease, are still being discovered. Clearly, these reports demonstrate that we still have illness in our society, but emphasizing the exceptions obscures the rule.

THE DECLINE IN INFECTIOUS DISEASE

Tuberculosis is a typical example of changes in health in the United States in the twentieth century. In 1840, tuberculosis was the leading cause of death, and in 1900 it ranked only slightly behind cardiovascular disease as the major killer. Moreover, tuberculosis affected individuals earlier in life than did the diseases of the heart, the number of years of life lost due to it was higher than that of any other disease at the turn of the century. In 1900, the death rate from tuberculosis was 194 per 100,000 individuals per year (Figure 2–1). By 1925, the death rate had declined by half; by 1940, by half again; by 1950, by half again; by 1955, by half

---

*Adapted from *Vitality and Aging: Implications of the Rectangular Curve* by James F. Fries and Lawrence M. Crapo. Copyright © 1981 by W.H. Freeman and Company. All rights reserved.

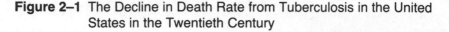

Figure 2–1 The Decline in Death Rate from Tuberculosis in the United
States in the Twentieth Century

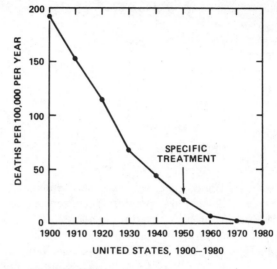

Source: U.S. Bureau of Health Statistics.

again; by 1960, by half again; and again by half in 1970. In sum, mortality from
tuberculosis has decreased over 99 percent in this century! Because of an additional shift of tuberculosis into older age groups, the number of years of life
shortened by tuberculosis has decreased by 99.5 percent. This incredible drop in
the death rate from tuberculosis was due to many factors, including pasteurization
of milk, inspection of cattle, reduction in urban overcrowding, improvement in
national nutrition, and isolation of tuberculosis cases.

Epidemiologists are fond of pointing out that about nine-tenths of the present
improvement had occurred even before the discovery of any drugs that could kill
the tuberculosis germ. Streptomycin was the first such drug, and it was first used in
the late 1940s. Other drugs were developed during the 1950s and 1960s. However,
there is no doubt that availability of these drugs allowed us to consolidate the
previous gains, to treat difficult cases, to shorten greatly and often eliminate
hospitalization, and to achieve a continued decline in the death rate from this
disease.

The United States Department of Public Health regularly publishes statistics on
the major causes of death, almost all of which are included in 14 categories. An
analysis of these categories can highlight past trends and current status.

Of the 14 categories, there have been spectacular mortality declines in 9. Six of
these are now officially listed as zero mortality, meaning that their occurrence as a

cause of death is now less than one in every 200,000 individuals every year (Figure 2–2). Smallpox is eliminated entirely. Paralytic polio, diphtheria, tetanus, typhoid and paratyphoid fevers, and whooping cough have been reduced to negligible levels. Deaths from measles and from streptococcal infections have been eliminated, even though the diseases themselves still occur. Most of these diseases disappeared because of social changes, public health measures, and immunizations. The beneficial effects of curative medical treatment are most obvious with syphilis, which declined dramatically only after the discovery of penicillin and its eventual distribution beginning about 1945. Death from syphilis is today almost entirely limited to the older individual who developed the disease before the antibiotic era, and thus syphilis deaths are now rapidly disappearing. All these conditions have declined over 99 percent, and in some cases, 100 percent!

The only exception to the virtually complete eradication of major infectious diseases is the category of pneumonia/influenza. Here, the reduction has been only 85 percent. However, this statistic hides an equally dramatic result. Pneumonia and influenza deaths now occur almost exclusively among infirm, very old, or already ill individuals. Such deaths, which are attributed to a germ, in fact result from diminished defense mechanisms and lost organ reserve. Deaths from these conditions in otherwise healthy individuals in the early and middle years of life have declined by the same 99 percent as the other infectious diseases.

Figure 2–2 The Decline in Death Rate from Some Acute Infectious Diseases

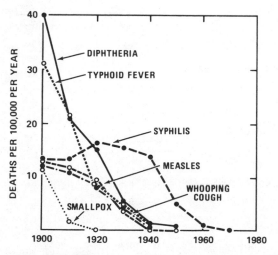

Source: U.S. Bureau of Health Statistics.

THE SHIFTING THREAT TO HEALTH

With the elimination of the acute diseases, other illness categories are now the major causes of death (Figure 2–3). Diseases of the heart and circulation and various forms of cancer have shown the largest increases as causes of death in this century. Diseases of the heart and circulation now account for over half of all deaths, and cancers account for about half the remainder.

The major reason for this increase is not an epidemic; rather, it is a result of the success in virtually elminating infectious diseases. Survival from the diseases that used to kill early in life allowed the illnesses that occur later in life to increase in frequency as a cause of death.

Figure 2–4 shows the major illness categories that have not declined. Among them, a new major cause of death has appeared in this century that is of considerable interest. In 1900, there were a very small number of motor vehicles and no deaths from motor vehicle accidents. The rate of accidental death increased

Figure 2–3 Changing Pattern of Mortality in the United States

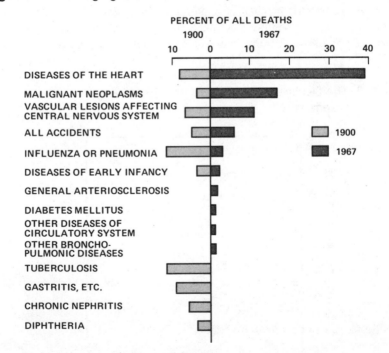

Source: Redrawn with permission from Donabedian et al., *Medical Care Chartbook,* Fifth Edition, Bureau of Public Health Economics, University of Michigan School of Public Health, 1972.

Figure 2–4 Increased Mortality Rates from Chronic Diseases and Accidents

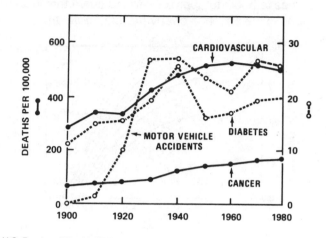

Source: U.S. Bureau of Health Statistics.

substantially as more and more people drove automobiles; motor vehicle accidents now rank third nationally as a cause of death. Even more important, such accidental deaths occur mostly at young ages. Their effect on decreasing the quality and quantity of life is nearly equivalent to cardiovascular disease in terms of years of life affected.

THE SHARP DOWNSLOPE OF NATURAL DEATH

The elimination of premature disease in the United States in this century is reflected in the sequence of human survival curves shown in Figure 2–5. At the 50th percentile, it is obvious that the median age at death is higher for each successive period; people are living longer and longer. Far more important, however, is the change in the shape of the curve. In 1840, deaths occurred at a nearly constant rate throughout the natural life span, after a high death rate in the first year. In 1900, there was still a high rate of infant mortality, but the curve was beginning to bend slightly upward. At later time periods, the first part of the curve becomes flatter and flatter, and the last part becomes steeper and steeper. The curves for all years converge at about the same point, with very little difference among eras as the tail of the survival curve is reached. The curve is becoming rectangular. The ever-sharper downslope represents the barrier to immortality; it illustrates graphically the upper limit of the natural human life span.

Figure 2–5 Sequential Survival Curves in the United States. The
progressive elimination of premature death allows these
curves to begin to approximate the curve that would be
found in the absence of any premature death.

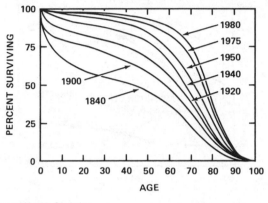

Source: U.S. Bureau of Health Statistics.

Implications of the Rectangular Curve

The rectangular curve is a critical concept, and its implications affect each of
our lives. This curve is not a rectangle in the absolute sense, nor will it ever be. Its
changing shape results from both biological and environmental factors.

Many biological phenomena follow what is often called a normal distribution
along the familiar bell-shaped or Gaussian curve. If one studies the ages at death in
a well-cared-for and relatively disease-free animal population, one finds that the
ages are distributed on both sides of an average age of death, with the number of
deaths decreasing in frequency in both directions as one moves farther from the
average age at death. If one plotted a theoretical distribution of ages at death in
humans, it would take the shape of the curve shown in Figure 2–6. This simple
bell-shaped curve, with a mean of 85 years and a standard deviation of 4 years,
might exemplify the age at death of an ideal, disease-free, violence-free human
society. The sharp downslope of the bell-shaped survival curve is analogous to the
sharp downslope of the rectangular curve.

Therefore, the rectangular curve has an initial brief, steep downturn because of
deaths shortly after birth; a very slow rate of decline through the middle years; a
relatively abrupt turn to a very steep downslope as one nears the age of death of the
ideal Gaussian curve; and a final flattening of the curve as the normal biological
distribution of deaths results in a tail after the age of 90.

A society in which life expectancy is believed to increase at every age and in
which one becomes increasingly feeble as one grows older is a troubled society.

Figure 2–6 Ideal Mortality Curve in the Absence of Premature Death. The average death occurs at age 85, with a standard, deviation of about a year. Ninety-five percent of all deaths occur between the ages of 77 and 93.

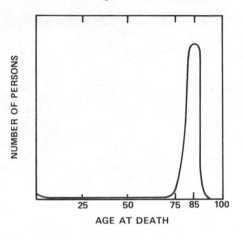

Source: U.S. Bureau of Health Statistics.

Yet, society moving according to the curves of Figure 2–5, as our society is, is moving toward a world in which there is little or no disease and individuals live out their natural life span fully and vigorously, with a brief terminal period of infirmity. The social implications of this shifting pattern are discussed in later chapters; here the authors intend to indicate its origin. Dramatic changes in mortality patterns result in equally dramatic social changes.

The Ideal Human Life Span

The concept of the ideal human life span can now be explored. As the curves of Figure 2–5 are extended yet a few more layers, we reach the top curve of Figure 2–7. The resulting natural or ideal curve has an average age at death of 85 years. With the assumption that violent death will still occur, the ideal curve will have a slow early decline, with the form shown in Figure 2–7. The precise shape and location of this curve may be calculated statistically in several ways using existing knowlege of mortality trends and the knowledge of the limits to the life span already discussed. Figure 2–8 provides data for such calculations.

Since 1900, in terms of years of life saved, we have already progressed the great majority of the distance toward this ideal curve. Disregarding traumatic and violent death, progress in eliminating premature death since 1900 has, by 1980, removed about 80 percent of the area between the ideal curve and the 1900 curve.

Figure 2–7 Ideal Survival Curve Resulting from the Elimination of Premature Disease in the United States. By 1980, over 80% of the area between the curve for 1900 and the ideal curve had been reduced.

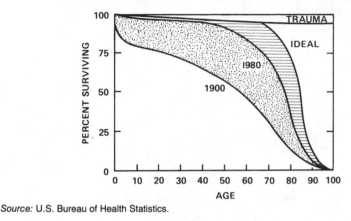

Source: U.S. Bureau of Health Statistics.

Moreover, the greatest change has occurred in the earlier years of life; most remaining premature death is concentrated in the years over age 60 and is due to chronic illnesses.

These changes are dramatic. In 1900, the average individual died 38 years prematurely; in 1950, the average individual died 17 years prematurely; and in 1980, the average individual died only 12 years prematurely. White females in 1980 died on the average only 7 years short of the theoretical limit. Of the remaining years of average premature death, three of them are accounted for by violent death. Clearly, the medical and social task of eliminating premature death, from this point of view, has been largely accomplished.

Another way to look at the natural life span is to consider trends in life expectancy. This is a slightly different statistical representation and is shown in Figure 2–8. The average length of life in the United States has increased from approximately 47 years at the turn of the century to over 73 years today, an increase of more than 25 years. Life expectancy for white females is now 78 years and, for white males, 70 years. The steady rise in life expectancy in the early years of this century leveled off to a relative plateau after about 1950, but the increase has resumed over the past 6 or 7 years. These data, shown as the top line of Figure 2–8, are familiar to many people, and they serve as the basis for predictions about the increasing numbers of individuals over age 65 in our population as the result of previous baby booms and for often erroneous projections of the type and number of medical facilities needed in the future.

A critical look at these data, however, shows that the increase in life expectancy results from the elimination of premature death, rather than the extension of the

Figure 2–8 Change in the Life Expectancy in the United States during the Twentieth Century. From birth, life expectancy has risen from 47 years to 73 years. In contrast, from age 75, the increase has been only from 8 years to 11 years. The greater the age from which life expectancy is calculated, the less has been the improvement.

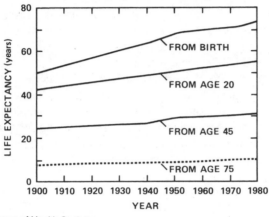

Source: U.S. Bureau of Health Statistics.

natural life span. When life expectancy is calculated from particular ages, the higher the age, the lower the increase. From age 40, life expectancy has increased relatively little. From age 75, the increase is barely perceptible. Beyond the age of 85, an increase cannot be confidently determined at all.

A few uncertainties with these data should be discussed, although the arguments above do not depend on them. The human life span might not be absolutely fixed, but rather might be slowly increasing, perhaps as much as a month or so each century. The data are consistent with the possibility of such an increase. Also these estimates should not be construed too literally. There will always be some illness and accidental and violent deaths. Also, there will be some point of diminishing returns beyond which our medical care delivery system will make it very hard to move farther toward the ideal life-span. However, there is the potential to reduce greatly the mortality from the currently leading causes of death, and the authors expect that, during the next several decades, there will be continued progress toward the ideal rectangular curve.

CHRONIC DISEASE

To develop strategies for decreasing mortality from chronic disease, one must first understand the nature of these illnesses. There are striking parallels among the major chronic diseases, and there are striking differences between these and the previously formidable acute diseases. There also exists a third class of major diseases, which are neither acute nor encountered by most individuals.

A chronic disease has characteristics far more important than duration, and definition of chronic in terms of time has little value. Although "duration greater than six weeks" or similar expressions often have been used to define chronicity, the authors suggest that more important insights are that these diseases tend to (1) be incremental, (2) be universal, (3) have a clinical threshold, and (4) be characterized by a progressive loss of organ reserve. In many ways, these diseases are similar to normal processes of gradual loss of function with age, but the disease processes cause such loss to occur at an accelerated rate.

These universal conditions—perhaps universal is a better term than chronic— begin relatively early in adult life. They start with minor changes in the cells of a particular organ, gradually cause microscopically visible damage, progress until they can be determined in presymptomatic form by various tests, and eventually emerge as disease symptoms in the patient. From this point, the process continues as a set of worsening symptomatic problems and eventually culminates in disability or death.

The most important chronic disease, atherosclerosis, serves as an example of this process (Figure 2–9). Atheroma can be detected at autopsy following accidental death in many 20-year-olds and by x-ray arteriograms in many asymptomatic individuals in their thirties and forties. Both the development of atherosclerotic plaques on the inside walls of arteries and another process, the fibrous-tissue scarring of medial muscular arterial coats, begin in early adulthood. As the artery becomes narrower and the wall itself becomes more rigid, the passage of blood becomes more difficult. Higher blood pressures may be required to force blood through the passage, and the higher pressures may increase the rate of damage to the arterial walls. Passing platelets may adhere to the damaged areas, and clots (thrombosis) may occur, completely blocking the blood flow. If the clotted artery supplies a critical body part, death or severe symptoms may occur instantly at the time the clot forms. If the process has developed in a single location, such as, the left anterior descending coronary artery—the "artery of sudden death"—then death can occur, even though the rest of the arteries have not been compromised. If the process has progressed relatively evenly in many arteries, the first symptoms may be those of inadequate circulation, such as, chest pain (angina pectoris), intermittent leg pain (claudication), or abdominal discomfort. Sometimes an aneurysm (ballooning) of the aorta may cause the first symptoms, and sometimes hemorrhage from a damaged artery into the brain is the first manifestation.

The sequence depicted in Figure 2–9 is of course greatly oversimplified. The actual events underlying arterial degeneration are more complex and often controversial. They include development of atheromatous plaques (atherosclerosis), high-blood-pressure-associated lesions in the smaller blood vessels (arteri-

Figure 2–9 The Clinical Course of Atherosclerosis. Atherosclerosis may progress relatively evenly, or it may result in a sudden catastrophic event such as heart attack or stroke. Both the decrease in vessel caliber and flow and the probability of catastrophe proceed incrementally and progressively. The other major chronic illnesses show similar progressions.

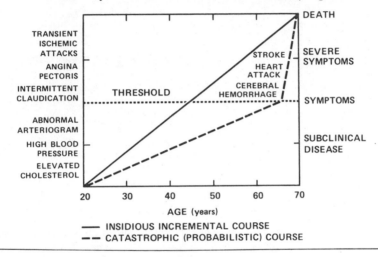

olosclerosis), degeneration of the medial layer of the arteries, and an increase in fibrous tissue with a decrease in elasticity that appears to be age-related. Conceptually, however, problems with arterial reserve illustrate well the principles underlying universal incremental illness. The process long antedates the first symptoms of disease. The clinical threshold may be passed either abruptly, as with a heart attack or stroke, or slowly, as with the several syndromes of arterial insufficiency and their associated pain due to oxygen starvation. As the disease progresses, the time at which the first irreversible symptom will be felt comes nearer, and the probability of a sudden catastrophe increases. These principles are expressed to some degree in each of the major chronic illnesses (Figure 2–10).

Unseen passage toward illness or the probability of catastrophe can also occur in diabetes, cancer, osteoarthritis, emphysema, and cirrhosis, as well as numerically less important diseases of other organs. The parallel progressions are listed in Table 2–1. For example, in noninsulin-dependent (Type II) diabetes, one may initially detect elevated fasting blood glucose; sugar in the urine, followed by diabetic complications of the eye, nerves, and kidney. With osteoarthritis, first the joint cartilage has different staining characteristics; later, a narrowed joint space and some bone spurs can be seen on x-ray. Precancerous states show irritated and aberrant-appearing cells. The preemphysematous lung first loses some alveolar septal walls, and the patient manifests difficulty in expelling air with normal flow

Figure 2–10 The Clinical Course of Chronic Disease. The universal, chronic diseases begin early in life, progress through a clinical threshold, and eventuate in disability or death. An important strategy for their control is to alter the rate (slope) at which they develop, thus postponing the clinical illness or even "preventing" it.

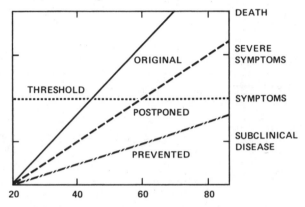

rates. The precirrhotic liver first enlarges, with fatty infiltration and inflammation. In each of these conditions, many people with the early stages never progress to the later stages during their lifetimes, and many people do not progress smoothly through all these stages. Yet, the conditions, often influenced by environmental or self-induced insults to the organ, can be considered schematically to be universal. Only the rate of their development is different in different people.

Each of these conditions is manifested in accelerated loss of organ reserve—in the arteries, the joint cartilage, the lungs, the liver, and the organs that are the sites of the various cancers. These are the major illnesses of today.

Some important, long-lasting diseases without these characteristics constitute a third group of conditions that are neither acute nor universal. Examples of this third group are Hodgkin's disease, ulcerative colitis, insulin-dependent (Type I) diabetes, rheumatoid arthritis, psoriasis, multiple sclerosis, muscular dystrophy, and schizophrenia. These conditions are not universal, they are not incremental in the same sense, and they act much more similarly to acute illnesses. That is, it often seems as though one may "catch" them, they spontaneously disappear on occasion, they may reverse impressively after medication or surgery, or in some instances they may even be cured. These conditions do not parallel the natural aging process, and thus they are not included in the classification of chronic, universal diseases.

Arteriosclerosis is hard to classify, as it is not universal in all countries. Arterial degeneration, referring broadly to loss of elasticity, in the vessel wall and development of fibrotic change, probably is a universal condition.

Table 2–1 The Increments of Chronic Disease

Age	Stage	Atherosclerosis	Cancer	Osteoarthritis	Diabetes	Emphysema	Cirrhosis
20	start	elevated cholesterol	carcinogen exposure	abnormal cartilage staining	obesity	smoker	drinker
30	discernible	small plaques on arteriogram	cellular metaplasia	slight joint space narrowing	abnormal glucose tolerance	mild airway obstruction	fatty liver on biopsy
40	subclinical	larger plaques on arteriogram	increasing metaplasia	bone spurs	elevated fasting blood glucose	X-ray hyperinflation	enlarged liver
50	threshold	leg pain on exercise	carcinoma in situ	mild articular pain	sugar in urine	shortness of breath	upper GI hemorrhage
60	severe	angina pectoris	clinical cancer	moderate articular pain	hypoglycemic drug requirement	recurrent hospitalization	ascites
70	end	stroke, heart attack	metastatic cancer	disabled	blindness; neuropathy; nephropathy	intractable oxygen debt	jaundice; hepatic coma

This distinction between chronic, universal conditions and other long-lasting diseases is critical, even though it is arbitrary; some workers might classify certain diseases differently. Regardless of classification differences, three points hold: (1) Currently, the universal diseases are by far the greatest health problem in the United States. (2) The best strategy for control of the chronic diseases that represent accelerated aging is to attempt to slow the rate of their progression. (3) The medical tradition of searching for primary cure remains particularly appropriate for long-lasting diseases, but not for universal diseases.

We do not know the aggravating or risk factors for all universal diseases, and thus we cannot assume that all such diseases may be affected by environmental changes. For example, some cancers, such as, cancer of the prostate, are not reliably associated with modifiable factors. Currently, a popular estimate is that about 50 percent of cancer is already known to be due to hazards in the environment, either personal smoking, industrial pollution, alcohol, medications, coffee, or other substances. Some of the remaining 50 percent of cancer cases may also be environmentally caused. Yet, the chronic diseases for which we strongly suspect causes in the environment or personal behavior greatly outnumber those for which we do not.

The major health problem, then, is the universal, chronic, incremental, accelerated loss of organ reserve, occurring under many disease guises, which we call by different names and which affect different organs. The solution is to postpone these diseases—not to "cure" them, but to slow them down. For most such diseases, we already know how to decrease the probability of occurrence, the incremental growth, or both. We have identified the risk factors, and from these we are able to formulate a strategy for better health.

Strategy

If the rate at which universal diseases progress can be slowed, then the time of their clinical appearance can be delayed; that is, the time when the symptomatic threshold is passed. If we sufficiently delay this passage, symptoms will not develop during the natural life span, and the disease will have been "prevented." Actually, the disease process will not have disappeared, but its accelerated characteristics will have been lost, and from the standpoint of the affected individual, it is as if it never occurred.

Figure 2–10 shows the nature of prevention in these conditions. The process is slowed, not prevented, and the clinical threshold is postponed, not prevented. However, because of our finite life span, this process appears as though it were actually prevented.

Chronic disease is postponed by removing those risk factors associated with acceleration of the process. There are a number of well-established risk factors, and the success of this strategy has been shown with many but not all of them. The risk factors include cigarette smoking, excessive alcohol consumption, excessive body weight, excessive consumption of fatty foods, inadequate exercise, exposure to environmental toxins, inadequate use of mature psychological defense mechanisms, and living in the psychological state of helplessness, without options for major life choices and decisions.

The Role of Personal Choice

Removal of many of these risk factors requires personal choice, and the very process of making the choices may itself have positive health benefits. To a large extent, society shapes the choices of the individual. Societal incentives have often ignored health consequences, as in the subsidization of tobacco crops and incentives that have fostered a litigious society. Our personal choices are influenced by many factors, and society should ensure that individuals are encouraged to make decisions that improve health.

Moreover, concerted effort is required to minimize many of the risk factors that threaten health. Drunken driving penalties, air pollution standards, mandatory protections from toxic chemicals, and objective information sources for the consumer are part of a rational strategy to improve health. The individual in our modern democracy has a voice and a vote, but often faces powerful special-interest lobbies, so that political campaigns are often necessary to achieve even self-evident consumer improvements.

One may ask whether strategies based on behavioral change and personal choice have any likelihood of success. Often, we hear of disappointing results from such efforts. The failure of national antismoking campaigns, the lack of medical success with treatment of obesity, the recalcitrance of alcoholism, and the inability to change teenage driving habits are frequently cited as evidence that "you just can't change human nature." These observations, however, arise from misplaced expectations and impatience, rather than from accurate analysis. Changes indeed have been slow, but signs of improvement can be seen.

For example, there have been substantial changes in smoking behavior in the 15 years since the first Surgeon General's report on the harmful effects of cigarette smoking. Per-capita tobacco consumption has decreased by 26 percent, and cigarettes with less tar and better filters account for a greater proportion of total tobacco consumption. Among college-educated persons and young adults, the changes have been greater. And for those closest to the data—physicians—the percentage of smokers has declined from a large majority of 79 percent to a small minority of 14 percent.

There has also been a decline of about one-third in per-capita consumption of saturated fats. We have a five-pound leaner national body weight per person, despite a slight increase in the national average height. Aerobic exercise programs have been adopted in school athletic programs, and the national road running phenomenon is too obvious to need much mention; there are now some 30 million joggers.

In making health projections, we should expect that these changes will be reflected in greater well-being, but they will only affect the rate of development of universal disease after the lag period required for intervention. Thus, lung cancer in men should peak in frequency in the early 1980s and will then decline slowly, the decline from the peak frequency being greater than the 26 percent decline in per-capita cigarette smoking. Emphysema statistics should follow a similar curve. For women, the peak of the curve will be reached about five years later, but the same decline will follow. We are currently reaping the bitter harvest of increased cigarette smoking by women, and it will be a few years before the recent decreases are fully reflected in the frequency of disease above the threshold. At present, the decline in cigarette smoking in both men and women is accelerating, giving hope that the ultimate effect will be far greater than can be presently projected. Yet, a 25 percent decrease in the two major chronic lung illnesses still will represent a spectacular achievement.

The prospects are even better for arterial disease. For the first time, improvement in a progressive universal illness has been recorded. The incidence of all cardiovascular disease has declined steadily over the past decade. Age-adjusted overall mortality from ischemic heart disease declined by 20 percent between 1968 and 1976. The decline in cerebrovascular disease, including strokes, has been the most marked, with about a one-quarter decrease. There remains controversy about the cause of this great improvement, with advocates of diet, exercise, decreased cigarette smoking, and improved treatment of hypertension all willing to receive the credit. No single factor seems to explain the decline very satisfactorily, and it seems likely that a combination of influences has been important. Yet, the improvement is there; change is possible.

The Compression of Infirmity

Given the preceding definition of our major health problem and the probable effectiveness of the remedial strategy, we can now look at the results that are likely to be obtained if a systematized effort to reduce health risks is undertaken. The most obvious result is the postponement of chronic, universal illness itself. Figure 2–11 shows this phenomenon for an individual. On the top line, the present occurrence of illness over a typical lifetime is portrayed. A serious disease, such as pneumonia, might occur early in adult life. If the person survives, a later illness, such as heart attack at age 50, might occur. Survivors of such episodes move farther along their lifeline to other diseases, such as, emphysema, stroke, and lung cancer. Finally, the survivors of all these illnesses reach the time of natural death.

Notice the effect of increased survival from premature illness in unmasking the later diseases. The individual may have several illnesses, and they are much more

Figure 2–11 The Compression of Morbidity. The ability to postpone chronic disease, taken together with the biological limit represented by the life span, results in the ability to shorten the period between the clinical onset of chronic disease and the end of life. Infirmity (morbidity) is compressed into a shorter and shorter period near the end of the life span.

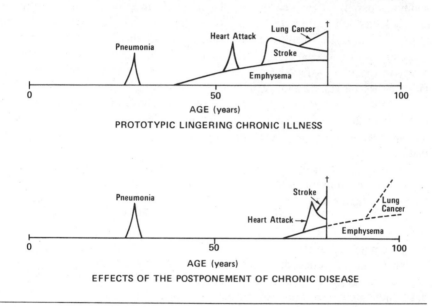

likely to be chronic, expensive ones, rather than brief, acute ones. Illnesses occur more frequently with age, and several may coexist at once. The exchange of acute disease for chronic illness and the increase in the average life expectancy have resulted in a dramatic increase in medical costs and in an increase in the number of years of impaired health per person. Lingering illness has become much more common in our society than in previous years.

A dramatic reversal, however, is about to occur. A phenomenon that the authors term the "compression of infirmity" will appear as the postponement of chronic illness continues. If the maximum life span is fixed, then as the age at onset of illness increases, the period of illness must become shorter. Illness will then become less lingering, not more. The bottom line in Figure 2–11 shows this effect. With chronic illness delayed—in some cases, so delayed that the illness will not occur within the life span—the period of adult vigor is prolonged.

Moreover, illness at the end of the life span will prove more refractory to treatment, more inevitable, less possible to cure, and increasingly less reasonable to treat. As we evolve toward these illness patterns, there should be an acceleration of the already visible trends toward living wills, hospices, home care, and generally more humane attention to the dying. If society responds to these opportunities in a rational way, there should be need for fewer medical services, less intensive care for the terminally ill, fewer hospitalization days, and decreased national medical costs.

The authors have emphasized the progressive nature of chronic disease for an additional purpose: to make clear that the effect of illness on the quality of life is closely linked to its effect on the duration of life. Disability precedes death, and infirmity is linked to death over a period of slowly increasing disability. The consequences of this linkage are predictable. As the mortality curve becomes nearly rectangular, a hypothetical morbidity curve must also become more rectangular. Rectangularization of the curve representing the end of the period of adult vigor, not only the curve representing the end of life, must occur. The rectangular curve implies that living longer than the maximum species life span is not possible; but it also implies that it may be possible to live well until the end of that life span.

Figure 2–12 shows the life expectancy in 1950 and an ideal projection. This ideal curve is simply a different representation of the rectangular curve; both represent a population of individuals. As the curves shift to the right, all individuals live longer. However, life expectancy increases more for earlier ages than for later ages; life expectancy from age 20 increases more than does life expectancy from age 70 or 80.

Over the next decades, the difference in increases in life expectancy from birth and from age 70 will not be nearly as apparent. The great majority of premature deaths now occur over the age of 60, and most occur over the age of 70. The typical

---

Figure 2–12 The Shift in Life Expectancy. Life expectancy increases at all ages, but the increase becomes less with advancing age.

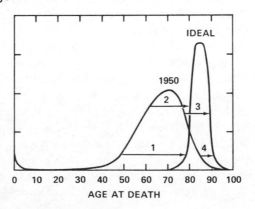

individual in an ideal society would live 10 or 12 years longer than at present, and most of these additional years would be lived following age 70. So, life expectancy from age 70 will increase as chronic disease is postponed and almost as fast as life expectancy is increased from age 20. Life expectancy from 80 or 85 will increase also, although very much less. Life expectancy above age 90 will remain nearly constant, but it still will increase slightly. Already, the decline in cardiovascular deaths in the last few years is having these effects on life expectancy.

There is another way to look at this critical phenomenon. At the turn of the century, death occurred at an average age of 47, after an illness of only a few days. Less than 1 percent of the average life span was spent in terminal illness. Gradually, with the emergence of chronic disease, this figure has increased, so that a terminal illness taking up 10 percent or more of a life span is not unusual. With the compression of infirmity, this percentage will again begin to decline.

CONCLUSION

Disease need not necessarily be a prolonged part of the aging process. The average human life span is fixed at approximately 85 years. Our current greatest health problem is the prevalence of chronic, universal diseases, which account for a relatively long period of infirmity toward the end of life. Although there is little hope for cure of these diseases through the traditional medical model, the onset of these diseases may be postponed through modification of risk factors, many of which are possible to control, either personally or socially. As the onset is delayed to older ages and approaches the limit of the human life span, we can envision a society where everyone can expect to live in vigorous health to close to the average life span and then die after a brief period of illness.

Chapter 3

Health Promotion and the Elderly: A Critical Perspective on the Past and Future

Meredith Minkler, Dr.P.H.
Rena J. Pasick, Dr.P.H.

Recent concern with health promotion and disease prevention in the elderly provides a sharp and welcome contrast to the traditional medical model approach to the health needs of this nation's fastest growing minority.[1] At the same time, however, many current health promotion programs carry their own set of biases and assumptions that bear careful examination.

Several major problem areas in existing health promotion programs are addressed in this chapter. First, the micro- or individual level focus of many of these health promotion programs provides a smokescreen for other structural problems that often underlie unhealthy behaviors and life styles, especially among the elderly poor. Second, the narrow selection of appropriate change targets frequently has the effect of ignoring the critical role that providers, decision makers, and other segments of society can and should play in helping to create environments conducive to health. Third, the "youth bias" inherent in many health promotion programs leads to the relative neglect of the elderly as a potential target group. Finally, major limitations in research and evaluation contribute to the slow development of effective intervention in health promotion for the elderly and other groups. Based on the interrelationships among these issues, a broader conceptualization of health promotion, one more responsive to the needs of older Americans, is suggested.

INDIVIDUAL LEVEL FOCUS

Health promotion programs for the elderly, as for other groups in society, have to date tended to focus on the isolated individual as the appropriate target for behavior change efforts. By implicitly suggesting that health and disease are largely determined by individual behavior choices, these programs deflect attention from some of the basic sociostructural factors that heavily influence individual health practices. Poverty, racism, sexism, and ageism, occupational hazards, and environmental pollutants—all of these "social pathogens"[2] are ignored by many current health promotion programs.

In short, the focus of current health promotion on individual *responsibility* for health is not accompanied by a focusing of attention on individual *response-ability*[3]—the capacity for responding effectively to one's personal needs and challenges posed by the environment. Response-ability for the elderly may involve such diverse issues as the acquiring of skills in self-management of a chronic illness, increased access to transportation or to a broad array of community-based programs and services, involvement in a supportive network conducive to health maintenance and health promotion, or the nursing home resident's being encouraged and enabled to engage in personal decision making to the maximum extent possible. On a more basic level, individual response-ability necessitates and implies a minimum level of economic health, without which efforts at health promotion may be fruitless. For the 36 percent of the elderly Americans living at or near the poverty line,[4] ensuring economic health must be considered a fundamental prerequisite to more conventional health promotion efforts.

Ironically, many current health promotion programs for the elderly do describe, as part of their *raison d'être,* the multifaceted problem of aging in American society. However, following an often sobering account of the parameters of the problem—for example, high rates of poverty, inadequate housing, and social isolation—such programs focus almost exclusively on helping individual elders adjust creatively to losses by learning to "manage" stress and develop effective coping mechanisms in other ways. Their emphasis is not on attacking the underlying causes of poverty, ageism, deprivation, and social isolation, but rather on facilitating coping and adjustment to these and other problems as if they were immutable givens.

Major components of such programs, including health monitoring, nutrition, exercise, and stress management, emphasize such objectives as increasing participants' ability to improve their diets, to exercise, and to cope effectively with stress. Although often quite comprehensive in their discussion of the specifics of desired behavior changes, however, such programs, as noted earlier, focus only minimally on the need for structural changes in the underlying social conditions that keep so many of the elderly impoverished, socially isolated, and otherwise disadvantaged.

For example, elders are told of the importance of walking, but not how they can *safely* walk if they live in high-crime, inner-city neighborhoods. They are told what nutritious foods to eat, but not how to afford them if they are living on small, fixed incomes. Most disturbing of all, they are taught to identify and to manage stressors in their lives, but generally are not encouraged or helped to work individually or collectively toward the eradication of the root causes of stress.

Such approaches to health promotion remove the individual elder from the context of his or her environment, implicitly suggesting that the onus for and possibility of health promotion rest with individual life-style choices over which the individual has almost unlimited control. It is in this spurious assumption that the unintentional victim-blaming of such approaches often lies.

The importance of differentiating between unhealthy individual behaviors and the root causes of those behaviors is shown in Table 3–1. For each of six major health promotion areas, this table first lists conditions associated with aging that are most widely regarded as alterable, most likely to have adverse health outcomes if not altered, and considered most amenable to behavioral intervention. The second row of Table 3–1 lists the behaviors most frequently targeted for intervention in efforts to reduce the conditions in the first row. Although alleviation of these specific conditions could serve not only to prevent disease but also to promote health, vigor, and well-being, these objectives cannot be realized if the underlying causes of the behaviors and conditions go unchecked. The third row, which lists several such causes, demonstrates that intervention into environmental causes requires an entirely different level and type of effort than that which is traditionally devoted to behavior change. The sources and consequences of ignoring the underlying causes of health problems are examined in greater detail in the research and evaluation section of this chapter. As fundamental causes of health problems, these underlying environmental and related factors must be directly confronted not only by policy makers and city planners but also by health professionals concerned with the creation and maintenance of environments conducive to health promotion.

Several of the health promotion programs described in later chapters of this book do combine a focus on individual health behavior with broader efforts aimed at helping elders bring about changes in their physical, social, and political environment. The Seattle-based Wallingford Wellness Project described in Chapter 14 thus works to increase the responsibility of elderly participants with a strong emphasis on environmental awareness and advocacy training. Similarly, the Tenderloin Senior Outreach Project (TSOP) in San Francisco (Chapter 20) has involved inner-city elders in crime reduction efforts in their neighborhood through the establishment of several dozen "Safehouses" or refuges where community residents can receive immediate aid in an emergency. Through the mechanism of weekly support/social action groups, elderly TSOP members also have attacked the problem of malnutrition, establishing a senior-run minimarket and beginning to develop cooperative food purchasing clubs to increase food access and affordability.

Such programs as these differ greatly from those health promotion efforts that focus solely on life-style choices in such areas as diet and exercise by assuming a level of response-ability that many elders in our society are effectively denied. By

Table 3–1 Immediate/Behavioral and Underlying/Environmental Causes of Alterable Health-Related Problems Associated with Aging

	Nutrition	Smoking	Stress Control
Alterable Conditions Associated with Aging	Reduced calcium absorption Loss of lean body mass Loss of bone mass Inadequate levels of Vitamin K, Vitamin D Muscle weakness and tetany Hypertension Obesity/overweight Impaired glucose tolerance Hypercholesterolemia (low level of high density lipoprotein) Osteoarthritis	Decreased standard pulmonary function Respiratory inefficiency Irregular drug metabolism Decline in body weight Reduced bone mineralization Reduced muscle strength Loss of taste capacity	Isolation/loss of social support Reduced self-esteem Decreased sense of control/dependency Depression Sleep disturbances
Immediate/Behavioral Causes	Inadequate caloric intake Little variety in diet Lack of knowledge of proper nutrition Over-consumption of processed foods Inactivity Drug therapy Alcoholism Salt added to foods Excessive food consumption Consumption of high fat/high caloric density foods	Cigarette smoking Cigar smoking Pipe smoking	Retirement Bereavement Poor health Inactivity Other stressful life events Lack of coping skills

Underlying Causes			*Misuse of Alcohol and Drugs*
Dietary adequacy declines with income and with illness Apathy toward food due to loss of social context for eating Difficulties in food preparation Lack of transportation to food supplies and eating centers Cultural influence Marketing and food production Appetite stimulation from drug Disability/illness	Socioeconomic status Personality dimensions determined by heredity Addiction to nicotine Influence of smoking relatives and friends Mass media Sex role	Cumulative poverty Poor housing Poor transportation Institutionalization Negative cultural attitudes Crime victimization Mass media portrayal of the helpless elderly Age discrimination at work Status and role change	Use of multiple drugs at once Addiction to drug Use of too much drug Use of too little drug

Alterable Conditions Associated with Aging	*Accident Prevention*	*Exercise and Fitness*
	Osteoporosis Muscle weakness Impaired coordination Gait disturbance Depression/apathy Loss of confidence Impaired vision/hearing Decline in posture control Arthritis Increased reaction time	Reduced muscle strength Reduced muscle endurance Loss of lean body mass/increase in body fat Poor posture Reduced coordination/agility Reduced joint mobility Reduced balance Reduced cardiorespiratory endurance Reduced tendon strength Reduced flexibility Loss of bone mass Hypertension Reduced oxygen intake Obesity Anxiety and depression Reduced reaction time/decreased thinking ability

Table 3–1 continued

	Misuse of Alcohol and Drugs	Accident Prevention	Exercise and Fitness
Immediate/ Behavioral Causes	Incomplete/inaccurate/inappropriate diagnosis by physician Lack of physician familiarity with geriatric pharmacology, physiology, psychology Depression/stress Chronic pain User's lack of information on appropriate drug use and possible side effects Prescription of confusing and extended drug regimen Drug side effects Impaired activity and dexterity	Insufficient dietary calcium Inactivity Drug therapy Cardiac arrhythmia Organic mental disorder	Inactivity Lack of knowledge on necessity for exercise and what constitutes safe and sufficient exercise
Underlying Causes	Ageism in medical care Cost of drugs/poor insurance coverage Social isolation	Substandard living conditions related to poverty Reduced estrogen from time of menopause in women Inattention to safety hazards in interior design Insufficient maintenance of building interiors Poor lighting Lack of safety features such as ramps and handrails Inattention to specific needs of elderly in pedestrian accident prevention	Loss of social stimulus Shrinking peer group/isolation Retirement Disability Fear of crime Negative image of elderly Lack of stimulating activities and environment

Source: Adapted from *Health Promotion for the Elderly: A Critical Perspective* by A. Pardini, R. Pasick, and P. Franks, Aging Health Policy Center, University of California, San Francisco. Report prepared under Administration on Aging Grant #90–AP0003, 1984.

considering the social context within which health-related decisions are made, such programs as TSOP and the Wallingford Wellness Project may make inroads toward solving the root causes of the problems they seek to address. Moreover, they may avoid the inadvertent victim-blaming that occurs when programs operate as though the individual is personally responsible for health problems that in reality are often caused, or exacerbated by, forces over which he or she may have little control.

TARGET GROUP SELECTION

The individual behavior change focus of most current health promotion efforts has resulted in a narrow defining of target groups that is counterproductive to improving the health of our society. By focusing disproportionately on the individual elder as the target of educational programs, for example, health promotion efforts for older Americans have tended to ignore the often critical role that policy makers, care providers, the media, and other segments of society can play in helping to create health-promoting environments. To ignore that role is not only to render narrowly focused health promotion efforts less effective but also to suggest implicitly that substantial individual-level change can be achieved without concurrent health-promoting changes in the broader sociocultural environment.

Although numerous examples could be cited of the need to expand the targets of our health promotion efforts for older Americans beyond the individual elder, the following instances illustrate the point.

Policy Makers

For 15 years, Medicare and Medicaid have been the nation's largest health care reimbursement systems. Yet, the focus of both programs has remained steadfastly on disease, rather than health, and on acute, institution-based care, rather than on prevention and community-based alternatives to institutionalization. Until policy makers can be convinced to "shift gears" on these programs so that they begin to reimburse adequately for services and programs conducive to preventive health maintenance and health promotion, it is unlikely that such services will receive the attention and support necessary for their effective implementation.[5] Such change can best be achieved through pressure from an informed public and the professional community.

Health Care Providers

Effective health promotion for the elderly is not likely to take place without substantial changes in the attitudes, interest, and knowledge base of providers working with older persons. A prominent focus on the elderly should be included in the education of physicians, dentists, pharmacists, nurses, and other health professionals. In addition to studying such areas as nutrition and the elderly and the physiological changes with age, health care providers should be helped to appreciate the goal of reducing functional dependency in the aged and should, as part of their training, become acquainted with the various community and other social supports that might be called on in helping meet that goal.

Transportation Systems

For many older persons, access to transportation can mean the difference between functional independence and dependency. Both improved public transportation and more affordable private transport—for example, lowered taxi rates for seniors who rely heavily on this means of transportation—are needed to facilitate general mobility and to enable older persons to gain access to other health-promoting services and programs. Volunteer transportation services, such as those provided through the Retired Senior Volunteer Program (R.S.V.P.), also should be encouraged and facilitated (e.g., by the adoption of policies providing reimbursement for fuel for those elders, often on fixed incomes, who provide this service).[6]

Food Manufacturers

Numerous researchers have documented problems of inadequate nutrition among the elderly, particularly among those living alone.[7] Although many factors, including depression-induced apathy toward food and inadequate income, may contribute to this problem, the multibillion dollar food industry also must bear part of the responsibility. Food manufacturers need to be made aware of the demographics of aging and to be persuaded to produce nourishing, acceptable foods in small packets or containers and at prices affordable to the elderly on fixed incomes. "Campbell's" low sodium, one-serving soups, developed for and advertised to the elderly, provide a good example of movement in this direction, but much further progress is needed.

Mass Media

Television in the United States is more heavily watched by the elderly than by any other age group. Yet, with the notable exception of some public education and cable network programming and of such programs as the recently discontinued "Over Easy," little television programming is directed specifically at this age group. Great Britain is experimenting with the provision of nutrition and fitness information on radio and television directed at the elderly. In the United States, such efforts would be a welcome supplement to the heavy advertising of laxatives, arthritis remedies, vitamin supplements, and other products geared at an older audience that are not always conducive to wise health care decision making. Additionally, and of at least equal importance, such efforts as those by the Gray Panthers "Media Watch" committee to end the negative portrayal of the elderly in television programming, films, music, and greeting cards should be considered a critical health-promotion activity geared at this important and influential target group.

THE "YOUTH BIAS"

Victim-blaming and focusing on the individual are not the only problems with health promotion programs. They also tend to have a built-in youth bias and, indeed, often equate being healthy with being young or youthful. Frequently, such a bias is grounded in negative societal images of aging as a period separate from one's productive life that is characterized by decreased social worth, loss and decline, and an accompanying loss of health and beauty.[8] These negative images have hampered the development of health promotion programs for older people and indeed have often "rendered the idea of health promotion for the elderly inimical."[9]

Dr. Donald Iverson, director of Health Promotion/Disease Prevention at Mercy Medical Center in Denver, Colorado, and former Senior Assistant to the Deputy Secretary for the Department of Health and Human Services (DHHS), has argued that the elderly have "simply been forgotten" as a target of public and private sector health promotion programs.[10] He states, "All too frequently, the goal of these programs is to reduce the overall risk of individuals to premature death. This goal tends to exclude the elderly whose risks of premature death are less than those of individuals who are in the 35–55 age range."

When one realizes that an estimated 86 percent of older Americans have at least one chronic disease,[11] the need for health promotion programs that take into account the special needs and circumstances of this age group becomes apparent. By focusing narrowly on primary prevention and the avoidance of premature aging and premature death, many current health promotion programs not only fail to address the needs of the elderly but also unwittingly may contribute to gerontophobia,[12] or the cultural dread of aging so pervasive in our society. The de facto exclusion of the elderly as a focus of concern in many health promotion efforts ignores the potential for substantial health improvement in this age group. Further, it overlooks the significant positive health effects that can occur, often in a short period of time, when particular health-promoting activities are undertaken. When it is recalled that a woman reaching age 65 has, on the average, 18 years of life remaining and a man has close to 14 more years,[13] the importance of extending our health promotion concerns to this age group is underscored.

Relatively little attention has been devoted to smoking cessation among the elderly, for example, on the assumption that the habit has become intractable over the individual's lifetime and that largely irreparable damage has already been done. However, several immediate benefits are to be realized through cessation, even after decades of smoking. Because smoking aggravates hypertension, elimination of the habit can aid in lowering heart rate and blood pressure within a matter of days.[14] For most smoking-related cancers, there is a decline in risk over time, occurring most rapidly during the first five years after smoking cessation.[15] The risk of dying from ischemic heart disease decreases even more rapidly.[16]

Ironically, the focus on younger age groups that is characteristic of many health promotion programs may have been encouraged inadvertently by the federal government through its national guidelines for health promotion. The 1980 "Objectives for the Nation"[17] developed by the Office of Disease Prevention and Health Promotion in the DHHS defined four settings as being pivotal for health promotion activities: (1) the workplace, (2) schools, (3) clinical settings (e.g., hospitals), and (4) the community.

Although it is both appropriate and cost-effective to focus major health promotion efforts on worksites and schools where large numbers of people can be reached and early risk reduction efforts can be initiated, this choice of settings automatically excludes most all elderly persons. The third setting focus—the hospital—is also a logical and appropriate choice, and hundreds of hospitals now offer health promotion programs, usually for a set fee. Hospital-based programs, however, the major goals of which often include attracting individuals to the hospital in the community, seldom target the elderly in these activities. Further, some of the programs offered—for example, smoking cessation—are mistakenly held to be irrelevant to older persons.

Finally, the fees connected with hospital-based health promotion programs, however modest from the standpoint of middle-income workers, may effectively prevent participation by large numbers of elderly persons living on small, fixed incomes. These individuals may have to balance $35 for an 8-week stress management or fitness course against the costs of such necessities as food, housing, or needed health care items not covered under Medicare or Medicaid. When such trade-offs have to be made, health promotion programs are not likely to emerge the winners. Reduced fees for elders interested in attending hospital-based health promotion programs and, ideally, Medicare reimbursement for such courses could go a long way toward increasing the accessibility of such programs to those elders for whom financial barriers may otherwise preclude attendance.

The final setting for health promotion—the community—has also failed for the most part to reach or reach out to older population groups. This failure may be attributed in part to the heavy reliance of most community-based health promotion efforts on the mass media. Although somewhat effective in stimulating immediate, short-term interest and disseminating information, health promotion programs using the mass media are ineffective in creating sustained behavior change, particularly when compared with more personal communication approaches.[18] Most health promotion media spots, moreover, seem to be targeted primarily at younger age groups or subgroups (e.g., pregnant women). Indeed, in an effort to move away from the traditional public service announcement format, such spots have increasingly taken on the characteristics of glossy and competitive television and radio advertisements; the young and the beautiful are portrayed—usually in comfortable white middle to upper-middle class settings—and the implicit message ties health and health promotion to youthful physical attractiveness, the dominant ethnic culture, and economic well-being.

There are, of course, some important exceptions to these generalizations. The President's Council on Physical Fitness has developed two television spots on exercise for the elderly, the National Institute on Drug Abuse has mounted a mass media campaign designed to decrease medication misuse among older Americans, and the National High Blood Pressure Education Program has developed a component targeted specifically at the elderly. Overall, however, few government-sponsored health promotion programs currently in the planning or implementation stages have identified the elderly as a target group.

On a more positive note, examination of the promotional materials of many city park and recreational departments indicates that many of their exercise programs and general social activities *are* directed at the elderly. Yet even in this area there is need for concern. With the recent budget cuts in the Department of the Interior's Bureau of Heritage, Conservation, and Outdoor Recreation (BHCOR), this promising avenue for reaching diverse segments of the elderly community may become less viable.

That federal monies for health promotion are diminishing, rather than increasing, and that programs in the private sector continue to focus primarily on worksite and hospital settings further suggest that health promotion efforts will be less, rather than more, likely to reach out to the elderly in the foreseeable future.

RESEARCH AND EVALUATION

The behavioral and environmental issues in Table 3–1 reflect one of the greatest flaws in health promotion: Rarely is rigorous investigation applied to the unraveling of complex relationships among immediate and underlying causes of disease or disease precursors.[19] Targeted behaviors are usually identified through short-term, cross-sectional studies. These studies provide measures of statistical association that are frequently used as if they were definitive causal paths. In reality, however, we do not know if many specific biological or psychological conditions prevalent among older people are appropriate for or amenable to intervention that would result in significant improvement in health and well-being. Second, in those cases where evidence does support the alterability of certain conditions, we do not know if affordable mechanisms can be developed or would receive the political commitment necessary for the initiation and maintenance of such changes across large population groups.

Table 3–1 summarizes dominant views on which behaviors and conditions are important in the promotion of health for the elderly. However, causal paths are not specified nor quantified because of the lack of data on the strength and nature of these relationships. In addition, some items appear under one area of health promotion as a cause and in another as an effect. This underscores the interrelatedness of all the factors under discussion and further explains the conceptual confusion surrounding these issues.

Bickman[20] concisely describes this problem as "lack of theory." In his discussion of conceptual barriers to the evaluation of social prevention programs, he examines many issues that apply to health promotion as well. For example, as he notes:

> Not only do we lack good theories of specific problems but we have difficulty in defining the nature of social problems . . . we need to integrate our concepts, borrowed and otherwise, across different areas of prevention. . . . Such integrative efforts might infuse some much needed conceptual vitality into this field.

The ever-present obstacle that impedes the generation of valid and reliable data about health promotion in general and for older people in particular is the continuing lack of follow-up and evaluation. Because existing programs generally were established on a small scale and with limited budgets, available resources are more than consumed by program development and maintenance. When some form of evaluation is undertaken, it is often only sufficient to uncover short-term results such as altered behavior. Rarely is there a commitment to and the resources necessary for the long-term and broad-based follow-up that would be necessary to determine health outcomes.

A vicious circle thus emerges: Funding for evaluation is compromised by the incomplete and complex nature of the scientific data base, and evaluation that would help to refine that evidence is impossible without substantial investment of time and money. As a result, the little evaluation that is done focuses more on short-term outcomes, changes in behavior, and/or on conditions associated with behavior. Conclusions about actual health effects are usually then drawn by implication, rather than by verification.

A related problem is that limited resources and narrow research foci often lead to the development and testing of interventions on an isolated and singular basis. The inadequacy of this approach was pointed up by Kane et al.[21] when they noted that:

Multifactorial chains make the efficacy of any single intervention difficult to determine. Conversely, some behaviors may contribute to several different diseases or problems. Their role in any one disease may be
minor, yet the summative effect of their contribution may justify
advocating the behavioral change.

The importance of refining research and interventions extends beyond implications for participants in the programs themselves because a far larger sphere of
people and problems can be affected. As Milio[22] has noted in *Promoting Health
Through Public Policy:*

> People's health is primarily the result of environments in which they live
> and the patterns of behavior they follow. Those patterns are shaped by
> environments, and environments are shaped by public policy. Finally,
> public policy is shaped by the information that is available to the
> policymakers as well as the material interests of those who are organized
> to assert their claims.

If research in health promotion continues to focus on individual behavior changes,
public policy will reflect this emphasis, and the major preventable health problems, especially for members of the elderly population, will go unabated.

DIRECTIONS FOR THE FUTURE

When the first Surgeon General's Report on Health Promotion and Disease
Prevention was released in 1979, its purpose was described by then-Secretary of
Health, Education, and Welfare Joseph Califano as "to encourage a second public
health revolution in the United States."[23] The purpose of this "second revolution" was, of course, to reduce dramatically morbidity and mortality from the
major chronic diseases. Ironically, however, although these diseases are most
often found among the elderly, it is precisely this group that has been most
neglected in policies and programs aimed at achieving health promotion and
disease prevention.

Real success requires that we combine our focus on individual behavior choices
with an appreciation of the need for *social* choices, which would include, for
example, providing those health and social supports on the individual through the
national levels without which health promotion efforts may be of limited
usefulness.

In order for health promotion to address adequately the needs of the elderly, the
concept of health itself must be recast. As Filner and Williams have suggested,
health thus might be defined as the ability to live and function effectively in society

and to exercise self-reliance and autonomy to the maximum extent feasible, but not necessarily as total freedom from disease.[24]

Critical to this definition is the interdependence of traditional perceptions of health—physical and mental health—and broader social and economic considerations. The ability to "live and function effectively in society" thus is seen as being related as importantly to having a sufficient income on which to live as it is to the state of one's physical or mental health. Similarly, the exercising of "self-reliance and autonomy" may depend as much on the availability of adequate transportation, social supports, and community-based health and social services as on one's physical condition or psychological and cognitive functioning.

Just as traditional conceptions of health must be refined and broadened to have greater relevance to the elderly, so must our definitions of health promotion be expanded. Such a broadening of focus is encompassed in Green et al.'s[25] definition of health promotion as *"any combination of health education and related organizational, political and economic interventions designed to facilitate behavioral and environmental changes conducive to health."* This definition is more sophisticated than conventional conceptualizations in its implicit awareness of the complex of social, cultural, economic, and other factors that influence health and health behavior. It further lends itself to what has been termed "system-centered education," which aims at altering the social or cultural structure of a community "in such a way as to provide better conditions, opportunities, supports and incentives for improving the health of individuals in the community."[26]

System-centered education geared toward health promotion for the elderly may involve:

- increasing the problem-solving capacity of the elderly group or community (e.g., through advocacy training and legislation that protects and promotes the rights of older persons)
- providing a comprehensive continuum of community-based health and social services conducive to health maintenance and self-reliance for older persons in need of such supports
- helping elderly individuals gain access to knowledge, skills, and other resources that may be used in meeting personal health goals and objectives.

By focusing on the broader system as the target of change efforts, health promotion utilizing a system-centered educational approach is more likely to be more effective and ethically sound than health promotion efforts that are more exclusively oriented toward individual behavior change.[27]

Although the above-mentioned changes could go a long way toward improving the effectiveness of health promotion efforts, they will still be of limited usefulness unless they are combined with careful evaluation and research efforts that can demonstrate their efficacy and the generalizability of their findings. Because public policy is shaped in part by the information available to policy makers, only through the combination of research and evaluation with a broadening of focus can the true potential of health promotion for improving the lives of America's elders be realized.

NOTES

1. M. Minkler and J. Fullarton, "Health Promotion, Health Maintenance, and Disease Prevention for the Elderly" (Background paper for the 1981 White House Conference on Aging prepared for the Office of Health Information, Health Promotion, Physical Fitness, and Sports Medicine, Department of Health and Human Services, USPHS, Washington, D.C., 1980), p. 234.

2. R. Labonte and S. Penfold, "Canadian Perspectives in Health Promotion: A Critique," *Health Education,* April, 1981, pp. 4–9.

3. The authors gratefully acknowledge Eli Zimmerman, doctoral candidate at the University of Massachusetts, Amherst, Mass., for drawing this helpful distinction.

4. R.H. Binstock, "The Aged as Scapegoat," *The Gerontologist* 23, no. 2 (1983): 136–143.

5. Minkler and Fullarton, *op. cit.,* p. 234.

6. *Ibid.,* p. 234.

7. E.B. Feldman (ed.), *Nutrition in the Middle and Later Years* (Boston: John Wright, 1983), p. 5–8.

8. R.N. Butler, *Why Survive? Being Old in America* (New York: Harper and Row, 1975), p. 496.

9. Minkler and Fullarton, *op. cit.,* p. 234.

10. Dr. Donald C. Iverson, Director of Health Promotion/Disease Prevention, Mercy Medical Center, Denver, Colorado, September 2, 1982: personal communication.

11. E. Shanas and G. Maddox, "Aging, Health and the Organization of Health Resources," in *Handbook of Aging and the Social Sciences,* ed. R.H. Binstock and E. Shanas (New York: Van Nostrand Reinhold Co., 1976), pp. 592–618.

12. D.H. Fisher, *Growing Old in America* (New York: Oxford University Press, 1978).

13. H.B. Brotman, "Every Ninth American," in *Developments in Aging: 1980* (U.S. House of Representatives Special Committee on Aging) (Washington, D.C.: U.S. Government Printing Office, 1981).

14. U.S. Department of Health and Human Services, Public Health Service, *Smoking and Health: A Report to the Surgeon General* (Washington, D.C.: U.S. Government Printing Office, 1979).

15. R. Doll and R. Peto, "Cigarette Smoking and Bronchial Carcinoma: Dose and Time Relationships Among Regular Smokers and Lifelong Non-Smokers," *Journal of Epidemiology and Community Health* 32 (1978): 303–313.

16. J. Grabowski, psychopharmacologist, January 1984, Clinical Research Division, National Institute of Drug Abuse: personal communication.

17. U.S. Department of Health and Human Services, Public Health Service, *Promoting Health/ Preventing Disease Objectives for the Nation* (Washington, D.C.: U.S. Government Printing Office, 1980), p. 2.

18. L.M. Wallack, "Mass Media Campaigns: The Odds Against Finding Behavior Change," *Health Education Quarterly* 8, no. 3 (Fall 1981): 209–260.

19. For a fuller discussion of this subject, see A. Pardini, R. Pasick, and P. Franks, *Health Promotion for the Elderly: A Critical Perspective* AoA Grant 90–AP0003 (San Francisco: Aging Health Policy Center, University of California at San Francisco, 1984).

20. L. Bickman, "The Evaluation of Prevention Programs," *Journal of Social Issues* 39, no. 1 (1983): 181–194.

21. R. Kane, B. Kane, and S. Arnold, *Prevention in the Elderly: Risk Factors* (Background paper for the Conference on Health Promotion and Disease Prevention for Children and the Elderly: A Research Agenda, sponsored by the Foundation for Health Services Research, Washington, D.C., October 9–11, 1983), p. 3.

22. N. Milio, *Promoting Health Through Public Policy* (Philadelphia: F.A. Davis Co., 1981), p. 6.

23. U.S. Department of Health and Human Services, Public Health Services. *Healthy People* (Washington, D.C.: U.S. Government Printing Office, 1979), p. vii.

24. B. Filner and T.F. Williams, "Health Promotion for the Elderly: Reducing Functional Dependency," in *Healthy People* (Washington: D.C.: U.S. Government Printing Office, 1979), pp. 365–387.

25. L.W. Green *et al., Health Education Planning: A Diagnostic Approach* (Palo Alto, Ca.: Mayfield Publishing Co., 1980), p. 7.

26. U.S. Department of Health and Human Services, Public Health Service, Office of Health Information, Health Promotion, and Physical Fitness and Sports Medicine, *Toward a Health Community: Organizing Events for Community Health Promotion* (Washington, D.C.: U.S. Government Printing Office, 1980), p. 7.

27. Minkler and Fullarton, *op. cit.,* p. 234.

Chapter 4

Health Care and Social Policy: Health Promotion and the Elderly

Carroll L. Estes, Ph.D.
Sherry Fox, R.N., M.A.
Constance W. Mahoney, M.A., M.P.H.

Health promotion for the elderly cannot be separated from the larger issues of health care, of the society's policy choices in regard to aging, and the social, economic, and political environment in which these are a part. This chapter addresses the construction of social policy, the history of health care and social policy for the elderly, the changing social context, changing conceptual frameworks, and the expansion of the definition of health to include a focus on health promotion. Implications for health policy for the elderly and recommendations for future policy are also discussed.

THE CONSTRUCTION OF SOCIAL POLICY

In considering social policy and health care for the aging, one must first determine what is included under the term policy. In the broadest sense, social policy includes (1) mandated, legislative, or administrative actions or goals; (2) what is implemented; and (3) the consequences flowing from the implementation. Social policy is a dynamic process, continuously emerging and being negotiated within a social context that takes account of social, economic, and political conditions, as well as how needs are defined.[1]

Health policy for the aged is a complex undertaking because there is no agreed-on, measurable definition of health; definitions of health for the aged are even less clear-cut. In addition, definitions of the aged's health care needs have changed often, shaping policies and programs for the aged. Moreover, marked changes in demographic, epidemiologic, social, and economic conditions, and the shifting bases of political power over the past 30 years have affected health care policies. Finally, many of the problems faced by the elderly in the United States result from the dominant societal image of aging and the aged, rather than being an inevitable result of aging itself. What is done for and about the elderly, the provision of health care services, and our research-based knowledge about old age and aging are influenced by this image.[2]

For example, elders tend to be thought of as an unproductive drain on society, with little consideration given to the ability of many elderly people to remain productive at very advanced ages, given the opportunity. Instead, the elderly must contend with a shrinking job market, mandatory retirement, and age discrimination in hiring. Further, old age is commonly perceived as a process of inevitable biological decrement, decline, and decay. These stereotypes of the aged have subtly shaped our understanding of the relevant health policy issues, leading to consideration of the aged as sick and as a problem to society, rather than a focus on the broader issues involved in achieving healthy aging.[3,4]

Major health care policies for the aging population reflect the biomedical definition of health in which health is seen as the absence of disease, disease is seen as a deviation from a biological norm of a young and "healthy" society, and aging is seen as a biologically determined process of inevitable decline. Health maintenance is thus focused on treating these processes of disease and decline. Intervention, therefore, is based on a belief in the medical technological treatment of individuals.

The dominant view among policymakers then, is that services, especially high-cost, technology-based medical services, can solve the aging "problem." This medicalization of aging both denies the extremely significant role that social and economic factors play in determining the health status of the elderly and underplays the potentially significant role of health promotion. In addition, a large medical-industrial enterprise has been created to provide publicly subsidized, high-cost hospital and nursing home (institutional) services to the aged, which address only limited aspects of the health needs of the aged. Although the attention given to the biological and biomedical aspects of aging has been important and has contributed much to our limited knowledge about aging, this emphasis in the public mind, the media, and the allocation of public resources—both for research and services—has diverted attention from the importance of another growing body of research knowledge: the significant influence of multiple social, behavioral, and environmental factors on aging, in terms of an individual's experience of old age, his or her health status and place in society, and how society responds to the older person as a "problem."

HISTORY OF CURRENT POLICY

Public policy has been responsive to some of the most overt needs of the elderly, particularly income and medical care, through Social Security, Medicare, and Medicaid. Social services block grants and the Older American's Act also provide health-related services. These programs' major health-related contributions lie in the provision of acute illness care, modest income support, and nutritional assistance.

Social Security

In the broadest sense, Social Security can be considered the first legislated health care policy for the aged because, by providing a minimal level of income, it provided the opportunity for maintenance of proper nutrition, a healthy living environment, and independence. Social Security was created in the Depression era to provide a minimal level of retirement and death benefits to the elderly worker, widow, and family. This very important program raises two-thirds of older persons above the poverty level.

Health Care Insurance: Medicare and Medicaid

The federally sponsored health care insurance programs, Medicare and Medicaid, were enacted in the mid-1960s when equity and access to care were major social concerns. Both Medicare and Medicaid policies focus on disease and limit reimbursement largely to the institutional—hospital and nursing home—and physician service categories.

Medicare, the major federal program covering medical services for people 65 years of age and older, was designed to ensure access to needed medical service for the aged and to protect them against the high cost of care for hospital and physician services. Medicaid is a federally assisted, state-administered program that pays for basic medical care for the poor—both young and old—the blind, and the disabled. It is the major source of financing for long-term chronic illness. Although it was designed to offer relief to the poor for medication costs, doctors' bills, and nursing home (long-term) care, many elderly poor have been denied coverage under Medicaid because eligibility requirements are both stringent and vary from state to state.

With the enactment of Medicare and Medicaid, health care policies based on the biomedical model became the publicly financed mode of care. The Medicare dollar is largely absorbed by hospitals for acute-care treatment of catastrophic illness at the terminal stage,[5] whereas the Medicaid dollar for elders is absorbed by nursing home institutional care. In both programs, an enormous amount of public dollars is consumed by medical institutions serving a small percentage of older people in crisis. Further, these programs barely reflect the needs of many elderly for chronic illness care. Even the minimally health-promoting activities of physical check-ups are not paid for by Medicare, foreclosing potential opportunities for preventive health care.

Food Assistance Programs

National nutritional policies have evolved over the past 50 years with increasing attention given to the nutritional health of the population, particularly high-risk groups, such as the poor and elderly.[6] In the 1960s and 1970s, concern with the effect of poverty and malnutrition on health led to the enactment of special food assistance programs for the elderly.

The National Nutrition Program for the elderly—now covered under Title III of the Older Americans Act—was first authorized in 1965 as a research and development program providing congregate meals for persons 60 years of age and over and their spouses. In 1978, Title V of the Comprehensive Older Americans Act Amendments added separate funding for home-delivered meals. Preliminary data from program evaluation indicate that nearly two-thirds of all participants had annual incomes below $4000. By 1980, 20 percent of the 168.4 million meals served were home-delivered;[7] 1984 data indicate that the number and percentage of meals delivered to elderly confined to their home are rising due to earlier discharge of hospital patients and the general aging of the population.[8]

The Food Nutrition Service of the Department of Agriculture serves the elderly poor through two major programs: the Food Stamp program created in 1964 and commodities in lieu of Food Stamps. In 1982, about 9 percent of Food Stamp participants, or 2.5 million persons, were age 60 or over; 1.1 million of these were living alone.[9]

Although some elderly have received benefits from these nutritional policies, the efforts have not been comprehensive and far-reaching enough to be classified as a major resource in meeting the health promotion and disease prevention needs of the elderly.

Existing health policies for the elderly—Social Security income supplementation, Medicare and Medicaid health coverage, and food assistance programs in the form of low-cost congregate meals, home-delivered meals, and Food Stamps—have undoubtedly improved the health status of the elderly. However, these policies have been limited in their impact by their reliance on the narrow biomedical definition of health and on conceptions of the elderly as a "problem" population requiring individual medical interventions. Moreover, given the current political and economic conditions of fiscal austerity, these established policies for the elderly face uncertain futures.

CHANGING SOCIAL CONTEXTS

Definitions of health that form the basis for health policy are constructed and reconstructed by policy makers within a social context, which then shapes their formulation. The major health care policies that presently affect the elderly were developed within the socioeconomic context of the 1960s, in which equity and access to medical care were major social concerns and the understanding of health was limited largely to the cure of physical illness and injury. In the 1970s and 1980s, significant changes in demographic, epidemiological, social, economic, and political conditions have been instrumental in reshaping definitions of health and policies for the elderly. Some of these critical changes are elaborated below.

Demographic Conditions

Present and projected demographic changes have profound implications for the health and well-being of the elderly and for the entire U.S. population. Since 1960, the over-65 age group has grown more than twice as fast (55 percent increase) as the younger population (24 percent increase). The elderly now comprise 11 percent of the total population, an increase from 9 percent in 1960. The number of persons over 75 is growing more rapidly than any other age category, and the very old cohort of elderly is growing even more rapidly. For the 20-year period from 1960 to 1980, the number of persons aged 75–84 rose 65 percent, and those aged 85 and over rose 174 percent, from 1.0 million in 1960 to 2.6 million persons in 1980.[10] These dramatic increases, particularly in the oldest age groups, are expected to continue over the next three decades.

Epidemiological Conditions

Not only have the number and percentage of elderly in the population been increasing but also epidemiological data indicate that the mortality rate is declining and disease patterns are changing. The elderly, as well as the younger population, are experiencing significant declines in overall mortality levels. Heart disease, cancer, and stroke account for 75 percent of all deaths among the elderly population. Most of the overall decline in mortality among the elderly from 1950 to 1979 was a result of the decline in two of the leading causes of death—heart disease and stroke. Only death rates from cancer during this time have increased.[11] Although improvements in mortality are shared by both men and women, women have experienced a greater degree of improvement.[12] Most important, the rate of decline in mortality rates among the very old population has been accelerating. For persons aged 75 to 84 years, the decline in mortality between 1968 and 1978 was 13 percent, compared with an 8 percent decline in the previous 10-year period (1958–1968). For persons 85 years and older, the mortality decline was even more dramatic—a 25 percent decline in the 1968–1978 period.[13]

Changes in the incidence and prevalence of disease are another factor affecting the social context in which health is defined and health policy constructed. Although infectious and other acute diseases have been reduced through public health and medical efforts, chronic illness—heart disease, cancer, stroke, and arteriosclerosis—has emerged as the major cause of death and disability. In 1979, 46 percent of those 65 and over suffered from a chronic disease, and 30 percent of the noninstitutionalized elderly reported that their health is fair or poor.[14] Moreover, the percentage of persons reporting functional impairment is twice as high among the poor as among those with adequate incomes. Because the prevalence of chronic illness increases with age and causes a greater degree of disability, the very old have more need for assistance than the younger old. As noted above, the number of persons achieving the ranks of the very old is increasing dramatically, leading to a more disabled elderly population cohort.

Economic and Political Conditions

The projected rise in the numbers and longevity of older persons and the increase in the incidence of chronic illness and disability raise important economic and political issues. On the national level, spiraling health care costs, the growing proportion of the gross national product (GNP) that these costs comprise—now almost 11 percent—and the increasing burden of health care cost being borne out-of-pocket directly by the elderly are of concern.[15] The elderly—11 percent of the population—account for 29 percent of the United States health care expenditure.[16] In 1982, nearly 90 percent of short-term hospital expenses for the elderly were paid for by Medicare; the state and federally financed Medicaid program paid for 48 percent of long-term nursing home costs. Whereas a total of $15 billion were expended for nursing home care—for less than 5 percent of the elderly population that is institutionalized at any one time—only $1.6 billion were expended for home health care.[17,18]

In the 1980s, there has been a significant change in federal policy, with an abrupt halt in the willingness to continue the expanded federal role in health that was established in 1965 with the passage of Medicare and Medicaid. The economic effects of inflation, recession, unemployment, tax cuts, high interest rates, and increases in defense spending are vividly reflected in a new era of fiscal austerity.[19] The retrenchment in domestic social policy is dramatically illustrated by recent cutbacks in Medicare, Medicaid, and Social Security.

Despite the benefits of Medicare and Medicaid programs, individual older persons continue to face economic crisis in meeting health care needs. Medicare paid less than one-half of the cost of physician services for the average Medicare patient. When all health expenditures are counted, Medicare is estimated to pay for only about 44 percent of the total health care costs of the elderly. For those living on fixed incomes, which includes most of the elderly, direct out-of-pocket medical costs rose 64 percent between 1978 and 1982.[20] Older women are currently spending about one-third of their income on health care and because they comprise 60 percent of all Medicare enrollees, proposed changes in Medicare will disproportionately affect them.

Although many older persons are able to live out their lives in relative comfort, women, blacks, and other minorities continue to be most disadvantaged. About one-half of the elderly poor are single women living alone, and the highest rates of poverty are found among older Hispanic and black females.[21] Further, the income sources of the less advantaged elderly have been eroding. In 1981, the minimum Social Security benefit was eliminated for future beneficiaries, eradicating the income floor of $122 a month—already below the poverty level—provided to those who qualified for Social Security but whose employment, widowhood, or divorce did not qualify them for Social Security payments of at least the minimum level. The growing income disparities between those elderly who are well-off and those who are disadvantaged have been amply demonstrated.[22,23]

Similar problems have arisen for the elderly who are dependent on nutrition assistance programs. As participation in food assistance programs has increased, publicly financed costs for these programs have become a major concern, and controversy has emerged concerning fragmentation, duplication of benefits, inconsistent eligibility requirements, the lack of common goals, and failure to demonstrate improved nutritional or health status among recipients.[24] Food assistance programs were earmarked for expenditure reductions in 1981, and research in 1983 reported funding cutbacks for some nutrition programs, particularly in support services and transportation. These cutbacks led to the consolidation of agencies in fewer geographical sites, resulting in reduced access for many older persons.[25] Although Congress in 1983 refused to enact major spending cuts in the Food Stamp legislation, particularly as it affected the elderly, nevertheless, elderly Food Stamp recipients who received a Social Security increase in January 1984 experienced a cut of 30 cents in Food Stamp benefits for each additional dollar of Social Security received.[26]

Social Conditions

During the period of heightened social consciousness of the 1960s and 1970s and continuing into the 1980s, social movements emerged around such diverse issues as civil rights, consumer rights, wholistic health, fitness, self-care, feminism, and ageism. These popular movements grew out of and simultaneously fostered a new emphasis on individual rights and the role of society. There has been a resurgence of individualism as a social value, which has been adopted by private sector businesses and institutionalized as part of the mainstream political and economic system. In health care, emphasis has shifted away from the individual's rights to that care and society's responsibility for providing access to it toward the individual's responsibility for rising health care costs.

TOWARD A BROADER CONCEPTUAL FRAMEWORK

Health promotion signifies a shift from the biomedical definition and model of health and disease toward a broader biopsychosocial view that encompasses the social and physical environment, as well as individual life style and behavior.[27] This new model is exemplified by Green's[28] approach to health promotion, which calls for a combination of health education and related organizational and politico-economic interventions designed to facilitate behavioral and environmental adaptations that will improve or protect health.

The work of Dubos,[29] McKeown,[27] and Belloc and Breslow[30] have contributed to an overall understanding of determinants of health and an emphasis of the importance of the environment, social factors, and life style as major determinants of health status. Policy makers are paying increasing attention to this emphasis. The pioneering work of Dubos in enlarging the understanding of the individual's adaptation to the social and physical environment opened the doors to this new understanding of old ideas. McKeown pointed out the role of improved nutrition, changing personal habits, and sanitation in achieving the marked improvements in health status during the past 150 years, calling into question the strong belief that improved medical care and technology have been the major source of health gains. Belloc and Breslow demonstrated an association between life-style habits and physical health status, supporting the promotion of individual behavior change as part of preventive health principles. Physical health was measured in terms of disability, chronic conditions, impairments, symptoms, and energy level. Positive behaviors for health were sleeping seven or eight hours each night, maintaining normal weight, engaging in physical exercise, not smoking cigarettes, and drinking no more than four drinks at one time.

> In every age group those who reported all seven favorable health habits had, on the average, better physical health than those who reported six. With one minor exception (persons over 75 years of age) there was a consistent progression toward better health at each age as the number of good health habits increased. . . . (Furthermore,) the average physical health status of those over 75 who followed all of the good practices was about the same as those 35–44 who followed fewer than three. . . . In other words, the physical health status of those reported following all seven good health practices was consistently about the same as those 30 years younger who followed few or none of these practices. . . . These data are consistent with the idea, and the temptation is great to conclude, that a lifetime of good health practices produces good health and extends the period of relatively good physical health status by some 30 years.[31]

Fries and Crapo[32] note the increase in the incidence of chronic disease, as people are more likely to survive illnesses that used to strike early in life. Because chronic disease is now the major cause of death, the major emphasis of health care must shift from the treatment of acute illness toward the removal of risk factors associated with chronic illness. Because life style is a major risk factor associated with the onset of chronic illness and resulting functional disability, Fries and Crapo postulate that modification of life style and behavior to promote health can alter the process of aging; improve the physical, mental, and social functioning of the elderly; reduce disability normally associated with aging; and extend a vigorous life up to the end of what they describe as the natural biological life span.

Such findings were first translated into policy by an important report by the Canadian Minister of Health and Welfare, *A New Perspective on the Health of Canadians*.[33] La Londe suggested that providing access to health care and improving the quality of care were not the most effective ways to improve the health of the population. Instead, approaches should be geared to four major categories: human biology, environment (physical and social), life style, and health organization.

Applying these concepts to health promotion policy for the elderly would necessarily include attention to social, as well as individual, determinants of health for the aged. Dramatically reduced incomes, decreased power and social standing, the threat of economic and social dependency, chronic illness, and the loss of social support systems, as well as individual life style, are all powerful determinants of the well-being of the elderly in our society.

EMERGENCE OF HEALTH PROMOTION FOR THE ELDERLY

Although limited health promotion activities for the elderly have taken place within the established aging enterprise and the newly emerging fitness/health promotion network that includes small segments of the medical community, little health promotion activity has been initiated or undertaken by the elderly themselves.[34] The President's Council on Physical Fitness and Sports reports that, regarding the health promotion activity of exercise, older persons (1) believe their need for exercise diminishes and eventually disappears with age; (2) exaggerate the risks involved in regular exercise beyond middle-age; (3) overrate the benefits of light, irregular exercise; and (4) underrate their own capabilities and abilities to participate in fitness activities.[35]

Until recently, the elderly were not included in popular wellness or health promotion activity. According to Minkler and Fullarton,[36] the probable reasons for their exclusion are that health promotion programs (1) focus on life extension and the elderly are perceived as *not* having a future; (2) focus on reducing risk factors associated with premature mortality and morbidity, whereas many of the elderly have already lived beyond risk of premature death; (3) advocate youthfulness and the prevention of signs of aging; therefore "old folks" are unwelcome; and (4) focus on absence and avoidance of chronic disease, which is an irrelevant goal for most elderly who already have one or more chronic conditions that may or may not be limiting their level of functioning.

Somers, Kleinman, and Clark[37] also note that little attention has been paid to health promotion for the elderly because of attitudes shared by the public and professionals that, for people over 65, it is "too late" and that the elderly should enjoy what little time they have left without any outside intervention to change their life style or behavior. Acknowledging that public attitudes are changing, the authors advocate initiating health promotion and preventive services specifically for the elderly. Heiple[38] notes specifically that older women have been excluded not only from activity generated by the wholistic health movement but also from the humanistic health care changes brought about by the women's health movement.

Since the mid-1970s, health promotion has grown in visibility as a major policy issue in Congress, federal agencies, and at state and local levels of government. This effort has been aided by many groups outside government, including the Institute of Medicine of the National Academy of Sciences and a growing number of university and business interests. Private sector groups that have become active advocates of health promotion include voluntary professional health organizations, health and life insurance companies, fitness and health food industries, and many major employers.

An important stimulus in the development of health promotion for the elderly was the publication in 1979 of *Healthy People: The Surgeon General's Report on Health Promotion and Disease Prevention*.[39] This report highlighted specific quantifiable health status goals for various age groups, including, for the first time, national objectives for the health of older adults: "by 1990, to reduce the average annual number of days of restricted activity due to chronic and acute conditions by 20% to fewer than thirty days per year for people aged 65 and older."[40] This document laid out a conceptual framework for national health promotion activities focusing on individual behavior or life style as a major determinant of health and illness:

> Personal habits play critical roles in the development of many serious diseases and in injuries from violence and automobile accidents. . . . In fact, of the ten leading causes of death in the United States, at least seven could be substantially reduced if persons at risk improved just five habits: diet, smoking, lack of exercise, alcohol abuse, and the use of antihypertensive medication.

To date, health promotion policy has focused almost exclusively on the responsibility of the individual to make changes in his or her life style in the areas of (1) improved nutrition, (2) exercise and fitness, (3) stress control, (4) reducing misuse of alcohol and drugs, and (5) smoking cessation. It has not advocated public and private sector responsibility for initiating change in social institutions and the political and economic system to promote a healthier environment that would be supportive of healthy life styles.

One of the 14 committees of the 1981 White House Conference on Aging was devoted to promotion and maintenance of health; it recommended that "the health policy of the nation should be to a) improve the health of Americans, especially the elderly; b) curtail health care costs; c) focus attention on health promotion and disease prevention."[41] Special consideration was to be directed to benefits that the elderly could derive from behavioral and life-style modification under their control. One of the major conference recommendations urged increased governmental, voluntary, and private sector activity in health promotion and fitness for the elderly.

Increased governmental activity in promoting individual responsibility for improving the health status of the nation is planned, with the elderly as the targets of this new government policy. Programs to promote changing individual behavior and life style are ready for implementation. In 1985, the Department of Health and Human Services, through the Administration on Aging, and the U.S. Public Health Service has launched a two-year public information and education campaign for the elderly to encourage participation in specially organized fitness programs designed exclusively for older adults.[42]

POLICY ANALYSIS

Beginning in the late 1970s the health policy rhetoric has changed, with health promotion added as its focus. This new rhetoric reflects an expanded definition of health that recognizes life style or behavior as determinants of health. Nevertheless, major governmental policy in the form of legislation and funding for research and health care delivery continues to emphasize costly, end-of-life, acute-care "crisis" intervention based on the biomedical ideology and the dominance of the medical establishment. This paradox reflects the dynamic process of policy formulation in which conflicting ideologies are negotiated within the policy framework. The introduction of the health promotion ideology in the face of the dominant, strongly entrenched biomedical ideology of present health policy for the elderly can, therefore, be expected to lead to both intended and unintended consequences. In any event, change is likely to be incremental. On the one hand, governmental policy advocates health promotion to improve the health status of the growing elderly population and to reduce rising medical costs. On the other hand, it continues to subsidize the in-place medical system of high technology and fee-for-service care. Moreover, although placing responsibility for health on the behavior of individuals, government policy makes significant cutbacks in Medicare and Medicaid funding and makes restrictive changes in regulations that threaten the present health status of the elderly, especially the poor and the very old, most of whom are women. Although advocating individual change in behavior, governmental policy continues to support an economic system and social environment that profits from the promotion of unhealthy life styles. Governmental policy advocates increased commitment of family members for the care of the elderly, yet fails to provide supportive services, such as respite care, for those who become caretakers, most of whom are female.

Policy Considerations

The ideological groundwork for the importance of national health promotion activities for the elderly has been carefully developed, and yet, without secure policies and funding, there may be only rhetoric, rather than true substance, in the ideals. Health promotion policies for the elderly must recognize that an individual's health is shaped by a host of factors, including age, sex, race and ethnicity, language, physical and mental health history, income, employment status, occupation, education, religion, place of residence, living conditions, social and family support, and personal habits and values. An individual's health and the choices he or she makes about life style or behavior take place within a broad social context. Social values and customs, public policies—especially those that bear on the economy, the environment, and the financing and delivery of medical care, prevention, and social services—and the policies and practices of business and industry and the media all shape the context of the individual's life style and health. For the elderly, life style and health emerge over many years and thus reflect a life-course biography and history within a particular society.

Policy Recommendations

If the goals of health promotion are to improve health status and to reduce medical costs, health promotion policy for the elderly must be developed within a broader social-political-economic framework than has been undertaken to date. Future policy should incorporate the following recommendations:

- Health promotion policy must give credence to the social and environmental determinants of health, as well as behavioral or life-style determinants. To be effective in improving health status and in reducing health care spending in the long run, policy must provide for adequate income, decent housing, and a safe and secure environment. Making changes in one's life style is most difficult when basic needs for food, clothing, shelter, and medical care are unmet. Advocating individual responsibility for health is self-defeating, unless society also recognizes and takes responsibility for providing for the social determinants affecting health.

- Health promotion policy must avoid the narrow focus on health status of the elderly as they approach their end of a lifetime of behavior. Instead, health promotion policy must promote a healthy life style for the entire population, over an entire lifetime; this would avoid what appears, at the present time, to be a policy of blaming the elderly for their present health status and their consumption of medical services.

- Health promotion policy must advocate that the medical insurance reimbursement system be restructured to reward the promotion of health, not the promotion of sickness. Publicly funded Medicare and Medicaid must provide incentives for health prevention and promotion of healthy life styles, as must the private sector insurers and fee-for-service medical services. Health education and one-to-one medical counseling may do more to promote health than expensive medical technology; however, health promoting activities are presently not reimbursable expenses for health care providers.

- Health promotion policies must work supportively within a continuum of community-based, long-term care, social support services for the elderly. The present network of community social services must not be abandoned in an expedient effort to reduce medical expenditures by making the most healthy elderly solely responsible for their health behavior and isolating the older, frail elderly in their homes without access to community support services.

- Finally, health promotion policy must recognize that public policy is not separated from private sector policy. Although some companies have been quick to promote for-profit fitness centers and health food stores and still other corporations have taken steps within their own establishments to promote healthy life styles for their employees to reduce insurance costs, by and large, business and industry, with the cooperation of government, continue to promote unhealthy living through occupational and environmental pollution and the production and marketing of products that are dangerous to the health of consumers.

Sufficient research data have now been amassed that confirm the benefits of health promotion in reducing risk factors associated with chronic illness and disability. These data can provide a firm foundation for the development of a strong, national health promotion policy, not only for the elderly as an age-segregated population cohort, but for citizens of all ages. Such a policy will have profound implications for the financing, organizing, and delivery of health care services; research; private sector policy; and the health and well-being of the present and future generations of elderly citizens.

NOTES

1. Carroll L. Estes and Beverly C. Edmonds, "Symbolic Interaction and Social Policy Analysis," *Symbolic Interaction* 4, no. 1 (1981): 75–85.

2. Carroll L. Estes, *The Aging Enterprise* (San Francisco: Jossey-Bass, 1979), p. 12.
3. Robert N. Butler, *Why Survive? Being Old in America* (New York: Harper and Row, 1975), pp. xi–22.
4. Carroll L. Estes, L. Gerald, J. Zones, and J. Swan, *Political Economy, Health, and Aging* (Boston: Little Brown, 1984), p. 94.
5. Karen Davis, "Medicare Reconsidered," in *Health Care for the Poor and Elderly: Meeting the Challenge*, ed. Duncan Yaggy (Durham, N.C.: Duke University Press, 1984), pp. 77–97.
6. Marion M. Nestle, Philip R. Lee, and Jane E. Fullarton, "Nutrition and the Elderly," Policy Paper No. 2 (San Francisco: Aging Health Policy Center, University of California, 1983), p. 1.
7. *Ibid.*, p. 7.
8. Juanita B. Wood *et al.*, "Public Policy, the Private Nonprofit Sector and the Delivery of Community Based Long Term Care Services for the Elderly," Final Report, Year 2 (San Francisco: Aging Health Policy Center, University of California, 1984), p. 20.
9. U.S. Senate, Special Committee on Aging, "Developments in Aging: 1982," Volume 2, Appendix (Washington, D.C.: U.S. Government Printing Office, 1983), p. 5.
10. Alan Pardini *et al.*, "The Health of Older People: A Framework for Public Policy" (San Francisco: Aging Health Policy Center, University of California, 1983), p. 3.
11. National Center for Health Statistics, *Health: United States, 1982* DHHS Pub. No. (PHS) 83–1232 (Washington, D.C.: U.S. Government Printing Office, 1982), p. 34.
12. Dorothy P. Rice, "The Health Care Needs of the Elderly," in *Public Policy Issues in Long Term Care of the Elderly*, ed. Charlene Harrington, Robert J. Newcomer, Carroll L. Estes, and Associates (Beverly Hills, Calif.: Sage, 1984), pp. 41–66.
13. Alan Pardini, *op. cit.*, p. 3.
14. U.S. National Center for Health Statistics and P.W. Ries, "Americans Assess Their Health: 1978," Vital and Health Statistics, Series 10, No. 142, DHHS Pub. No. (PHS) 83–1570 (Washington, D.C.: U.S. Government Printing Office), 1983, p. 126.
15. Carroll L. Estes and Philip R. Lee, "Social, Political, and Economic Background of Long Term Care Policy," in *Long Term Care of the Elderly*, ed. Charlene Harrington, Robert J. Newcomer, Carroll L. Estes, and Associates (Beverly Hills, Calif.: Sage, 1984), pp. 17–39.
16. B. Filner and T.F. Williams, "Health Promotion for the Elderly: Reducing Functional Dependence," in U.S. Department of Health, Education, and Welfare, Public Health Service, *Healthy People: The Surgeon General's Report on Health Promotion and Disease Prevention: Background Papers*, DHHS Publication No. 79–5507, 25 (Washington, D.C., 1979b), p. 367.
17. R.M. Gibson, D.R. Waldo, and K.R. Levit, "National Health Expenditures," *Health Care Financing Review* 5, no. 1 (Fall 1983): 1–31.
18. U.S. Health Care Financing Administration (HCFA), Medicare and Medicaid Expenditures Statistics, unpublished data, (Baltimore: Md.: U.S. Department of Health and Human Services, 1982).
19. Carroll L. Estes, Robert J. Newcomer, and Associates, *Fiscal Austerity and Aging* (Beverly Hills, Calif.: Sage, 1983), pp. 17–39.
20. Carroll L. Estes and Philip R. Lee, *op. cit.*
21. Carroll L. Estes, Lenore Gerard, and Adele Clarke, "Women and the Economics of Aging," *International Journal of Health Services* 14, no. 1 (1984): 55–68.
22. Stephen Crystal, *America's Old Age Crisis* (New York: Basic Books, 1982).
23. Carroll L. Estes and Lenore Gerard, "Governmental Responsibility: Issues of Reform and Federalism," in *Fiscal Austerity and Aging*, ed. Carroll L. Estes, Robert J. Newcomer, and Associates (Beverly Hills, Calif.: Sage Publications, 1983), pp. 41–59.

24. Marion M. Nestle, Philip R. Lee, and Jane E. Fullarton, *op. cit.,* p. 6.

25. Juanita B. Wood *et al.*, "Public Policy, the Private Nonprofit Sector and the Delivery of Community Based Long Term Care Services for the Elderly," Final Report, Year 1 (San Francisco: Aging Health Policy Center, University of California, 1983), p. 40.

26. U.S. Senate Special Committee on Aging, "Developments in Aging: 1983," Volume 1 (Washington, D.C.: U.S. Government Printing Office, 1984).

27. Thomas McKeown, *The Role of Medicine: Dream, Mirage or Nemesis?* (London: The Nufield Provincial Hospitals Trust, 1976), pp. 79–90.

28. L.W. Green *et al.*, *Health Education Planning: A Diagnostic Approach* (Palo Alto, Ca.: Mayfield, 1980), p. 306.

29. Rene Dubos, *Mirage of Health* (New York: Harper and Row, 1979), pp. 1–292.

30. Nedra B. Belloc and Lester Breslow, "Relationship of Physical Health Status and Health Practices," *Preventive Medicine* 1 (1972): 409–421.

31. *Ibid.,* pp. 418–420.

32. James F. Fries and Lawrence W. Crapo, *Vitality and Aging: Implications of the Rectilinear Curve* (San Francisco: W.H. Freeman, 1981), pp. 59–67.

33. Marc La Londe, *A New Perspective on the Health of Canadians: A Working Document* (Ottawa: Ministry of National Health and Welfare, Government of Canada, 1974), pp. 31–34.

34. Pat Franks, Philip R. Lee, and Jane E. Fullarton, "Lifetime Fitness and Exercise for Older People," Policy Paper No. 4 (San Francisco: Aging Health Policy Center, University of California, 1983), p. 46.

35. President's Council on Physical Fitness and Sports, "Exercise and Aging," *Physical Fitness Research Digest,* 7, no. 1 (April 1977).

36. Meredith Minkler and Jane E. Fullarton, "Health Promotion, Health Maintenance, and Disease Prevention for the Elderly" (Background paper for the 1981 White House Conference on Aging, Washington, D.C.: 1980), pp. 1–2.

37. A.R. Somers, L. Kleinman, and W. Clark, "Preventive Health Services for the Elderly: The Rutgers Medical School Project," *Inquiry* 19 (Fall 1982): 190–221.

38. Pamela J. Heiple, "Health Care for Older Women: Toward A More Humanistic Approach," in *Aging and Health Promotion*, ed. Thelma Wells (Rockville, Md.: Aspen Systems, 1982), pp. 51–59.

39. U.S. Department of Health and Human Services, *Healthy People: The Surgeon General's Report on Health Promotion and Disease Prevention, 1979,* DHEW Publication No. (PHS) 79–55071 (Washington, D.C.: U.S. Government Printing Office, 1979).

40. *Ibid.,* p. 71.

41. White House Conference on Aging, 1981, *Final Report* (Washington, D.C.: U.S. Department of Health and Human Services, 1982), pp. 100–103.

42. Alan Pardini and Constance W. Mahoney, "A Resource Guide for Fitness: Programs for Older Persons" (San Francisco: Aging Health Policy Center, University of California, 1984), pp. 1–111.

Chapter 5

Education and Training in Wellness for Health Care Providers

Philip G. Weiler, M.D., M.P.H.

The field of health promotion, disease prevention, and wellness for the elderly has been gaining increasing support over the past decade and is emerging as one of the principal program development areas for educational institutions during the 1980s. In order to discuss education and training programs in this area, it is necessary to consider first some of the reasons for the interest in wellness and the elderly and the current research issues that are framing the discussion.

INCREASING INTEREST IN HEALTH PROMOTION

The increased interest in health promotion is due to several events, including the publication of Marc La Londe's report *A New Perspective on the Health of Canadians*[1] in 1974, followed by *Healthy People; The Surgeon General's Report on Health Promotion and Disease Prevention*[2] in 1979.

The publication of the Canadian report was a watershed event that focused attention on the view that the principal killers and cripplers of the day could be attacked more effectively by redirecting resources to diminishing self-imposed risks and improving the environment. The report developed the health field concept that attributed the major causes of death and disease to four broad elements: human biology, environment, life style, and health care organization. Life style was reported to account for 50 percent of the overall mortality, human biology for 20 percent, environment for 20 percent, and health care organization for only 10 percent. The health field concept has been a very powerful tool for analyzing health problems and developing service and training programs to meet those needs. For the first time, it provided a method of assessing health problems that highlighted their health promotion and disease prevention aspects. However, the report did not specify health goals for different age groups.

The Surgeon General's report,[2] which built on the La Londe report, focused attention in this country on our "slow-motion suicide" and set specific, quantifiable health goals for various age groups, including, for the first time, national objectives for healthy older adults. It emphasized maintaining independence, self-sufficiency, and quality of life, rather than just longevity. The report also stated that health surveillance and health maintenance for the elderly are most effective when incorporated into a comprehensive, integrated system of geriatric services. Some of the measures recommended by the report for promoting health in the elderly were programs for immunizations (i.e., influenza and pneumococcal), nutrition, exercise, safe and affordable housing, recreational activities, in-home services, ready access to health services, and health information.

In addition, interest in health promotion has been growing within the aging network as well. For example, the 1981 White House Conference on Aging[3] devoted one of its fourteen committees solely to promotion and maintenance of wellness. Specifically, the Committee on Promotion and Maintenance of Wellness recommended that:

> 1) Accrediting bodies for programs for the training of certain professionals (i.e., physicians, nurses, therapists) and others require courses that cover geriatrics and health promotion. 2) Emphasis should be placed on developing and disseminating educational materials for the elderly, as a component of health promotion efforts by Federal, State and local governments, as well as private entities. 3) The health policy of the Nation should be to: (a) improve the health of all Americans, especially the elderly; (b) contain health care costs, and (c) focus attention on health promotion and disease prevention. 4) Additional consideration needs to be given to the benefits the elderly can derive from behavioral and lifestyle modifications within individual control. Information regarding appropriate patterns and probable benefits need to be made a part of health education for the elderly and for those who serve them. 5) The health care delivery system be restructured so that preventive medicine and wellness are primary objectives and immediate action be taken to place temporary limits on the rate of increase in hospital costs. 6) Emphasis should be given to a comprehensive review of prevention-oriented screening procedures for the elderly to determine their medical efficacy. In addition, attention should be given to the cost-effectiveness of such procedures. Results of that review need to be widely disseminated to the elderly and to health professionals, to better target prevention efforts and to provide the basis for considering what services are cost-effective from the viewpoint of the individual, the health service delivery system, and third-party payers.

These recommendations form an excellent framework for future development of training, research, and service programs in the field of health promotion for the elderly. In the final report of the White House Conference, disease prevention for the elderly was one of its four major recommendations.

Impact of Demographic Change

The demographic shift is another factor adding momentum to the interest in geriatrics and prevention. One of the major demographic changes of the twentieth century is the increase in the percentage and number of people reaching age 65. Although the elderly over 65 were only 4.3 percent (4 million) of the population in 1919, they comprised 11.4 percent (18 million) of the population in 1980 and will make up over 20 percent (55 million) in 2030. The fastest-growing segment in the elderly population is the 85-years-and-over group, which will increase over 500 percent between the years 1950 and 2000, as compared to a 135 percent increase of those 65 years and over. As a group, the elderly use health resources to a greater extent than other adults. In 1980 for example, their personal health care expenditures represented about 29 percent of the total for all Americans, and by 2040 this figure will be 45 percent. Furthermore, it has been estimated that, by the year 2000, 50 percent of the average physician's time will be spent in the care of the elderly. In a 1981 publication, the Rand Corporation estimated a need for about 7,000 to 10,000 geriatricians by the year 1990.[4] Yet despite the growing number of elderly, an American Medical Association (AMA) survey of physicians in 1982 reported fewer than 700 physicians with a primary interest in geriatrics; this number has only increased slightly in recent years.[5] Although substantial efforts are being made by medical schools to develop geriatric programs, these efforts are relatively recent and are occurring at a time when medical schools are under severe fiscal and other constraints. The first department of geriatrics was not established until 1982 at Mt. Sinai Medical Center. In contrast, the first department in pediatrics was established at Johns Hopkins University in 1912.

Redefining the Goals

In recent years, there has also been a growing concern that a large proportion of the care received by the elderly follows the acute care model and is predominantly of an acute medical and/or institutional nature that may be inappropriate and even deleterious for the elderly population. Although the emphasis in this model is on disease diagnoses, there is a general consensus that, for the older adult, functional independence, not the specific disease diagnosis, is a critical indicator of health and quality of life. The goals of health care need to be redefined to include functional independence as one of the primary goals. In large part, an individual's degree of functional independence is a product of his or her ability to have a variety of social and health care needs met. These needs are best met through a continuum of care, ranging from the home to the hospital, and building on community-based social/health services, multifunctional assessment, and case management. This redirected focus of care for the elderly also helps formulate the types of preventive programs that are needed in each of these settings.

Effectiveness of Prevention

Lastly, another impetus for the growing interest in health promotion and aging is the documentation[6] of its successes. Some attribute these successes to the extensive development of wellness programs and health education efforts. There has been both a reduction in cardiovascular disease and in certain risk factors, such as smoking, diets high in cholesterol, lack of exercise, and untreated hypertension. For example, between 1960 and 1977, the heart disease rate for women 65 and over fell 18 percent, whereas for men it fell 14 percent. The percentage of decline for older men equaled that for all men. The percentage decline for older women was greater than for all women. Between 1964 and 1975, there was a 22 percent reduction in per capita consumption of tobacco. For the period from 1963 to 1975, the per capita consumption of milk, cream, butter, and eggs fell over 13 percent. The percentage of adults who exercise daily increased 92 percent from 1961 to 1980. The number of untreated hypertensives in the United States fell 10 percent between 1962 and 1974. Specific programs, such as the Stanford Heart Disease Prevention Program, Well-Elder clinics in California, and numerous others throughout the nation, have been successful in preventing disease, detecting and treating problems before they become major handicaps, and promoting a higher level of wellness among the elderly.

RESEARCH ISSUES

Recently, several large-scale research efforts have focused on the general area of preventive health services for older persons. In 1977, the Institute of Medicine of the National Academy of Sciences recommended that "projects should be initiated to determine the effectiveness of specific preventive services and programs for the elderly, such as screening for chronic disease, preretirement counseling and nutrition education. These projects should be aimed at avoiding the occurrence or minimizing the extent of functional dependency."[7]

Also during 1977, Breslow and Somers proposed a "Lifetime Health Monitoring Program" for incorporating preventive measures in a more effective way into the personal health services of 10 different age groups, the last 2 of which were comprised of the elderly (60 to 74 years and 75 years and over).[8] In contrast to many previous recommendations, these authors made explicit those services that would likely achieve the health goals of each group. For example, for the age group 60 to 74 years, they recommended the following: professional visits every two years for the healthy adult at 60 years of age, with tests for specific chronic conditions; professional counseling regarding changing life style related to retirement, nutritional requirements, absence of children, possible loss of spouse, probable reduction in income, and reduced physical resources; annual immunization against influenza; annual dental prophylaxis; periodic podiatry treatments as needed. The following year another Institute of Medicine report,[9] this one sponsored by the Ad Hoc Advisory Group on Preventive Services, incorporated these recommendations. This report was more specific in certain areas, adding vision and hearing tests and breast (women) and rectal examination for the physical examination. The laboratory tests recommended were the Pap smear (women), blood sugar, hematocrit, urinalysis for sugar and protein, and stool guaiac. Counseling for cigarette smoking, alcohol and other drug use, sexual adjustment and family life, and accident prevention was also recommended. In 1979, the Canadian Task Force on the Periodic Health Examination[10] further refined the recommendations by noting the optimum frequency with which specific services should be delivered for separate conditions afflicting women and men 65 years of age and older.

In discussing the results of previous research, an important distinction must be made. As Breslow and Somers[8] have explained, the term "prevention" is seldom defined and has quite different meanings for various interest groups. Particularly relevant to this discussion is the distinction between prevention of institutionalization and prevention of disease. To date, most attention has focused on the former; the results of some of the early demonstration projects on the prevention of institutionalization have been published, and reviews of that work have appeared.[11,12] Unfortunately, the prevention of disease, particularly primary prevention (services delivered before the onset of observable signs or symptoms) and secondary prevention (diagnosis and treatment of presymptomatic disease), has seldom been a major or even secondary goal of these projects.

Yet, there has begun to emerge a significant body of literature investigating the effectiveness of specific preventive health services. Immunization for certain diseases (pneumococcal or influenza infections), screening for various types of cancer, blood pressure screening to detect hypertension (both diastolic and systolic), and other medical and social services had been judged useful in reducing morbidity and mortality among older persons. However, few studies have examined large clinical programs that can deliver comprehensive preventive service packages on a state-wide or multistate basis. Considering that a high priority has only recently been placed on determining the effectiveness of preventive services delivered in such programs, it is not surprising that few studies of this type have yet been completed. However, because of the widespread interest in the area now, particularly from the Department of Health and Human Services (DHHS), data from studies of preventive services should be available soon. The DHHS is planning initiatives in health promotion for the elderly that emphasize four major areas: nutrition, drug use, accident prevention, and alcohol abuse.

The Lifestyle Preventive Health Services (LPHS) Study, originally conceptualized by Breslow and Somers,[8] is a project financed by insurance companies to investigate the feasibility of including age-specific preventive health services in primary medical care covered by health insurance.[13] Six group practice sites—three experimental and three control—are included in this quasiexperimental investigation of the effects of physician-delivered risk reduction services (periodic health examinations and counseling on life-style changes) on the preventive care practices, health attitudes, and risk behavior of the experimental group. The experimental group's outcome will be compared to that of a control group that does not receive these services. Two of the patient groups, those aged 60 to 74 years and 75 years and over, are of special interest in the present context.

A similar effort is being conducted by the Department of Family Medicine at Rutgers Medical School in New Jersey.[14] The Prevention and Health Maintenance Demonstration Project, jointly funded by the Hartford Foundation and Blue Cross of New Jersey, is investigating the effects of preventive and health maintenance services on healthy individuals aged 65 to 70. Health attitudes and behavior of matched experimental and control groups are being examined through self-reports and third-party utilization records. Participation in the group is voluntary, and the control group will apparently not be included in the pretest. The services to be provided include two-hour health education sessions, ongoing management services, and an initial assessment consisting of a complete physical, Pap smear, tonometry for glaucoma, a podiatric exam, a chest x-ray, a battery of lab tests, and a social assessment.

A third study is being conducted by the Health Care Financing Administration (HCFA). As a major insurer of health care services to the elderly through the Medicare program, HCFA has a significant interest in prevention projects. Through the Cooperative Health Education Project (CHEP), HCFA is investigating the effects of a health education program delivered within a health maintenance organization (HMO).[15] Risk behavior, health attitudes, health status, and utilization of HMO services are being examined to determine whether HMO services improve the health and reduce the costs of Medicare beneficiaries. HCFA has also requested proposals to evaluate the cost-effectiveness of HMO programs.

Compression of Morbidity

Another interesting aspect concerning the effectiveness of preventive services has recently been raised. James Fries[16] postulated that the average human life span is fixed at about 85 to 90 years of age and that morbidity would be compressed if chronic disease could be postponed. Therefore, according to Fries, it is not necessary to eliminate chronic disease to improve the functioning of the elderly but only to delay the onset of its clinical manifestations (see Chapter 3). However, a review of a study of the elderly in Massachusetts reported by Schneider and Brody[17] indicated that there has been a lengthening of survival, with no real lessening of the percentage of the life span taken up by the morbidity period. In other words, the average period of diminished functioning seems to be increasing. There are several explanations for that phenomenon. First, recent health promotion efforts may not yet have had a chance to affect morbidity in this older age group. However, as the younger cohorts that have been more involved in health promotion grow older, the period of morbidity may indeed lessen due to the delay and/or prevention of chronic disease. Second, high-technology medical care may be having a disproportionate impact on mortality and the increasing life span by prolonging of death through extraordinary methods. With greater emphasis in health promotion and humane death, we may begin to see data showing a reduction in the period of morbidity.

The issues for the elderly population, then, are (1) what are the objectives for a preventive program and (2) how can they be measured. Should the objective be to achieve a high level of wellness, or is it better to define the objectives less broadly as being able to function independently in the community or as postponing or preventing disease or disability? In trying to reach an appropriate objective, one should be cautious. The dilemma in dealing with health promotion outcomes for the elderly is trying not to expect too much nor hope for too little.

TRAINING AND EDUCATIONAL PROGRAMS

The extent of training and education programs in the area of aging and wellness is glaringly inadequate, and information about such programs is not readily accessible. One problem in obtaining data about these programs is determining the extent of the aging network's involvement in this area.

Current estimates that there are at least 1 million professionals and paraprofessionals in the field of aging are based primarily on demands for personnel for programs serving the institutionalized elderly. There are an additional 10,000 or more professionals and paraprofessionals in community-based programs serving the elderly that are supported by the Administration on Aging.[18] Moreover, the concept of wellness includes more than the usual physician, nurse, and therapists. The health care team has been broadened to include recreational directors, physical education specialists, social workers, nutritionists, public health workers, and others. For example, there are about 500,000 persons involved in public health activities of some kind (however, few of these are involved in working primarily with the elderly); 25,000 of these are health educators, and 2,000 are nutritionists.[19] Other relevant occupations include behavioral scientists, dentists,

optometrists, podiatrists, pharmacists, physician assistants, and nurse practitioners. Some 200 skills and occupations are pertinent to the field of aging, and the
number is still growing.

Another difficulty in finding information on educational programs is the diversity of funding agencies dealing with either health promotion or aging education.
Federal support for training in health promotion as part of public health dates from
1956. It has included formula grants to schools of public health, grants to
departments and students of preventive medicine in medical schools, and short-
term training grants ($1.8 million a year since 1971). Since fiscal 1978, the Health
Professions Education Assistance Act has provided, through various means, the
principal support for the education of mid-level and senior personnel in the field of
public health. In addition, the federal government spent over $12 million a year
from 1975 to 1978 on training for health professionals, primarily physicians and
nurses, specifically in the field of aging.[19]

Medicine

Several grants from the Administration on Aging (AoA), such as the continuing
education/technical assistance grants and the Title IV-A training grants, have also
stimulated interest in the field of gerontology. Since 1970, the AoA has directly
supported medical education projects for the elderly in medical schools. AoA also
gives some support to more than 200 colleges and universities in 43 states, which
has resulted in more than 560 courses in aging.[18] The percentage of these courses
that include an emphasis on or element of health promotion may be increasing, but
no hard data are available to support that assertion. It is also not possible to
determine the popularity of these courses. Furthermore, institutions doing this
training have been extremely slow to emphasize health promotion and aging. The
professionals most often involved are those who either control health care
resources or provide direct care services, such as physicians, nurses, and social
workers.

Although off to a slow start, physician education in the field of aging is making
significant headway since the establishment in 1974 of the National Institute on
Aging (NIA) and the 1978 report of the Institute of Medicine, *Report of a Study:
Aging and Medical Education.*[20] In 1976, only about 3 medical schools out of a
total of 126 required undergraduate courses in geriatrics and gerontology, and only
15 had separate geriatric programs of any type. By 1981, over 86 medical schools
had geriatric programs at the undergraduate, graduate, or fellowship level and it is
anticipated all medical schools will develop programs in the next 10 years.[21]
Moreover, students have expressed their interest and support for geriatric programs through the American Medical Student Association. A recent survey by
Simson and Wilson[22] of medical schools found 484 different courses with a
prevention content, 143 courses with some content on aging, but only 20 courses

with both a prevention and aging content. In all the areas of prevention and aging, wellness and health promotion was listed as a top priority by 74 percent of chairpersons surveyed. According to Simson and Wilson, the major reason given for not including more prevention and aging courses in medical school was the curriculum was so full it did not allow new course content. Other reasons could include the bias against aging topics in professional schools that reflects ageism in society and the lack of a strong economic and basic science base for health promotion and aging. It is also noteworthy that a small but significant percentage—8 percent—of the medical school respondents did not think the area of prevention and the elderly was necessary in the education of physicians. Interestingly, numerous studies have demonstrated that physicians do spend a considerable proportion of their time in practice on patient education and counseling—about 25 percent of patient care time in general,[23,24,25]—and a large portion of this time will be with the elderly.

The Long-Term Care Gerontology Centers funded by the AoA and the "Teaching Nursing Homes" funded by the Robert Wood Johnson Foundation and NIA are both stimulating more academic programs in aging and, it is hoped, in health promotion. The teaching nursing home concept is based on the model of the teaching hospital-medical school affiliation as defined by Sheps[26] and as applied to other medical school affiliations, such as the teaching health department.[27] It is a formal affiliation between health professional schools (primarily medicine and nursing) and a health facility for the purposes of accomplishing mutual goals of teaching, patient care, research, and community service. Epidemiologic research and prevention should be major components of the program. At the present time the teaching aspects of these programs have not been as strongly emphasized as their research or health services delivery aspects. More needs to be done to support teaching, as well as to develop wellness components to these programs in both the institutional and community settings.

Nursing and Social Work

Perhaps because of their interest in the social components of health, nursing and social work have made considerably more progress than medicine in developing aging programs. Nursing has provided significant leadership in the study of gerontology, and in 1984 there were 38 geriatric nurse practitioner programs. Simson and Wilson[22] surveyed all 131 four-year programs in nursing that awarded baccalaureate degrees. They found 190 courses with content on prevention, 39 courses with a content on aging, and 25 courses with a content on both aging and prevention. Nursing programs place wellness and health promotion as the top priority area in prevention. In contrast to medical schools, in which 93 percent of the aging courses and 66 percent of the prevention content courses were elective, 76 percent of the aging courses and 88 percent of the aging and prevention courses were required in nursing schools. Several schools of social work also have well-developed aging and health promotion programs, although there are no data that are as specific as for nursing and medical schools. The Health Promotion with the Elderly Project at the School of Social Work at the University of Washington is one excellent example of a service program that demonstrates social work initiatives in this area and also provides outstanding teaching opportunities.

Physical Education

Colleges of physical education are becoming more interested in aging and wellness because of the changing demographics, increased interest in fitness and wellness by the student body, and more emphasis on health. One example is the training program in gerontology and adult health at the University of Maryland. This joint project between the university's Center on Aging and its College of Physical Education, Recreation, and Health is an intergenerational program emphasizing exercise, nutrition, and health promotion. The program, which lasts for nine weeks, has three parts: training, therapeutic activities and play, and health education. In the health education component, such topics as nutrition, sexuality, coping with stress, bereavement, communication, well-being, and life satisfaction are discussed.

Public Health

Given that the broad World Health Organization definition of health as "a state of complete physical, mental and social well-being and not merely as the absence of disease or infirmity" has served as a goal for public health, it is remarkable that schools of public health and departments of preventive medicine have not taken more of a leadership role in developing programs for health professionals in aging and health promotion. In a report on public health personnel in the United States by the DHHS,[19] none of the 23 schools of public health reported aging and health promotion as a major area of interest as determined by a review of their school catalogues. However, a surveyed conducted by the Association of Schools of Public Health revealed that 8 of 23 schools had some courses in gerontology. The content of the courses was not specified. There are also few departments of preventive medicine in medical schools—of which there are about 80—with an interest in aging and health promotion. One notable exception is the prevention and health maintenance for senior citizens project at the Rutgers Medical School, Department of Family, Community, and Environmental Medicine. Among other objectives, the program is attempting to increase and strengthen academic programs in geriatric care and preventive services. Another example is the Department of Community Medicine, School of Primary Medical Care, University of Alabama, which operates a health education program at 30 elderly nutrition sites.

Continuing Education

Although the authors have emphasized the education of health professionals beginning their careers, continuing education (CE) programs are crucial to the development of a cadre of experts in the area of aging and health promotion. For most professionals already in practice, but without special training in these areas, it can provide the opportunity to expand their knowledge and skills. For example, CE can provide an opportunity for those doing health promotion (without an emphasis on the elderly) and for those working with the elderly (without an emphasis on health promotion) to fill in the gaps in their training and skills. It also provides professionals the opportunity to keep abreast of the state-of-the-art developments in this rapidly expanding special interest area.

The National Center for Health Education and the Kellogg Foundation are involved in a joint project, the School and College Initiative, which could have a major impact in this area.[28] Its purpose is to stimulate the training of health professionals in health promotion. Recently, the Health Resources and Services Administration of the DHHS funded Geriatric Education Centers at the University of Michigan, Harvard Medical School, State University of New York, and the University of Southern California. These Centers are designed to serve as prototypical regional resources to train multidisciplinary faculty in the field of aging. Yet another program is the Western Gerontological Society's Community Education in Aging Project. This program develops CE programs in partnership with local sponsoring agencies.

Lastly, informal education sources for CE need to be mentioned, especially in light of the paucity of formal academic education programs. Volunteers, students, or those working in rural areas may not have access to CE programs, or the costs may be prohibitive. For those individuals, journal clubs, self-help groups,[29] conferences, self-instructional programs, and publications[15,30,31] may be helpful.

Principles of Education Programs

Despite the paucity of educational programs in this area, there are many innovative service programs and several excellent publications that address the major principles that should underlie these educational programs.[15,29,31] Because health promotion and wellness cuts across disciplinary lines, the following principles apply to all programs, including those for physicians, nurses, behavioral scientists, social workers, and other health professionals.

Health promotion and wellness training should address all those components that affect the quality of life of the elderly (Table 5–1).

There are three levels of prevention: primary, which prevents the development of the disease or disability; secondary, which detects the disease at a very early stage before signs and symptoms develop; and tertiary, which limits disability and

Table 5–1 Components of a Comprehensive, Wellness Concept

LEVELS OF PREVENTION	GOALS	SETTINGS
Primary	High Level of Wellness	Home
Secondary	Preventing Disease	Worksite
		Community-wide
Tertiary	Limiting Disability	Institution
	Humane Death	

loss of independence. Other less traditional goals of wellness need to be also considered. A high level of wellness promotes productivity, self-actualization, self-respect, and self-determination, as well as continued personal growth. In addition, the specific goal of preventing disease addresses the concept of screening for specific diseases, as well as reducing risk factors for diseases. These risk factors may be specific for certain diseases (i.e., smoking for cardiovascular disease) or may contribute to the decrease in host resistance to disease, thereby increasing susceptibility to a wide range of disease[32] (i.e., dementia, infection, arthritis). Next, the goal of limiting disability focuses on preventing the loss of independence and promoting functioning in the least restrictive environment. These areas need particular attention because the so-called trivial problems may render the elderly person's life miserable and may cause more suffering and disability than major problems (e.g., hypertension, diabetes). Finally, the goal of a humane death prevents unnecessary suffering. Unfortunately, it is frequently overlooked as an area where the principles of prevention still apply.

The setting for wellness programs includes all areas where the elderly live. Much can be done even after a person enters an institution where iatrogenic problems become a major problem.

Programs should emphasize that the student has as much to learn from the elderly as to teach. In teaching about health promotion, the teacher and pupil—be they faculty, student, or elder—must be able to change roles and learn from each other. This mutual bonding or counseling strengthens the beneficial effects of the interaction. It is also a key factor in the development of community programs. Participants must feel that they are part of the program and have developed some "ownership."

Students need a role model for healthy old age, such as the "one-hoss-shay" model of Oliver Wendell Holmes, in which chronic disease is either postponed or eliminated so that one dies of old age with a high level of functioning near the end of the maximum human life span. Once students dissociate aging from chronic disease and a long dehabilitating terminal disease, they have a model both for themselves and for elderly patients or participants.

Because they work in a society that is both antiaging and antihealth promotion, students need to understand their own feelings and self-image of aging and their own wellness. Therefore, programs should provide some exposure to techniques in self-imaging and "instant aging." These techniques provide methods by which the student begins to feel and understand his or her own aging, through a process of guided imaging (i.e., a script read by an instructor while the class listens with their eyes closed) and by using various props to simulate the loss of various senses during aging (i.e., the student puts on dark glasses to simulate cataracts and tries to follow instructions on a package). These are excellent methods of getting the student in touch with his feelings toward his or her own aging and the actual impediments of the aging process to see how he or she deals with these. The student also needs to be an active participant in the behavior patterns she or he will teach or advocate for others. One does not need to be a health promotion "saint," but one should at least actively strive toward improving one's own health habits.

Both aging and health promotion require the student to acquire community development skills; wellness for the elderly is a community affair. It involves advocacy, community organization, and public information. Programs and benefits result from organized community efforts.

The organization, financing, and delivery of health and social services are important subjects with which the student should be familiar. This is important because the elderly person must know how to obtain, use, and interact with the social/medical complex in the most efficacious fashion in order to maintain the highest level of functioning. For example, he or she should know how to derive the most benefit from an encounter with a health care provider, such as a nurse or physician—the so-called activated patient concept.

Specific health topics that need to be covered vary in number and extent, according to the different professional groups. However, in general, content should cover such topics as stress reduction, nutrition, physical fitness, retirement planning, environmental awareness, self-care, and safety, all of which affect the susceptibility to poor health and contribute to a lower level of wellness. Because the emphasis is on wellness, diseases must be approached from a preventive aspect. The ones most commonly discussed are senile dementia, hypertension, heart disease, diabetes mellitus, arthritis, and pulmonary disease. Problem areas, such as falls, drugs iatrogenesis, and sexuality, also need to be covered. Also included should be information about such ethical issues as withdrawal of life supports. The students should also become familiar with the model of disease causation that examines the role of general patterns of behavior to all-cause mortality.[32]

Evaluation is a critical part of any wellness program. It is important that accurate data be collected for both evaluation and epidemiologic studies. Students should be made aware of the importance of this information so that we can also learn more about the well elderly and the normal aging process.

Many teaching techniques should be used, including didactic presentations, site visits, conferences, and direct clinical involvement in a variety of community settings: hospitals, nursing homes, social centers, private homes, congregate housing, and the worksite.

Education should not be limited only to new content or technology but should also include sensitivity to the needs and concerns of the elderly for health promotion. This can be done through professional organizations, as well as the lay press.

Turf and Payment Issues

If we permit them to, the issues of professional turf and how to separate wellness from medicine can impede the future development of wellness programs for the elderly. For example, licensing leads to more fragmentation in the field and more battles over turf. Payment for services on a fee-for-services basis both encourages further licensing and stimulates inflationary cost increases. Instead, payment could be through private sources, prepayment programs, or the public health system. Local initiatives should be allowed to flourish as they have, and programs should remain flexible and nonthreatening. A full range of service providers, including currently licensed (e.g., physicians, nurses, pharmacists), and unlicensed personnel (e.g., self-help groups, community organizers, people interested in exercise and nutrition) should participate in wellness programs. The skills and knowledge that need to be taught should be incorporated into existing professional categories in a broadened aging network.

CONCLUSION

Education and training in wellness have developed remarkably in the last several years, but are still terribly inadequate, particularly in some professional groups. There needs to be a tremendous effort made in continuing education to assist in closing the gap between need and supply until more professionals are trained.

At the present time, service programs in wellness and aging are far more developed than the educational programs, but they should provide the needed impetus for the future development of those education and training programs.

NOTES

1. Marc La Londe, *A New Perspective on the Health of Canadians* (Ottawa: Minister of National Health and Welfare, Government of Canada, 1974), pp. 8–76.

2. U.S. Department of Health and Human Services, *Healthy People. The Surgeon General's Report on Health Promotion and Disease Prevention*. DHHS Publication No. 79–55071 (Washington, D.C.: U.S. Government Printing Office, 1979), pp. 3–155.

3. U.S. Department of Health and Human Services, *Final Report of the 1981 White House Conference on Aging*, Volumes 1, 2, 3 (Washington, D.C.: U.S. Government Printing Office, 1982), pp. 100–103.

4. Robert L. Kane, *et al. Geriatrics in the United States* (Lexington Books, Lexington, Mass., 1981), pp. 1–155.

5. Mary Ann Eiler, ed., *Physician Characteristics and Distribution Report* (Chicago: American Medical Association, 1982), p. 150.

6. U.S. Department of Health and Human Services, National Center for Health Statistics, *Health United States: 1980*, 81–1232 (Washington, D.C.: U.S. Government Printing Office, 1980), p. 75.

7. Institute of Medicine, *A Policy Report: The Elderly and Functional Dependency* (Washington, D.C.: National Academy of Sciences, 1977), p. 80.

8. L. Breslow and A.R. Somers, "The Lifetime Health Monitoring Program: A Practical Approach to Preventive Medicine." *New England Journal of Medicine* 296, no. 11 (1977): 601–608.

9. Institute of Medicine, *Perspectives on Health Promotion and Disease Prevention in the U.S.* (Washington, D.C.: National Academy of Sciences, 1978), p. 55.

10. "Report of the Task Force on Periodic Health Examinations," *Canadian Medical Association Journal,* 121 (1979): 1–45.

11. R.L. Kane and R.A. Kane, "Alternatives to Institutional Care of the Elderly: Beyond the Dichotomy," *The Gerontologist* 20, no. 3 (1980): 249–259.

12. J.J. Collahan, "How Much, For What, and For Whom," *American Journal of Public Health* 71, no. 9 (1981): 987–988.

13. Health Insurance Association of America, *Industrywide Network for Social, Urban and Rural Efforts,* "The INSURE Project on Lifecycle" (Washington, D.C.: Preventive Health Services), p. 38.

14. W.D. Clark, "Prevention and Health Maintenance for Senior Citizens Less than Seventy" (New Brunswick, N.J.: Rutgers Medical School, Department of Family Medicine, 1981).

15. K.G. Bauer, *Improving the Chances for Health: Lifestyle Change and Health Evaluation* (San Francisco: National Center for Health Education, 1980, Mimeographed), p. 35.

16. J.F. Fries, "Aging, Natural Death, and the Compression of Morbidity," *New England Journal of Medicine* 300 (1980): 130–135.

17. E.L. Schneider and J.A. Brody, "Aging, Natural Death and the Compression of Morbidity: Another View," *New England Journal of Medicine* 398 (1983): 854–855.

18. M. Sicker, "Manpower Needs," in A.N. Exton-Smith and J.G. Evans, eds. *Care of the Elderly: Meeting the Challenge of Dependency* (London: Academic Press, 1977), pp. 225–234.

19. U.S. Department of Health and Human Services, Health Resources Administration, *Public Health Personnel in the United States, 1980,* HRP–0904085 (Washington, D.C.: U.S. Public Health Service, 1982).

20. Institute of Medicine, *Report of a Study: Aging and Medical Education* (Washington, D.C.: National Academy of Sciences, 1978).

21. A.S. Robbins *et al.,* "A Study of Geriatric Training Programs in the United States," *Journal of Medical Education* (February, 1982): 79–86.

22. S. Simson and L. Wilson, "Medical School and Nursing School Education in Disease Prevention, Health Promotion, and Aging" (Presentation at the Annual Scientific Meeting, Gerontological Society of America, San Francisco, 1983).
23. A. Bergman, et al., "Time-Motion Study of Practicing Pediatricians," Pediatrics 38 (1966): 254–263.
24. H.M. Parrish, et al. "Time Study of General Practitioner's Office Hours," Archives of Environmental Health 142 (1967): 892.
25. H.E. Payson, et al., "Time Study of an Internship on a University Medical Service," New England Journal of Medicine 264 (1961): 439–443.
26. C.G. Sheps, "Medical Schools and Hospitals: Interdependence for Education and Service," Journal of Medical Education (1965): 40.
27. P.G. Weiler and D.K. Clauson, "Medical Schools and Public Health Departments: A New Alliance for Progress," Journal of Medical Education 54 (1979): 217–223.
28. National Center for Health Education, "The School and College Initiative, National Center for Health Education" (San Francisco: NCHE), p. 10.
29. S. Fallcreek and M. Mettler, A Healthy Old Age: A Sourcebook For Health Promotion with Older Adults (Seattle, Wa.: School of Social Work, University of Washington, 1983 Mimeograph), p. 105.
30. Chiyoko Furukawa, and Dianna Shomaker, Community Health Services for the Aged (Germantown, Md.: Aspen Publication Corp., 1982), pp. 3–359.
31. Center for the Study of Aging, "Futures After Fifty Program" (Albany, N.Y.: Center for the Study of Aging), pp. 1–3.
32. L.F. Beckman and D.L. Wingrad, "The Impact of Health Practices on Mortality in Human Population Laboratory for Epidemiologic Studies" (Berkeley: Nurigraph, Human Population Laboratory, California Department of Health Services, 1980), pp. 1–86.

Chapter 6

Funding Health Promotion for Elders

Martha Holstein, M.A.

As with many other worthwhile efforts, health promotion must compete for limited financial and other resources. The fund raising required to establish a wellness program in the nonprofit sector requires infinite patience; a deep belief in your project; an ability to hear "no" frequently without becoming too discouraged; the "digging" talents of an archeologist; clarity about your goals, objectives, and program implementation plans; and community support. However, fund raising for health promotion has one major advantage over many other programs: As a health-related effort, it may be reimbursable by third party payers.

Potential sources for program funding include public programs (federal, state, and local), foundations, corporate foundations, corporations, individual donors, fee-for-service, third party reimbursements, fund-raising events, and for-profit businesses. In addition to actual cash support, a considerable array of in-kind sources of program support can be obtained by diligent managers, as can opportunities for barter.

IDENTIFYING SOURCES

Federal Resources

From 1965 to 1980, the federal government provided significant sums for programs serving the elderly. In addition to age-based entitlement programs, such as Medicare and Social Security, a large number of demonstration or model projects received start-up, short-term grants. Many of these projects were health-related.

By 1984, this source of funds had dried up considerably, making the search for federal support more difficult and often less successful. Yet, the effort is still worthwhile, particularly if you discover the appropriate agency to fund your project. Moreover, the timing is right for health promotion programs. Philosophically, the federal government has joined the ''wellness revolution'' and favors prevention and health promotion. A health promotion strategy also conforms to the post-1980 attitude adopted toward elders—that they are relatively well off, need few services, and are capable of taking considerable responsibility for their own well-being.

A 1979 landmark study, *Healthy People: The Surgeon General's Report on Health Promotion and Disease Prevention*[1] contains a comprehensive statement on the federal attitude toward disease prevention and health promotion, including a chapter on ''Healthy Older People.'' It suggests that the broad, long-term goal of a health promotion strategy for elders must be an independent and rewarding life in old age, unlimited by the health problems that are within the individual's capacity to control. Increasing longevity without attention to the quality of life is not sufficient. A specific objective contained in the report is, to reduce the average annual number of days of restricted activity due to acute and chronic conditions by 20 percent, to fewer than 30 days per year for people 65 and older by 1990.[2] The most compelling health promotion need is to provide integrated and comprehensive services to the elderly.

More explicit and quantifiable goals are contained in the 1980 report of the Department of Health and Human Services (DHHS), *Promoting Health/Preventing Disease: Objectives for the Nation*.[3] This document addresses the health problems of all age groups. For elders, they include high blood pressure control, immunization, toxic agent control, occupational health and safety, accident and injury prevention, dental health, infectious disease control, smoking and health, misuse of alcohol and drugs, nutrition, physical fitness, and stress. The report focuses on education and information, as well as on services, technology, and evaluation.

Developments in Aging, 1981, Volume I,[4] a publication of the Special Committee on Aging, United States Senate, also addresses health promotion and the elderly. Carrying forward the DHHS 1976 ''Forward Plan for Health,'' this report emphasizes the quality of life based on improvements in health habits and home and work environments.

The report of the Technical Committee on Health Maintenance and Health Promotion for the 1981 White House Conference on Aging[5] also provides a succinct review of federal initiatives. It recommends a broad-based approach to health promotion that includes the guarantee of an adequate income to maintain a decent standard of living; nutrition education through the Older Americans Act and coordination of other federal programs; dental care coverage under Medicare; assessment centers to provide preventive health care and multidisciplinary health assessment; creation of self-care and mutual help groups through public and private efforts; development of a National Senior Health Corps to serve in the areas of health education, counseling, and outreach; and Medicare coverage for health promotion activities.

Since 1980, the Administration on Aging (AoA) has funded some excellent health promotion projects, generally in the range of $100,000–$125,000 annually. Some projects combine research, program development, and implementation in the areas of health education, health screening, and health promotion as related to chronic illness.

In late summer 1983, AoA and the Public Health Service (PHS) in the Office of the Surgeon General signed a formal Memorandum of Understanding that mandates that both agencies support health promotion activities for elders. The initiative's intent is to stimulate low-cost, relatively simple efforts in four target areas: drug use and misuse, injury prevention and control, nutrition, and physical fitness and exercise. Current plans propose that state units on aging, area agencies on aging, and divisions of the PHS work cooperatively in these target areas. These multiple access points will facilitate ease of entry into the information system, which will be enhanced further after each governor designates a state-level lead agency. For this, as with any federal program initiative, it is important to establish a personal contact from which you can obtain current information.

Other federal agencies and offices address health promotion and wellness issues as well, although with limited amounts of funding. The Office for Disease Prevention and Health Promotion within the Office of the Assistant Secretary for Health, DHHS, develops school, community, worksite, and clinical programs and may provide joint funding with the AoA. The National Institutes of Health and the National Center for Health Services Research are interested in prevention. The Food and Drug Administration and the Centers for Disease Control (Center for Health Promotion and Education) are other federal sources of interest and support, most likely for major research and demonstration grants over $100,000 annually. Because health promotion is closely linked to health care costs, the Health Care Financing Administration should also be contacted. Finally, the Institute of Medicine has a Committee on Health Promotion and Disease Prevention, but it lacks a clear direction.

The monumental *Catalog of Federal Domestic Assistance*[6] is the basic investigative tool for exploring federal funding sources. For health-related programs, titles under DHHS are likely starting places for your search. In addition, use its functional and subject indices to identify less obvious sources. Examine the *Catalog* carefully and critically, reviewing every program description that may be relevant. Summarize potential sources and create a minicatalogue for your own use. Additional suggestions of how to make the *Catalog* work for you are contained in an excellent article, "The Catalog of Federal Domestic Assistance,"[7] by Timothy Saastra published by the Grantsmanship Center in 1976.

Watch the daily *Federal Register*[8] and the *Commerce Business Daily*[9] for specific requests for proposals. Both are available on subscription, at federal regional offices, or in the documents section of most libraries. These and the *Catalog* can be purchased from the Government Printing Office.

After obtaining as much information as possible from the appropriate written sources, write the agency for further information and keep in contact by telephone. It may take some time and persistence to reach the person who can actually help you, but the effort will result in greater clarity and detail about possible program initiatives. You may also anticipate public announcements of program funding while increasing your familiarity with the funding sources' less visible agendas.

State Funding

State units on aging, through local area agencies on aging, have funded some health promotion programs. For example, the North Carolina Division on Aging sponsored "AHOY (Add Health to Our Years)" on a statewide basis. The "Growing Younger" program was sponsored by the Boise Council on Aging with funding from the Centers for Disease Control and the state of Idaho. Review state and local planning and service area plans to determine the approach appropriate to your community.

In addition to its agency on aging, become familiar with your state's department of health and health agency network. Although the fiscal crises experienced by many states have resulted in reductions in programs and services, you may discover untapped resources or help create future interest in funding programs in health promotion. Let the relevant agencies become familiar with the health promotion strategy, your efforts, and the reasons why, in the long run, these efforts may help them save money. The health network may become even more important following initiation of the AoA–PHS initiative.

Parent Agencies

Many programs receive direct support from a parent agency, such as the Red Cross or the YM/YWCA. This support may be the most secure route to permanent program funding. If you are not currently involved with a voluntary agency that is likely to sponsor a health promotion project, you might want to volunteer to serve on a committee or perhaps even on a board of such an agency. With patience and persistence, you may be able to interest that agency in health promotion for elders. The Wisdom Project—American Red Cross in Greater New York and the Queens Hospital Center—is a good example of a project initiated by the Red Cross with in-kind hospital support (e.g., staff nursing time donated to conduct a preprogram participant assessment). Because the Red Cross' contribution to the demonstration phase represents a commitment from its core budget, there is a good chance that support will continue in future project years for those portions of the project not covered by other sources.

Another advantage of being "adopted" by a respected parent agency is the credibility it may offer to a fledgling program. Even if the agency offers no funding, it may assist you to obtain resources through its expertise, name recognition, and contacts. It may take an established connection to convince a funding source of your program's merits.

Foundations/Corporations

Background

Foundation and corporate resources can become an important source of program funding and research support if you do your homework carefully. Approximately $6–7 billion are provided annually by these sources; this amount is divided about equally between corporations and foundations. The major difference among funding sources is their degree of professionalism. The more professional the program, the more information about it will be public and available, and the easier it will be to obtain that information. The review process will be clear, limits will have been established, and program guidelines will be available. The foundations of some corporations (about 10% nationally), such as Levi Strauss (San Francisco), Dayton-Hudson (Minneapolis), Exxon (New York), Atlantic Richfield (Los Angeles), and Syntex (Palo Alto) are as professional as the established foundations; they are professionally operated, respected units within the corporate structure.

With a smaller, less sophisticated program, you will have greater difficulty obtaining useful information about its program goals, previous grantees, giving levels, contact person, dates for submittal, and the review process. It will also be more difficult to reach an informed person by telephone because there rarely is a professional staff member.

Both foundations and corporations may only fund programs within strict geographic limits. Corporations, community, and smaller foundations often prefer to give in communities where they maintain offices or have plants. Bear in mind that the vast majority of foundations are small, family operations whose members like to see directly how grantees use their money.

An effective corporate and foundation fund-raising strategy depends, in part, on your understanding of why the funding source supports nonprofit programs. Most private foundations were created for a combination of altruistic and tax purposes. Their directions for the dispersal of funds may be quite explicit and, to the outside observer, often capricious. Or they may be very vague; many foundations support "health and welfare." Until you discover how that guideline translates into actual support, you have no way of knowing if your program is appropriate.

Companies, on the other hand, have no legal obligation to support nonprofit organizations although they too derive tax benefits from charitable contributions. Those companies that are actively philanthropic give money for a variety of reasons, in a variety of ways. They may believe that giving is a community investment and a way to respond to broader social concerns. More often, however, giving is linked explicitly to corporate needs (e.g., producing a pool of trained individuals who are potential employees, supporting services that benefit employees and their families, providing public recognition or prestige for the company, improving the market for the company's products, supporting the interests of senior management or groups in which employees are involved, responding to peer pressure). Assume that the narrowest concerns motivate corporate giving and use that knowledge to your advantage. For more information on corporate giving, see Sam Sternberg, *National Directory of Corporate Charity, California Edition*.[10]

Fortunately, health promotion/prevention programs respond directly both to narrow corporate interests and to broader societal concerns. Decision makers in both government and the private sector face profound dilemmas as they confront the rapidly rising costs of medical care. Employers now pay over one-half of the nations's health care bill; they obviously have a major interest in programs that may reduce the costs of health care. The changing relationship between Medicare and company health benefits for older workers, a result of 1982 legislation, may be an added incentive for companies to think positively about supporting health promotion projects for elders.

As you plan your program, think of creative ways that it might respond to the concerns about rising health care costs. Health promotion has the luxury of appealing to humanitarian and economic interests simultaneously. Use this dual appeal to your advantage.

Developing a Prospect List

The first step is to develop a list of potential corporate and/or foundation supporters (the prospect list). Directories provide the most accessible route to the names and priorities of the larger foundations and corporations. Smaller funding sources can be identified by analyzing your personal networks, or through discussions with managers of similar programs.

Select funding sources for further study based on their program and subject priorities—for example, health, elders, direct service, training—and their geographical focus. If your program is community-based, identify supporters in your local area because the most important and stable benefactors of your program will probably be local businesses and perhaps foundations. If your program is national in scope, your best source may be the larger national entities.

To find these national funding sources, review state foundation directories, the national *Foundation Directory*,[11] the *Foundation Center Source Book Profiles*,[12] the *Foundation Grants Index*,[13] and other related guides. Specialized directories are also useful; check *The Directory of Grants for Health*[14] and *Foundations that Provide Support for Health and Human Services*.[15] Foundation Center Libraries of the Council of Foundations are located in cities across the country; each branch has a staff that can direct you to the Foundation Center's *Comsearch Printouts*[16] (available in many subject areas for a charge; written request accepted), to the *National Directory of Corporate Charity*, IRS Forms 990, publications of the Council of Financial Aid to Education, and numerous other useful directories. Many directories are also available at university and good, general libraries.

For the names of companies with headquarters or plants in your community, turn to state industrial and business directories, Chamber of Commerce membership lists, and *Standard and Poor's Register of Corporations, Directors and Executives*,[17] which also provides very useful information about the background of the companies and their personnel. In these initial efforts, obtain information about the average size of grants, review schedule, names of board members or contribution committee chairs, annual number of new grantees, preferred means of contact, contact persons, phone numbers, plant communities, and availability of written materials.

Then consider several questions that may help you narrow your choices. Which type of company would have a logical interest in this area because of the nature of its work? Do any companies of this type have offices or plants in your community? Do you know anyone who works for them? Does a company have a particular interest in wellness or health promotion as displayed in internally supported promotion activities? You can identify some of these companies through the Washington Business Group on Health (922 Pennsylvania Ave., S.E., Washington, D.C., 20003). Major companies, such as IBM, Xerox, Pepsico, and General Dynamics, have invested in wellness programs and also have thoughtful giving programs.

Further, which type of company can benefit from a public relations standpoint by supporting disease prevention projects (e.g., drug companies)? Which companies have supported compatible programs? The answers to these questions not only focus your prospect list but also help form the basis of your personalized approach to each company. A particularly good prospect is a company with a vested interest in what you are trying to do and that is located in your community.

In addition, ask whether any of your participants, board members, or friends are involved with a corporation. Remember that some companies like to fund projects that involve their personnel. Others make decisions purely on the basis of personal interest; someone excited them about a program. For this reason, many fund-raising consultants suggest that the quickest route to obtaining corporate resources is to talk to as many people as possible to identify as many "inside" contacts as you can.

Start this process in small groups by "brainstorming" lists of contacts. People often do not realize how many corporate leaders they actually know. Personal introductions are terribly important. Highlight all companies where you have a possible contact.

Investigate several other information sources as well. Health promotion programs similar to the one you propose may be willing to share information about funding sources. If you approach them, obtain as much detail as possible, including the amount of time between submittal and award, any special problems with the funding source, and any particular interests of the source. Community foundations in your area often are willing to provide project consultation. Even if they are not an appropriate funding source they can advise you or speak about your project to any grantmaking group in which they participate.

Many communities have formal alliances of grantmakers, known by the acronym RAGS—Regional Association of Grantmakers—whose staff person is frequently an excellent source of advice. Other areas have more informal associations for grantmakers. Obtain the names of representatives to these groups, and ask for their assistance in recommending potential funding sources and in advocating for your program.

In addition, the formally organized, New York-based group, Grantmakers in Health, may be willing to explore potential funding sources. The less formally organized group, Grantmakers in Aging, also meets regularly to share ideas, educate themselves, and explore the possibilities of joint funding.

A few private or corporate foundations that have expressed an interest in health, elders, or health promotion are:

- the Kaiser Family Foundation (Menlo Park, CA)—emphasis on prepaid health care
- John Hartford Foundation (New York, NY)—major research and demonstration projects in health care financing
- the Kellogg Foundation (Battle Creek, MI)
- Florence Burden Foundation (New York, NY)
- Kimberly Clark Foundation (Neenah, WI).

Once you have searched the appropriate directories and printouts, brainstormed for potentially responsive companies and for personal contacts, sought help from comparable programs, and eliminated sources with priorities and geographical constraints that make them an unlikely funding source, you should have a fairly extensive prospect list. The hardest work comes next—obtaining first-hand information that allows you to narrow your list even further to the most likely prospects.

There is no standard procedure to obtain the first-hand information needed because grant programs are administered in many different ways. Sometimes, you may easily identify the contact person who can provide you with all the information you need. In other cases, a substantial effort is required to locate the correct person, and then the information you obtain may be vague. Or you may have to depend solely on written materials, such as annual reports, guidelines, application procedures, or lists of previous grantees. In all cases, your objective is clear: to obtain as much detailed information as you can about the funding source to guide your proposal development and to enhance your chances of a positive funding decision.

For example, in the area of health promotion, you need to know if the prospect funds direct service programs—the most common type of program—research, evaluation studies, training, or films. Do they have a history of funding in health promotion or if they fund in health, are they willing to entertain a proposal in this area?

With the more formally organized foundations and corporations, first contact them by telephone to request guidelines and further information. The call allows you to discuss the relevance of your idea to their funding priorities and to update any written material that you may have. Before you call, however, know exactly what you want to ask and why you have chosen this prospect for further investigation. If the funding official is unwilling to discuss a project on the phone, request whatever information they have for public distribution.

Obtaining comparable information from the corporation or foundation with a less formally organized giving program may present a considerable challenge. The first task is to identify the office or the person who makes funding decisions. Try starting with the public affairs department; among major companies, a little more than one-third of the direct giving programs can be found in the public affairs department. Giving programs might also be located within personnel, public relations, urban affairs, or administration departments. Many companies have corporate contributions committees and a secretary who organizes requests but has little actual authority. With some degree of diligent searching, you may find the person who handles corporate giving. Ask that individual about the company's general funding priorities, if it has ever funded a health promotion or aging project, and for the application guidelines and deadlines. Before you end the conversation, find out who you are speaking to, the exact name of the department, and the correct phone number. This information will be helpful at a later point.

For many smaller companies, it is not possible to obtain even this much information because funding decisions rest almost solely with the chief executive officer (CEO) or other top-level officials. In this case, giving tends to be closely tied to the personal preferences of management, and often unsolicited proposals are not considered. Do not give up, however, because you may be able to develop the appropriate contacts to make your program the president's personal favorite. On the other hand, do not put this company high on your list.

To develop an even greater understanding of the company's interests and directions, talk to the members of its public relations department and to its employees. Try to find out what the company's major concerns are and if it has any internal health promotion program. Read the business pages of your local newspaper or the national business publications. Review grantmaking and foundation magazines, such as *The Grantsmanship Center News*[18] or *Foundation News*.[19] Once you feel that your list is complete, that you have honed down your selection to those sources that clearly favor projects of your kind, you are ready for the application phase—communicating information about your project in written form to a receptive audience.

PROPOSAL DEVELOPMENT

The type of proposal you write depends largely on the intended recipient. For example, the federal government or a professionally staffed foundation generally requires a more detailed proposal than a corporate program where the CEO makes all the decisions.

For most federal programs, a full, detailed proposal, following carefully outlined guidelines that they send to you, is the only acceptable route. Other federal agencies, such as AoA, have started to use the 10-page concept paper as a screening device. Many foundations and corporations prefer a two-page letter of intent. If they are interested, they then ask for a full proposal.

No matter the approach selected or required, a few basics are essential: absolute clarity about your program or research plans, a belief in its purposes and methods, a clear understanding of why you want to undertake it, and an explanation of how your plans differ from or build on what others have done. Remember also, you are "selling" an excellent program, giving the funding source an opportunity to participate in a high-quality, worthwhile project that addresses major societal or community needs. Write as if you believe they need you, rather than the reverse. Listing a minimum of 10 key program benefits and 10 reasons why the project is unique may help you sell the program. Finally, meet with colleagues, discuss all program components, and be certain that you are filling a real need.

Your proposal is simply a logical explication of the program that you know so well and care so much about. There is nothing mysterious about it. Write in simple language, without jargon; be honest and direct. Once you have a basic proposal carefully developed and written, you may vary it for any number of purposes.

Many foundations and corporations request a letter of intent as the preliminary step. Clearly and briefly—in no more than two pages—describe your organization and the need for your project; explain what you propose to do to meet this need and why your organization is the best one to do the job; inform them about other project supporters, why you have selected that particular company or foundation, and why they would benefit from supporting your program. The fruits of your information gathering research should be contained in that last section. Depending on the project's budget and the funding source's particular giving patterns, select a specific dollar amount to request. Do not ask for full funding for a program with an annual budget of $60,000 from a source whose giving range is from $2,000 to $7,000. In that case, you may ask for the maximum amount they give and inform them that you plan to request comparable amounts from other sources; list these sources and any sources that have already contributed to the program.

At the close of your letter of intent, indicate when you will call the prospect for follow-up. The funding source thus expects your call, and for many, that knowledge provides an added impetus to review the proposal. Generally, a month between the time of submittal and the phone call is an appropriate time period. In the interval, you may receive a letter from them indicating the procedures that they will follow to handle your proposal; let that notification be your guide to future action.

If the funding source is interested in your proposal, it may request a full proposal, which is a more detailed version of the letter of intent. Again, keep that proposal short and logical. It should contain a cover letter, title page, table of contents, abstract, introduction (to the organization), statement of the need for the program, objectives, methods, evaluation, future funding plans, budget, and appendices. Generally, the appendices include a copy of your 501 (c) (3) ruling establishing your nonprofit status, a list of your board of directors and staff, resumes of project staff, your annual report—this report can be a very simple document—a list of other contributors, support letters for the project or testimonials regarding your organization, and any examples of your programs that will help establish your credibility. Actual proposal writing can be a very satisfying experience, if you are prepared. If you have not written proposals before, it may be wise to review books or articles on proposal writing.

POSTAPPLICATION PHASE

After submitting the proposal, call one month later if the recipient has not yet contacted you. Try to arrange for a personal visit to discuss your proposal; this step is more appropriate for corporate and foundation sources than for the federal government. In this way, the funding source has an opportunity to meet you and to develop additional confidence in your organization's ability to undertake the tasks outlined in the proposal. The personal visit has another advantage; despite the formal procedures that you have followed, many decisions rest on that elusive personal connection. After the visit, the program becomes tied to you as an individual.

Assume that this visit is the only meeting you will have. Know exactly how many people will be present; prepare simple handouts that summarize your proposal and the budget. Highlight your organization's strengths and provide a list of corporate sponsors. Encourage questions and ask ones that help you understand the other person's thinking. Listen intently. If possible, relate your program to their interests. Acknowledge the toughness of their decision-making process, with so many excellent but competing proposals, but sell your idea. Ask for a specific amount of funding. If the meeting goes well, also ask for introductions to other possible funding sources. When you walk away, they should know exactly why your organization, your staff, and your program represents an unmatched opportunity for them.

If the response is positive, you are embarking on what you hope will be a long-term relationship with the funding source. You both now have a stake in the program's success. Let the grantor know how you acknowledge contributors generally, and ask if it desires any other forms of recognition. An immediate thank-you letter is appropriate. Provide regular reports; sent it copies of your newsletters and publications. If any of your leadership will be on radio or television, alert the funding sources. It is important for you to continue building credibility. But more than anything else, you must do the job that you set out to do. In many cases, once you have received funding from a source, particularly from corporations, and have performed satisfactorily, the source will become your advocate with other foundations and corporations.

If a prospect refuses to fund your proposal and if its letter does not explain the reasons for the denial, call to request that information. It will be useful in future contacts with that and other funding sources. Additionally, it is gracious to write and thank the prospect for taking the time to review your proposal. Be persistent; it may take years to get funding from a particular funding source.

A carefully developed proposal that meets well-defined needs, matched with an equally diligent search for the most appropriate funding sources, yields the most positive results. As you explore the somewhat elusive world of corporate and foundation funding, keep four thoughts in mind: (1) Do not accept no from a person who is not authorized to say yes, (2) seek an introduction from within the funding source, (3) try to arrange for a personal meeting, and (4) make every minute of that meeting count. And if the source says no, despite your best efforts, do not become too discouraged. You still have a program worth funding and an organization to back it up. Keep trying.

OTHER SOURCES

Federal, state, local, foundation, and corporate funds are not the only sources of financing. Corporations may also donate in-kind benefits, which are often easier for them to provide than money. You must know exactly what items you need and identify those companies that have that precise resource. Remember, however, to treat requests for in-kind support as seriously as you do actual cash requests.

For instance, a company legal department may help you incorporate, and the public relations or marketing departments can help you package your program. Larger companies have the resources to help you develop a slide show or videotape. Or they may lend you videotaping and playback equipment so that participants have the opportunity to view themselves engaging in program activities. These audiovisual resources are useful in selling your program to outsiders and in maintaining participant enthusiasm.

Printing, postage, office space, supplies, function space, research assistance, and duplication services can all be donated. Some companies might consider putting the program director on their payroll and then "loan" him or her back to the community to operate the program. In this way, the cost of a salary is supported.

Another cost-saving strategy is to "piggyback" on corporate purchases of supplies and equipment. Because companies often buy in large quantities, they obtain considerable discounts; even after reimbursing the company for the cost of your supplies, you will save money.

Cooperative arrangements may be worked out with a company medical department that might provide preprogram screening and may continue with follow-ups. Their facilities might offer a home for your program in off-hours. Many businesses have gyms or health facilities that are underutilized, particularly at certain times of the day. Yet 10 A.M. might be the best time for your program to be scheduled.

Continue thinking of ways you can obtain help from businesses without a direct transfer of funds. You might be surprised at the results.

Fee for service (partial or whole) or donations are also valuable sources of income. It is important to recognize that many potential clients are both able and willing to pay for services. By charging a set amount or setting fees on a sliding scale, you can generate enough resources from people who are able to pay to support those who have greater difficulty. Low-cost memberships, with scholarships available, are also a reasonable way to develop broad-based funding. In view of the experienced health promotion efforts, it is particularly important to find ways to encourage the participation of people with more limited resources; too often, and largely inadvertently, health promotion programs have attracted members of the middle class who have the inclination, the background, and the resources to adopt healthier life styles. They have experienced the power of controlling their own lives and see health promotion efforts as one more step in that direction. Some change agent foundations may find targeting low-income or minority elders for your program with support from other participants' fees to be very attractive.

Consider bartering goods and services. For example, in exchange for facility usage, project staff may offer training to company employees. Recreation centers are good possibilities for such an exchange, but do not ignore businesses. You may help them establish their own wellness programs or invite company personnel to join your program.

The hospitals in your area may also be willing to exchange services. Some may donate staff to help with participant assessment or follow-up. If a physician is involved or if a medical diagnosis results in a recommendation for the activity provided by your health promotion program, third party payers may pick up some of the costs. Yet, reimbursement regulations are extraordinarily complicated. Medicare does not cover what is generally understood by the term prevention; it is biased toward acute-care. However, an arthritis program that is rehabilitative in nature may be reimbursable, if not by Medicare then by other payers.

Even if third party payment is unlikely, hospitals are useful contacts. They can benefit financially from certain wellness programs and may find health promotion to be even more in their self-interest as prospective payment programs and preferred provider agreements become more important. Affiliating your program with a respected hospital, for all the potential disadvantages of possibly medicalizing it, may open funding avenues that would otherwise be closed to you. Many sources typically fund hospitals when they say they fund in the area of "health."

The American Hospital Association has a Center for Health Promotion with four divisions: community health, employee health, patient education, and hospital, business, and industry, and a package of information about their activities that are made available on request.

An important and often overlooked resource for community programs is the individual donor who represents the single largest source of giving in the nation. This individual donor approach works best if your program has a natural constituency. Are there running clubs or senior organizations that have relatively affluent clientele or sponsors? Or consider individual business leaders or members of the Chamber of Commerce. Look to the community of very small business people as potential individual contributors. You can approach the donor either face-to-face or through a direct mail effort.

If you are soliciting funds from an individual donor in person—the most difficult aspect of fund raising for many people—follow a similar process to the one used to select possible corporate sponsors. With the assistance of your board and friends, target the people most likely to give, evaluate them as prospects, gather as much information about them as possible, cultivate their interests, find ways for them to develop a sense of ownership about your program, and ask for a donation. Understand why people give, and recognize that most people give because someone asked them. (For more useful information, see Susan Scribner and Florence Green, "Asking for Money," *Grantsmanship Center News*, March/April, 1983.)[20]

If you use the direct mail approach, your letter should state the most compelling reasons for supporting your program. Do not hesitate to be dramatic, or to do a "hard" sell. In your approach, your program must stand out from all the other appeals that the recipient receives. Try to keep the letter as short as possible but, at the same time, tell your story. Consultants recommend exceeding the one-page maximum, if necessary. Introduce the subject, then ask for money, and close with a reminder of the effect that the contribution will have on the older participant and, if you can do it reasonably, on the overall social costs of ill health. Use relevant statistics or case examples whenever you can relate them to your program's potential impact. In developing this letter, all the work that you did in preparing for your proposal writing will be very helpful; you restate why your program is unique, who it benefits, and why it is so important. No matter how you develop your lists, do not forget your board, staff, and even program participants. Participants may be particularly pleased to assist if they knew that the program needs additional resources to continue or to expand.

Enclose a reply envelope and a rate card with suggested contribution amounts. Some consultants maintain that the end of the year is a good time to launch a direct-mail campaign becauase people feel benevolent and need tax deductible contributions. It is probably best to avoid early January, when people confront holiday bills, and the summer, when so many people are traveling; good and bad arguments can be made for launching campaigns at most other times of the year. Direct mail can be expensive, particularly if you use a large mailing list and professional printing, but it may yield fruitful results, especially if your program is a national one. You may also consider using the service of a direct mail consultant. The *Grantsmanship Center News* (September/October, 1982) featured a very useful article, "A Primer on Mailing Lists."[21]

Another approach, which is costly in time, is the fund-raising event. Such events include testimonial dinners, shows, sponsored runs, lectures, or "slim-a-thons," the upbeat version of the walk or run in which sponsors agree to donate a certain amount of money for every pound lost. Time-consuming to organize, events work best if you have a natural audience. For example, you may decide to honor Mr. Smith who has run marathons every month for the past 65 years and is also CEO of the largest company in your town. Many people will come to your dinner simply because they cannot afford not to come. The hard job is first to convince Mr. Smith that he is willing to be so honored and, second, to round up a cadre of experienced volunteers to help ensure that the event is well organized and well publicized.

A different type of program is a simpler event, such as launching the "Friends of. . . ." You may still select someone well respected in the community to receive recognition, but the charge for the event is minimal. In this way, you can attract a large number of your peers who may spend $25 dollars for an event, but will not spend $100. These events are enjoyable, raise small amounts of money, and help give your program considerable local publicity. An event, moreover, may stimulate donations, especially if it receives press coverage. Other types of events are limited only by the constraints of your imagination.

It is important to explore combinations of funding or the imaginative use of volunteers that extends your capacity to provide services. Consider a "train the trainers" approach; this allows trained older people to conduct many aspects of wellness programs. An initial outlay of funds to develop or purchase training materials and to train a cadre of volunteers goes a long way to bring health promotion efforts into your community.

Lastly, the establishment of for-profit businesses to support your program opens a whole new realm of possibilities. To succeed in this arena, you need a good business sense and some assistance from an attorney. It requires a new way of thinking, but may be just the challenge needed to fund your program. *Enterprise in the Non-Profit Sector*[22] by James C. Cremmins and Mary Keil (1983) should stimulate your thinking.

CONCLUSION

Both societal and individual problems and attitudes favor your fund-raising efforts. Runaway health care costs affect both the private and public sectors. The focus on containing health care costs is turning public attention to wellness as a cost-reduction strategy. New public policies mandating prospective payment systems and preferred provider agreements are also reinforcing prevention efforts. The emphasis in the 1980s on personal responsibility and fitness and a shift in the nation's disease and population profiles, with chronic disease replacing acute diseases as the predominant cause of death and disability, should help you to obtain scarce resources. Your knowledge about the substantive area of health promotion and the techniques of fund raising, your commitment to your project's goals, and hard work are all further keys to your success.

NOTES

1. U.S. Department of Health and Human Services, *Healthy People: The Surgeon General's Report on Health Promotion and Disease Prevention* (Washington, D.C.: Government Printing Office, 1979), p. 71.

2. *Ibid.*, p. 71.

3. U.S. Department of Health and Human Services, *Promoting Health/Preventing Disease: Objectives for the Nation* (Washington, D.C.: Government Printing Office, 1980), p. 71.

4. United States Senate Special Committee on Aging, *Developments in Aging*, Vol. I (Washington, D.C.: Government Printing Office, 1981).

5. White House Conference on Aging, *Report of the Technical Committee on Health Maintenance and Health Promotion*, 1981. (available to delegates).

6. Executive Office of the President, Office of Management and Budget, *Catalog of Federal Domestic Assistance* (Washington, D.C.: Government Printing Office, Annual Updates).

7. Timothy Saastra, "The Catalog of Federal Domestic Assistance," *Grantsmanship Center News*, December-February 1976 (reprint), pp. 1–16.

8. *Federal Register*, Washington, D.C., U.S. Government Printing Office, daily.

9. *Commerce Business Daily*, Washington, D.C., U.S. Department of Commerce, daily.

10. Sam Sternberg, *National Directory of Corporate Charity* (San Francisco, Ca.: Regional Young Adult Project, 1981).

11. Council on Foundations. *Foundation Directory*, Washington, D.C., annual editions.

12. Council on Foundations. *Foundation Center Source Book Profiles*, Washington, D.C., regular updates.

13. Council of Foundations. *Foundation Grants Index*, Washington, D.C., bimonthly.

14. Public Management Institute, *The Directory of Grants for Health*, San Francisco, 1981.

15. U.S. Department of Health and Human Services, *Foundations that Provide Support for Health and Human Services* (Washington, D.C.: Government Printing Office, 1981).

16. Council on Foundations, *Comsearch Printouts*, Washington, D.C., regular computer updates.

17. Standard and Poor's, *Register of Corporations, Directors and Executives*, (New York: McGraw-Hill, 1984).

18. Grantsmanship Center, *Grantsmanship Center News*, Los Angeles, Ca., published bimonthly.

19. Council on Foundations, *Foundation News*, Washington, D.C., published bimonthly.

20. Susan Scribner, and Florence Green, "Asking for Money," *Grantsmanship Center News*, March/April, 1983 (reprint), pp. 9–17.

21. Susan Andres, "A Primer on Mailing Lists," *Grantsmanship Center News*, September/October, 1984 (reprint), pp. 15–30.

22. James C. Cremmins, and Mary Keil, *Enterprise in the Non-Profit Sector* (Washington, D.C.: Partners for Livable Places, and New York, NY, Rockefeller Brothers Fund, 1983).

Chapter 7

The Senior Center as a
Wellness Center

Joyce Leanse, M.P.H.

Senior centers have the potential to bring together a broad and varied program of services and activities that enable older persons to develop and maintain health-promoting behavior. In an accessible, nonthreatening, and supportive setting, senior adults can join with their peers to (1) learn information about life-style choices that promote good health; (2) practice behaviors that support good health (e.g., exercise, nutrition, and stress-reducing techniques); and (3) gain peer support to assist in learning and in maintaining healthy behavior. Senior centers not only offer resources that support self-responsibility in health care but also the breadth and nature of their programs in other areas enhance an older person's capacity to be responsive to his or her total range of personal needs.

In this chapter, the use of senior centers as wellness centers for older persons is discussed. This chapter defines their function in the community, describes the factors that led to their development and the federal support that encouraged their expansion, documents the health services currently being delivered, and provides examples of center programs to illustrate the rich mix of services and activities offered to support wellness.

THE ROLE OF SENIOR CENTERS IN THE COMMUNITY

Over the years the definition of a senior center has been refined and expanded. In 1975 the National Council on the Aging's (NCOA) National Institute of Senior Centers published the following definition in *Senior Center Standards*,[1] which reflects the field's representation of itself:

> A senior center is a community focal point on aging where older persons as individuals or in groups come together for services and activities which enhance their dignity, support their independence and encourage their involvement in and with the community.

As part of a comprehensive community strategy to meet the needs of older persons, senior center programs take place within and emanate from a facility. These programs consist of a variety of services and activities in areas such as education, creative arts, recreation, advocacy, leadership development, employment, health, nutrition, social work and other supportive services.

The center also serves as a community resource for information on aging, for training professional and lay leadership and for developing new approaches to aging programs.

There are over 10,000 senior centers in the United States in 1985—at least one in every major community and in most small towns—and they serve approximately one-quarter of the elderly population living in the community or about 6 million older persons. In 1970 the U.S. Administration on Aging published a directory listing only 1200 senior centers; four years later the NCOA published a directory of senior centers and clubs listing 4870 programs. Now, a number of states mandate senior center development, funding their initiation or expansion, and most local jurisdictions provide resources to assist their operation. This support ranges from providing full-funding for a comprehensive program to providing no-cost space rental or placing staff of related departments who augment center services. Senior centers are organized as public or private nonprofit agencies; some are part of larger organizations, others are independent, incorporated entities. Although not all of them meet the NCOA definition, most offer visible and accessible sites in which older people gather, obtain information, interact with peers, involve themselves in planned or informal activities, and obtain needed services. Their ubiquitousness, their identifiable relationship with older people, and the broad range of services they generally offer make them an especially viable locus for health promotion and health maintenance activities for older people. Indeed, many already are, and all could be, wellness centers for the mature adult.

Senior Center Origins

Senior centers began in this country in 1943 with the opening of the William Hodson Center in New York City under the auspice of the city's welfare department.[2] The Hodson Center was initiated in response to welfare workers' concern with their elderly clientele's constant seeking of information, which the workers recognized as quests for personal interaction. A few of these social workers initiated a group program where older people could interact with one another and also be introduced to meaningful ways to fill their unoccupied hours. The program soon expanded to include recreational and educational activities and then case work and personal services to assist "members" to maintain themselves in the community.

Other communities began to recognize the need for programs to serve the elderly as both a "client" group and a community resource. Under the sponsorship of private voluntary agencies or of city departments of social service, recreation, education, public health, or a combination thereof, senior centers were organized in a number of large metropolitan areas and even in a few smaller towns and suburban areas during the late 1940s and 1950s. Based on their location and their sponsorship, centers tended to serve either those with low or very limited income who primarily came for services or financially more comfortable elderly who attended for the recreational and educational opportunities. Few of either group admitted to their loneliness and need to link with peers, but all who attended regularly enjoyed the interaction that the activities facilitated. Furthermore, once linked with a senior center, participants could avail themselves of a broad range of activities and services.

From the beginning, center programming was geared to enable older people to form new relationships, learn new skills, gain a sense of achievement, and remain involved and contributing citizens of their communities. Self-government was encouraged and leadership training provided. Individuals seeking assistance with income, health, or housing concerns were given information and directed to appropriate resources; individuals seeking new roles and opportunities for achievement were enlisted as volunteers for the center or other community agencies.

Derived from the settlement house concept, senior centers were organized to serve the total person in a neighborhood setting. They sought either to bring to one location the multiple and varied services available in the community for older people or to assist older persons in becoming aware of those services and in obtaining them. Although arts, crafts, and music were offered, there were also luncheon clubs that taught "the essentials of nutrition and good eating habits"[3] and an Elders Council and other club activities that offered leadership training. The center also provided space for other agencies to offer their services to center participants, functioning as an early community focal point for services for the elderly.

Senior Center Expansion

Senior centers were the one local agency explicitly mentioned in the original Older Americans Act in 1965,[4] and their numbers increased as a result.[5] During the late 1960s the channeling of dollars into aging services by other federal agencies—for example, the Office of Economic Opportunity, Department of Housing and Community Development—enabled senior centers to expand their services and encouraged the development of special programs directed to minority group elderly previously unserved or underserved by largely activity-oriented programs. In 1972 services within senior centers expanded again as support for meals programs was added to the Older Americans Act.[6] Approximately 25 percent of the meals programs were placed in existing senior centers; the remainder created a base service in locations underserved or unserved by existing programs. Over the years many of these meal sites have become comprehensive multipurpose group programs for older persons; in effect, senior centers.

In 1973 a new Title V was introduced into the Older Americans Act specially for multipurpose senior centers, supporting alteration, renovation, and acquisition of facilities. Title V also introduced new language identifying a role for senior centers as "a focal point in communities for the development and delivery of social and nutritional services."[7] The 1978 Older Americans Act Amendments eliminated the separate funding authorized for Title V, consolidating senior center monies and their administration with previous resources and responsibilities of area agencies on aging under Title III.[8] The focal point concept, however, continues to be articulated in the legislation. Area agencies are now required to "designate, where feasible, a focal point for comprehensive service delivery in each community," and they are to give special consideration to multipurpose senior centers when making that designation.[9]

Federal and state legislation and wide-spread support from city and county government have resulted in an ever-increasing number of senior centers operating in the inner city, in suburban communities, and in small towns and rural areas throughout the country. The model of the senior center has even been replicated in Canada, England, Japan, Israel, Germany, and South Africa.[10]

A national survey conducted by NCOA in 1974[11] identified nearly 5000 senior centers serving approximately 5 million older people, nearly one-quarter of the elderly population in the United States at that time. Participants ranged in age from 60 to 95—a few were even older—and one-quarter were 75 years or older. They came from all economic backgrounds: 47 percent were blue-collar workers, 16 percent were white-collar clerical workers, and 16 percent were professionals or managers. Over one-half of the participants lived alone, and the great majority of these were women. Center facilities ranged from single-room storefront operations to multistory complexes complete with swimming pool, gymnasium, ballroom, and auditorium. Slightly over one-quarter of the centers had their own building, but many were located in churches or synagogues. At the time these data were collected, seven out of ten of the reporting senior centers offered at least education, recreation, information and referral, or counseling services. Nearly all of these—93 percent—also offered voluntary opportunities, and almost one-half of those or one-third of all senior centers also offered health services.

HEALTH PROGRAMMING—A ROLE FOR SENIOR CENTERS?

The philosophy of the senior center movement is based on the following premises: (1) Aging is a normal developmental process, (2) human beings need peers with whom they can interact and who are available as a source of encouragement and support, and (3) adults have the right to a voice in determining matters in which they have a vital interest. Senior center programming derived from these premises creates an atmosphere of wellness. It is geared to developing the strengths of older persons, addressing the need for building interdependencies among center participants and supporting unavoidable dependencies through services that are not only made more accessible but also made more acceptable to older persons and their special requirements.[12]

Over two decades ago at a 1965 NCOA conference, Sam Scheiner, director of the Adult Health and Recreation Center in Philadelphia, urged his fellow center directors to recognize that "the establishment and expansion of health services is the natural assumption and inherent responsibility of the Senior Center Program."[13] The Adult Health and Recreation Center, the first senior adult program to be sponsored by a city health department, provided, in addition to a wide range of activities and services, free annual physical examinations when members renewed their memberships. The center also offered:

- health education through discussions, classes, lectures, and films to alert individuals to symptoms, to allay fears, and to give practical information about nutrition, self-care, and the appropriate timing for medical intervention
- mental health counseling, especially to provide ego support
- self-help programs directed to individual concerns and providing opportunities for center participants to maintain therapeutic regimens prescribed by their physicians
- referrals to appropriate outpatient services and treatment centers

Scheiner's strong support for the center's role in health promotion was based on his own experience and work done by Kutner, Fanshed, Togo, and Lagner[14] in which they describe the relationship between the health setting and the individual's attitude toward health services:

Much of the motivation for seeking the means to curtail or remove health destroying processes is tied to social forces . . . indifference or apathy toward health and resignation to one's fate as seen in failure to show concern about health is associated with failure to use health facilities. . . . having others about [the older person] who give emotional support tends to make him more responsive to their urgings to seek medical care or take better care of his health.

Programming at the Adult Health and Recreation Center recognized the role of peer support and the unique potential of the center to structure and maintain peer support groups for older persons. It also built on a stated value of the senior center philosophy—that the older adult should be consulted about his or her needs. This value translated into involving older persons in the planning and implementation of the program. It also meant developing opportunities for lobbying efforts and strengthening their advocacy capacities so that they could play an active role in creating community support for needed services.[15]

Health Services in Senior Centers

Several studies conducted within the past decade clearly support the validity of Scheiner's notion that health services belong in senior centers. NCOA's 1974 survey of nearly 5000 senior programs[16] found that senior center health services ranged from complete professionally staffed clinics operated at center sites to planned discussions of health problems among participants. A more in-depth study on a smaller select group of senior centers was conducted by JWK International in 1980[17] for the Office of the Assistant Secretary for Planning and Evaluation, U.S. Department of Health, Education and Welfare. In the centers studied, health screening was offered by all of them; linkages with public health departments and mental health agencies were reported by 92 percent; with hospitals, 87 percent; with physicians, 80 percent; and with Visiting Nurses Associations, 67 percent.

The findings of a 1982 survey by NCOA of health services in senior centers[18] support the increasing role of centers in direct provision of health-related care. Although it is assumed that the centers that responded were those that offered a more extensive array of health services, that array included more direct service components than in the 1974 study. Health services by the responding centers— 728 of 3700 surveyed—are estimated to be provided on an average of about seven times for each health service participant during the course of a year. To a greater or lesser degree the responding centers provide the following health services:

- screening for hypertension—two out of three centers
- screening for diabetes—one out of two centers
- screening for glaucoma—one out of three centers
- screening for gynecological disorders—one out of four centers
- individual health counseling—two out of three centers
- mental health counseling—one out of four centers
- health education materials—one out of two centers
- exercise programs—one out of four centers
- physical examinations—one out of four centers
- transportation for medical appointments—one out of two centers

Some of these services are provided on a daily basis (exercise programs, screening for diabetes, nutrition education, physical examinations, transportation for medical appointments) and others on a weekly or monthly basis (individual health counseling, screening for hypertension and for glaucoma, mental health counseling). Almost three-fourths (532) of the responding centers indicated that no fee was paid for the health services they provide; about one out of eight centers (96) require or request a fee.

Hospitals and other health service agencies in the community provide important information and are referral links to the senior center. Hospitals and public health departments each have a linkage to about one-third of the centers; community mental health clinics and individual disease groups also provide information to about one-fifth of the responding centers. About 20 percent of the responding centers reported that hospitals referred older adults to the center for the center's health-related services, and a similar number of centers reported such referrals by social service agencies, public health departments, and nursing homes. These same agencies provided assistance in the training of center health personnel, with two out of every five centers reporting such assistance from public health and social service departments.

Although over 40 percent of the centers reported having space within their facility set aside for their health services, just over 8 percent actually had a clinic, and another 9½ percent reported an examining room. One-quarter of the reporting centers have a full-time nurse on staff, and one-half have a full-time nurse in the facility that is on the staff of another agency. Just over 10 percent of centers reported full-time physician specialists on staff; 5½ percent reported part-time physicians on staff; and over 45 percent reported physicians sent from other agencies. Some centers also reported full-time mental health counselors and physician assistants and part-time dentists on staff. Many more centers reported such personnel as outstationed from another agency or as independent vendors.

Examples of Senior Centers as Wellness Centers

Although the data support the extent to which a wide variety of health-related services are delivered through centers, brief descriptions of some actual programs may better demonstrate how health services fit together with other senior center programs to create senior wellness centers. These wellness centers address the general well-being of older persons—emotional and physical—which has long been the focus of senior center programming.

The Monroe Senior Citizens Center[19] which serves Monroe County, Michigan, "both at the center and in the home,"[20] seven days a week illustrates how the concept of wellness can permeate a center's orientation and its programming. As so many senior centers, it opened as a storefront; in 1985, 25 years later, it is housed in an attractive senior citizens apartment building, supported by the county's senior millage program (a county tax allocated to senior programming), the United Way, the area agency on aging, other public and private support, and monies generated from in-center programs.

The center's brochure notes:

> The philosophy of the Center focuses on the wholistic well-being of individuals, incorporating in its wide array of programming all aspects of being truly well—emotionally, physically, psychologically, and spiritually . . . . By offering recreational, health-promotion, and supportive programs and services, persons can not only remain self-reliant, but can remain contributing members of the community as well. The results are demonstrated in the current group of active, involved seniors who are erasing the stereotypes associated with aging.[21]

The center offers 19 recreational activities, 15 supportive services, 14 services for the homebound, and 12 health-promotion programs and services to "enhance overall wellbeing." These latter activities include daily, cooked-to-order breakfasts—a boon to men living alone who tend to skip this all-important meal—family-style noon meals served seven days a week, a walking club, exercise classes, and health screening. Assistance with Medicare and other insurance forms; a program for the hearing-impaired; transportation assistance; workshops on foot care, insurance, and housing; counseling; a sunshine committee that sends cards to ill or homebound individuals; friendly visiting, and dances and dance classes are also offered.

The Whistlestop Senior Center[22] in San Rafael, California, also offers an array of health-oriented activities and services during its seven-day week. Activities include exercise classes, folk dancing, square dancing, health insurance counseling, blood pressure screening, and a wide range of classes. For example, a vision health class promotes "holistic approaches to caring and improving eyesight . . . easy to learn and fun alternative forms of eye relaxation and vision health care techniques."[23] Another series of classes offers:

> a focus on exercise, activities, and body movements designed to maintain and improve flexibility, balance, and coordination, muscle strength and cardio-respiratory efficiency. Music, dance, and games will add to the joy of the sessions. Relaxation techniques will be taught and practiced for the purpose of assisting the individual to recognize and cope with symptoms of tension and stress. This class will provide an opportunity for everyone to develop his/her potential for comfortable and vibrant living.[24]

The Knowles Senior Center[25] in Nashville, Tennessee, illustrates how a center can augment its health resources by utilizing resources available in the community. One of the first senior centers to be funded by a department of mental health, it offers its services through two centers opened daily, an adult day care program, and 13 weekly clubs. A public health nurse is present at the center five mornings a week for blood pressure testing, counseling, and injections. There are monthly lectures by physicians and regular exercise classes, including water exercise classes. The facilities of the Marriott Hotel, Boys Club, and local high schools are used for these classes. A Senior Walk/Run is co-sponsored with the YMCA, and during May and June the center participates in the state-wide Senior Olympics at the county, regional, and state levels. Tennis, swimming, running, walking, and horseshoes are among the sports in which the center members participate. To ensure tasty as well as nutritious meals, student chefs from a local vocational school prepare the food. For the past 14 years the center has sponsored an annual health screening fair. In 1984 a health and fitness director was added to the staff to coordinate all the center's health programming.[26]

The Carrollton Hollygrove Senior Center[27] in New Orleans, Louisiana, which provides services to 110–125 elderly persons each day through its main center and two satellite facilities, also brings together community health resources to benefit older persons. There are two nurses on staff, one of whom is in charge of the adult day care program for frail and impaired older people. The other nurse supervises the health care program, which includes blood pressure monitoring, diet and weight control, and, as needed, the services of a dietician, pharmacist, dental hygienist, dentist, and podiatrist. The center's nurse schedules the appointments and sends out reminders to the participants. An escort service is available for medical visits. The center staff work closely with personnel of the community mental health center and the local hospital. There is a physical education instructor on staff. Congregate and home-delivered meals are provided with Title III funds.[28]

The Coordinating Council for Senior Citizens[29] in Durham, North Carolina, operates eight senior centers throughout the county. Two, which are open full-time, are located in senior citizen high-rise apartment buildings; six, which are open five days a week for four hours a day, are located in recreation department facilities and in a rural church. The centers form a network, designated by the area agency on aging as the county's focal point for service delivery to the elderly. Using the centers' resources for coordination, a comprehensive health program is made available both by utilizing community health resources and by orienting center activities and services to health-promotion in all the centers. Nursing students provide counseling, blood pressure testing, medical monitoring, and health education. The center's nurse coordinates these activities and arranges for additional health services. Each site offers exercise programs on different days of the week. The county health department arranges for health screening, provides a nurse on a regular basis, and arranges for volunteer nurses to assist with services to the 7000 older persons—one-third of the county's elderly—who participate in the centers' programs. Glaucoma, dental problems, and diabetes are screened throughout the year. A retired dentist offers his services regularly, and a podiatrist comes in once a year. Information on Medicare and Medicaid also is provided regularly.

The coordinating council also provides services that assist the frail elderly to remain in the community and that support their caregivers: adult day care, chore services, home health services, cleaning services, and telephone reassurance. The council also offers transportation for medical appointments (Medi-port); volunteer drivers are supplied by local churches. In 1984, the Council installed grabbars in the homes of frail persons to help prevent falls. All this community support comes only with considerable effort on the part of its board, participant leaders, and staff. One particularly effective mechanism for attracting community attention to older adults and their issues has been the annual Senior Citizens Speak Out, which the council coordinates. City and county decision makers tend to listen when so many voices are gathered together to praise or to instruct.[30]

The Palm Springs Senior Center,[31] located in a desert community in Southern California that attracts large numbers of retired permanent residents, as well as elderly winter residents, serves 5,000 older persons each month. In addition to educational and recreational activities and a Title III meals program, the center offers a variety of health services that the director views as basic to the program's primary purpose. Once a week, a Health Care Day is held, with physicians and paramedics offering services at no cost to center participants. Although the emphasis is on prevention, diagnostic services are also provided. Individuals needing further attention are referred to doctors who accept Medicare or Medical (Medicaid). Arrangements have been made with all three of the local hospitals to provide a low-cost health examination complete with lab tests for $40 that would otherwise cost $250. The examination includes blood tests, EKG, x-rays, urinanalysis, pap smear, and consultation with a physician. Special meals prepared under contract with one of the local hospitals are home-delivered through the center's "Cater-Cart" program. "Senior-cize" classes are offered to promote regular exercise among the participants. Peer counseling and adult day care are two additional services being established by the center; the latter is the only such program in the entire 14,000 square miles of the Cochella Valley. The entire program, including all its health activities, is administered by the center's director, although there is a special board of directors to oversee the health programming.[32]

The Future of Senior Centers and Wellness Programs

What all these examples convey is that almost any center can offer a health promotion/health maintenance program. Most do. And if they do not offer all the components that contribute specifically to health promotion—nutrition education, fitness and exercise programs, behavior modification, and support groups—they have the potential to do so. What some centers lack are adequate resources. Yet, as the examples illustrate, each community abounds with potential resources that centers can tap in unique and creative ways. There are volunteers, students of relevant disciplines, retired professionals, representatives of voluntary health-related organizations, and a host of other resources that can be brought together to create a health-oriented program for the elderly for delivery in senior centers. That part of a health program only requires some coordination; a more difficult but doable piece is establishing a wellness orientation that permeates all the activities and services offered by a center. Health programming should not merely be isolated events (even though offered regularly), but the health potential of every activity and service should be planned for, and each should support the other.

A model that warrants further attention is the linking of a senior center with a health maintenance organization (HMO), with each contributing its special services to promote and maintain the well-being of older people. Such a model might help senior centers fund their current services; it also would enable HMOs to offer a broad range of health promotion and maintenance activities to the elderly without acquiring new staff and probably at less cost than otherwise possible. Furthermore, the other services offered by senior centers—recreation, education, social services, and the support groups that naturally form or are easily organized in group programs—are not readily provided through HMOs but they are meaningful, and even necessary, to maintaining the wellness of older persons.

The current status of senior centers—their existence in nearly every community in the country, their popularity with local governments, and the extent to which hospitals and health professionals increasingly are making referrals or otherwise linking with them—attests to their viability and to the increasing role that they can be expected to play in the delivery of health-related services for older people. Health organizations that act on this potential will be able to address the health needs of large numbers of older persons, tapping and encouraging their self-reliance and the interdependent cooperation that senior centers maximize.

CONCLUSION

The senior center is an optimal setting for health promotion because (1) it offers a positive environment for learning, (2) it provides opportunities for applying and practicing newly learned healthful behavior through its varied activities and services, and (3) its entire program can be integrated around a health focus in a dynamic way.

Participation in a senior center is voluntary—people attend by choice—and is associated with socialization and recreation, as well as with seeking help for problems. In this nonthreatening and supportive setting, older people can easily gain knowledge and skills. The presence of peers who are interested in the same topics and in the same goal—improved health—provides strong reinforcement for learning and bolsters each participant's motivation to improve his or her health-related behavior.

Health-related services in senior centers are designed to foster good health habits, to integrate health and social services, and to make services more accessible to older persons. Because the health problems and needs of the elderly are often related to other needs—social, financial, nutritional, educational—a center's services in these areas have a strong influence on the success of center health programming. Minkler, in a critique of health promotion and health education programs,[33] introduces the concept of "response-ability," which she explains as "the capacity for effectively responding to one's personal needs and the challenges posed by the environment."[34] Senior centers enhance the response-ability of older persons. If we move beyond providing information and treating disease to a concept of healthful living, then it is apparent that a center's total program promotes health through enjoyable social activities, along with services that address needs and problems. Health promotion in such a setting is amplified: The information provided about healthy behavior is transmitted, reinforced, and exemplified.

NOTES

1. National Institute of Senior Centers, *Senior Center Standards* (Washington, D.C.: The National Council on the Aging, Inc., 1978), p. xi.

2. Joyce Leanse, Marjorie Tiven, and Thomas B. Robb, *Senior Center Operation* (Washington, D.C.: The National Council on the Aging, Inc., 1977), pp. ix-xiii.

3. *Ibid.*, p. xi.

4. *Older Americans Act of 1965*, Public Law 89–73, Sec. 301 and Sec. 401 (July 14, 1965).

5. Joyce Leanse and Sara B. Wagner, *Senior Centers: Report of Senior Group Programs in America* (Washington, D.C.: The National Council on the Aging, Inc., 1975), p. 12.

6. *Older Americans Act of 1965*, As Amended, Public Law 92–258, March 22, 1972, Title VII.

7. *Ibid.*, Public Law 93-29, May 3, 1973, Title V, Sec. 501(C).

8. *Ibid.*, Sec. 306(A)(3).

9. "Older Americans Act Rules and Regulations," *Federal Register*, 1321.3, March 31, 1980.

10. Unpublished report of Senior Center Session at the International Conference on Gerontology (Jerusalem, Israel, 1975).

11. Leanse and Wagner, *op. cit.*

12. *Senior Center Standards, op. cit.*, p. 5.

13. Sam Scheiner, "Expanding Health Services in Centers," *Second National Conference of Senior Centers* (New York: The National Council on the Aging, Inc., 1965), p. 46.

14. Bernard Kutner, David Fanshed, Alice Togo, and Thomas Lagner, *Five Hundred Over Sixty* (New York: Russell Sage Foundation, 1956), p. 172.

15. Scheiner, *op. cit.*, pp. 46–50.

16. Leanse and Wagner, *op. cit.,* pp. 30–32.

17. *An Exploratory Study of Senior Centers* (Virginia: JWK International Corporation, August, 1979), pp. 33, 35.

18. Betty Shepherd, ed., "Health Services in Senior Centers on the Rise," *Senior Center Report* 7, no. 2 (May/June 1984), pp. 1–2.

19. Monroe Senior Citizens Center, 15275 South Dixie Highway, Monroe, MI 48161.

20. Monroe Senior Citizens Center Brochure.

21. *Ibid.*

22. Whistlestop Senior Center, 930 Tamalpais, San Rafael, CA 94901.

23. Whistlestop News and Special Events Bulletin, November, 1983.

24. *Ibid.*

25. Knowles Senior Center, 1801 Broad Street, Nashville, TN 37203.

26. Charles Durland, executive director of the Knowles Senior Center, Spring 1984: personal communication.

27. Carrollton Hollygrove Senior Center, 3300 Hamilton Street, New Orleans, LA 70118.

28. Howard Rogers, program staff of the Carrollton Hollygrove Senior Center, Spring 1984: personal communication.

29. Coordinating Council for Senior Citizens, 807 South Duke Street, Durham, NC 27701.

30. Ann Johnson, executive director of the Coordinating Council for Senior Services, Spring 1984: personal communication.

31. Palm Springs Senior Center, 550 North Palm Canyon Drive, Palm Springs, CA 92262.

32. Mike Moran, executive administrator of the Palm Springs Senior Center, Spring 1984: personal communication.

33. Meredith Minkler, "Health Promotion and Elders: A Critique," *Generations* (San Francisco: Western Gerontological Society, Spring, 1983), pp. 13–15, 67.

34. *Ibid.,* p. 13.

Chapter 8

Wellness and Long-Term Care

Theodore H. Koff, Ed.D.

LONG-TERM CARE DEFINED

What does long-term care actually represent? Is the term indeed an appropriate title for the services it intends to describe? Brody[1] has referred to long-term care as:

> one or more services provided on a sustained basis to enable individuals whose functional capacities are chronically impaired to be maintained at their maximum level of health and well-being. The underlying values are that all people share certain basic human needs, that they have a right to services designed to meet those needs and to be furnished services when needs cannot be met through their own resources (social, emotional, physical, financial).

Health care traditionally has been oriented toward healing or overcoming illness and thus achieving wellness. In contrast, long-term care has connoted an irreversible continuation of illness, with expectations of increasing disability until death occurs. Such a sharp dichotomy of anticipated outcomes has led to an assumption that striving for wellness is not a component of long-term care. However, wellness need not connote only the absence of illness or disability. It also can mean the ability of the individual to function despite disability, of families to function in support of their members, and of communities to offer the most appropriate services to maintain and improve levels of wellness among their citizens.

Long-term care has been identified as chronic care because it deals with health problems that do not go away, but linger on, disrupting the individual's life style. Long-term care also is customarily perceived as being provided to residents of nursing homes or congregate housing for the elderly, although there is increasing recognition of the alternative of making services available to people living in their

119

own homes. Regardless of where it is delivered, long-term care focuses on the illness, disability, or limitations of the recipient.

Because most people who need long-term care have multiple problems, and because both medical and social supports are required for prolonged periods, design of a suitable care program is often more complex than treatment of an episode of acute illness or accident trauma. The concept of wellness is relative and is likely to vary, as well as to be interrupted by acute illnesses. The recipient of long-term care may need to go to a hospital more frequently than other persons, so that the interaction of the predominantly medical model of hospital care and the medical/social model of chronic care can result in additional psychological, financial, and policy-related complications.

Medicare, the major national health care program for the elderly, emphasizes care for acute illness and does not provide assistance in solving problems related to chronic conditions. As a consequence, inappropriate hospitalization sometimes occurs, and there is strong evidence that costs of hospital care are increased.

A more accurate system of determining the specific needs of persons who require long-term care and a broad spectrum of services that can be delivered in a manner that maintains for each individual the highest possible level of wellness are needed. What gerontologists have proposed as a continuum of care should be modified to encompass the wellness concept.

THE CONTINUUM OF CARE

Because wellness is not merely the absence of disease but is the ability of the individual to deal with problems of illness in the most constructive manner, health services for the elderly must connote expectations of wellness, regardless of where the person is served. The myths and stereotypes that suggest that aging is a downhill spiral of illness and deficiencies contribute to the absence of wellness in long-term care. The current view that all long-term care services should be organized into a coordinated continuum perpetuates this misconception by presenting the continuum as a linear progression from the home to the nursing home—a one-way downhill pattern—as illustrated below:

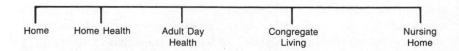

| Home | Home Health | Adult Day Health | Congregate Living | Nursing Home |

Nowhere in this continuum is it suggested that increased wellness is a possible outcome of intervention and change. Rather, it reinforces the stereotype of problems of aging as necessarily decremental and not subject to improvement.

A revised conceptualization of the continuum of care may be helpful in exploding the myth. Instead of being seen as a line, the continuum can be viewed as a circle, suggesting that there are different points of intervention and that intervention may be required only temporarily. If, in addition, services are represented as flowing freely in separate orbits around the person served, it becomes clear that there may be intersections at various times and places, for various lengths of time, depending entirely on the individual's needs. For example, most older persons remain at home all their lives and will not use a nursing home or other institutional care program. Many health problems of older persons, if diagnosed early and appropriately treated, can be subject to successful health care intervention.

Moreover, the problems seen in today's cohort of older persons may not necessarily be characteristic of future generations. Commitment to the value of altered life styles and a more equitable allocation of public resources to chronic problems could change the pattern of mortality and morbidity. This view is supported by the life-span perspective on development and behavior, which sees developmental changes in human behavior as occurring from conception to death and arising from a matrix of biological, psychological, social, historical, and evolutional influences.[2]

Incorporating Wellness into the Continuum

There are five important ways that wellness can be made an integral part of the continuum of long-term care; all focus on treating the capacities and capabilities of the person, rather than his or her frailties or disabilities. All also emphasize a wholistic approach that encompasses the whole lifetime of the individual, the total state of wellness at a particular time, the full range of resources of the family and social structure, the potential for creating supports in the physical environment, and the encouragement of self-determination.

Lifetime Preventive Health Care

Much of the need for long-term care could be eliminated by a better understanding of the effects of lifetime health practices.

The Center for Disease Control has estimated that about half the mortality from the 10 leading causes of death in the United States is strongly linked to long-term patterns of behavior (life-style). Such known behavioral risk factors as cigarette smoking, excessive consumption of alcoholic beverages, use of illicit drugs, certain dietary habits, insufficient exercise, reckless driving, noncompliance with medication regimens and maladaptive responses to stress are involved in the pathogenesis of cardiovascular diseases and cancers as well as accidental disabilities and other disorders.[3]

If a death to which any of these factors is a contributing cause could be preceded by a period of intensive health care—perhaps long-term care that focuses on wellness—then about half the number of persons who now receive long-term care might avoid or reduce the need for such care by voluntary compliance with a changed life-style.

The study of life-span development stresses the dual phenomena of constancy and change in behavior from birth to death. Some of the hypotheses that evolve from the life-span perspective are directly applicable to the development of a new perspective on wellness and long-term care:

- Neither aging nor development is limited to any particular time of life. Therefore the quest for wellness can assume different forms of expression throughout life, but the constant search for wellness can be maintained and nurtured.

- The multiple determinants of constancy and change in behavior express themselves interactively and cumulatively, thereby providing a multiplicity of opportunities for unique intervention strategies.

- Individuals are agents in their own development. As individuals differ, so do their life histories. Therefore, generalizations about people are difficult to formulate and should be subject to close scrutiny.

- Each new birth cohort ages through a different trajectory of life events, brought about by the impress of sociohistorical change and by individual reactions to it.

- Intervention efforts among the aged are effective in changing the course of development, even as they are in the young.

In addition, life-cycle behavior may, in fact, be a product of the expectations of society, rather than an inevitable feature of biological aging. It may very well be that the expectations of psychological and social withdrawal by the elderly—the lack of vitality, intellectual activity, and independence—are behaviors conditioned by societal expectations, which negate the value and competence of the older person.

Baltes and Baltes, in their study of intellectual functioning, suggest "that losses in neural functioning that the elderly suffer may not always impair intellectual performance."[4] However, because the social roles of the elderly in our society are often ill-defined or even absent, their abilities fall into disuse and deteriorate. "In more optimal environments, the trajectory of manifest capacities may continue to rise into old age, long after the latent capacities have peaked."[5]

Seeing the Person as a Whole

Generally, when older persons are assessed to determine their need for services—whether given in an institution or at home—the diagnosis is presented in terms of illness and limitations. When this is done, the individual is only partially described and, unfortunately, is presented in terms of handicap, rather than capacity. An individual could be described as accurately in the context of wholeness, as a person having potentials, goals, and capacity for wellness.

An illustration drawn from home-delivered services shows how these important services lend themselves to supporting wellness. The typical long-term care services offered at home, whether they be to the homebound or to the temporarily infirm, usually include nursing care; rehabilitative or therapeutic services, such as occupational or physical therapy; social work; and nutritional services. However, there are other home-delivered services that might at the same time promote wellness, such as cultural, artistic, and spiritual services unrelated to the person's sickness but that might strengthen the whole person. An example would be bringing spiritual services to an individual at home, not because the person is near death but because he or she continues to live. Opportunities to enjoy music, art, literature, or crafts also enrich daily life and promote wellness.

The best illustration of the presence of wellness in existing long-term care programs is hospice, a program that deals with people near death, especially with those dying of cancer. In fact, it is the concept of wellness that underlies the philosophy and program of hospice.

Hospice grew out of the concern for the way dying people were treated in our health system. Death was disguised, avoided, and dealt with as part of a conspiracy of silence. Health care workers aggressively sought cure, but when that was unattainable they frequently avoided continuing contact with the dying person and caring was discontinued. Death brought a sense of failure and of the impotence of the health care provider to maintain life, despite good intentions and the application of modern technology. Patients were inappropriately served—in the hospital instead of at home, away from family instead of with family, with continuing pain instead of free from pain. Instead of being treated as a window, as it is in less sophisticated societies than ours, death was viewed as a door.[6]

When these attitudes and values were communicated to the dying person, they were internalized by that person as evidence of his or her unworthiness to receive attention from the care providers. The trauma of impending death was exacerbated by the absence of caring, by pain—both physical and emotional—and by the absence of control over one's own life.

Death is unavoidable, but it need not be accompanied by iatrogenic illness, such as isolation, fear, and withdrawal, to which health care providers have contributed.

The basic value of hospice calls for the reduction or avoidance of the pain that so frequently occurs with cancer, especially in the final stages of life. The technology that has been successfully used to control pain has been part of the resources of health care for a long time, but long-standing constraints resulting from fear of addiction had been imposed on it.

In opposition to those constraints, hospice advocates for wellness by permitting the dying person to experience relief from pain through the appropriate use of medications. This relief provides more than physical comfort; it also helps the individual remain in contact with the social environment, the social network, and spiritual values so that a sense of caring and sharing gives meaning to the remainder of life, without respect to its duration. This hospice definition of wellness demonstrates dedication to the totality of the person.

Hospice also redefines the patient as the entire family, considering the unique interactions within the family as contributing to the wellness of the individual patient or to all the patients in the family. This conceptualization is in sharp contrast to conventional health care programs that isolate the individual by enforcing visiting schedules and by failing to understand the limits or capacities of family members to share in an important life experience.

Wellness also is embodied in the design of the physical space for hospice inpatient programs, which minimizes the influence of hospital design and the symbolism of sickness. Instead, home-like features are introduced, with separation of space for daytime activities from sleeping areas and the invitation for family members to "move in" to the hospice setting.

In addition, wellness is a significant component of the hospice home care program, which has demonstrated that an individual and family often can be supported at home, rather than having the patient move to an unfamiliar institutional environment. Permitting a person to die at home, especially with the absence of pain and in close contact with the family, maintains established patterns of living, such as meals, personal schedules, and contact with pets or important parts of the physical environment during the end of life.

Finally, wellness is maintained in hospice by respecting the individual's decision-making ability and capacity to remain in control, with the support of family and other care providers. Ownership of one's life is a possession jealously guarded throughout life. When health care providers attempt to usurp this ownership, they create dependency and reduce the individual's self-respect and autonomy. These usurping behaviors reinforce a sense of incompetence and illness, rather than foster wellness.

Family Involvement and Social Supports

There are many opportunities to introduce and support wellness in institutional care. Providers of nursing home care have much to learn from hospice care and can apply such knowledge without compromising the principles or programs of nursing home care. The issue of maintaining and supporting family ties is as important in nursing home care as it is in hospice, yet nursing homes in general do not support active family participation in the life of the institutionalized older person.

For any individual to whom family has been significant, wellness is not possible in the absence of family. Family can include blood relatives, those related by marriage, and others who have been closely associated in important relationships. It should be recognized, however, that disruptive families who neglect, fail to understand, or deny the importance of the older person cannot respond to that person's needs and may even contribute to the illness.

Many nursing homes do sponsor family nights and other events when families are invited to participate in some scheduled educational or social event. However, nursing home care is usually based on the transfer of responsibility for care from the family to the institution. For any of a variety of reasons, the family cannot assume ongoing responsibility for the care of an individual and contracts with the nursing home to provide care. Family involvement may continue in the form of paying bills, of providing some support, or, infrequently, of care planning. The nursing home assumes responsibility not only for care but also takes some control over the individual or the individual and family. This control may be seen in the establishment of a visiting-hour schedule or the making of decisions about care or selection of a roommate.

The dichotomy is established. The nursing home provides the care. The family will visit and be supportive, but rarely is continuing care a family responsibility. Now what would institutional care be like if, during the preadmission interview with family members and the applicant, the institution and the applicant negotiated which portion of the caring responsibility the institution would assume for the family and the extent of responsibility the family would continue to assume?

Although institutionalization is needed in most cases because the family is unable to maintain full responsibility to provide care for an individual, it need not be accompanied by complete delegation of care to the institution. Perhaps the family could assume responsibility for following a schedule of eating with the resident and assisting with feeding, if necessary. Perhaps the resident might spend one day a week in the home of relatives, or relatives might provide a weekly afternoon out, do personal laundry, or give a bath. The extent of the involvement could vary, as could the nature of the assignment, and the variables could be renegotiated on a regular basis.

Obviously, wellness relates to the continuity or the assumption of responsibility by the family and, concomitantly, the retention of control and authority by the family. Rather than taking over completely, the institution could assume a portion of the responsibility of caring for a person. Negotiating a sharing of responsibility would be as much a symbolic act as a reorganization of work assignments, representing retention of control by recipients of care, rather than transfer of control to the providers of care.

Family involvement, as with that of professionals and paraprofessionals, must not be superficial; it must take into consideration the capacity of family members to provide ongoing support and to handle stress and loss. Family members can be most helpful if they understand the changes to be expected, the anticipated course of events, and appropriate interventions. The ability of adult children to deal with significant changes in their parents' health and/or behavior may influence the capacity of the parents to benefit from the intended assistance.

Adult children often are physically separated from their parents for extended time periods, which begins when the children complete their education and leave home and continue until their parents' infirmity requires increased help. Many children respond with love and concern, but for a variety of reasons, which may include geographical distance and involvement in their own lives, arrange for the provision of services, rather than providing them directly and personally. Nonetheless, the family is involved as it relates to the actual caregivers and monitors the content and quality of care. This involvement reduces the loneliness or isolation of the parent and helps maintain a sense of wholeness and wellness.

Another consideration must be the possibility of augmenting family resources to support the older person. Availability of in-home services, day care, and respite care not only can postpone institutionalization but also can establish a cooperative relationship between families and service providers that can help provide continuity, should the move to a nursing home become necessary.

Through this continuity, an important communications link could be forged. Providers of long-term care often complain about the obstructive behavior of families, how their guilt is manifested in unreasonable demands and expectations, and the need to keep them away and uninvolved during difficult treatment periods. Every effort should be made to prevent the establishment of adversary positions between the family and the institution that these complaints reflect. Again, hospice provides ample opportunities to observe the potential for positive family involvement in long-term care and the wellness of family after a death.

Incorporating wellness into long-term care through such approaches not only would change the attitudes and organization of the institution but also would have an enormous effect on the public perception of institutional care. The role of the institution would change to become an extension of the family and home in which the emphasis on wellness would make possible the continuity of family relationships, responsibility, and control.

Sensory and Social Environment

In the Lawton theory of environmental press,[7] the critical aspects of the environment have greater consequences for those individuals who are most dependent on their environments. From this theoretical framework, the resident of an institution could suffer most from adverse aspects of the environment. Conversely, positive changes in the environment, even of the smallest dimension, can have a great effect on the institutionalized person. Imagine, then, the magnitude of the effect that a major emphasis on wellness would have on those who are homebound or are residents of an institution or congregate institutional environment. It is those who are most dependent who benefit most from supportive environments that stress wholeness and wellness. Those who are less dependent may have a response of lesser magnitude but still benefit from increased comfort and sense of wellness.

The presence of an unresponsive environment can be severely debilitating and as restrictive as a flight of stairs is to an older person in a wheelchair. An individual's disability can be exacerbated by an environment that does not provide proper supports; it can further incapacitate requiring the need for further supportive services. A properly designed and utilized environment, however, can both minimize the losses of the older person and give positive support. Elements of a properly designed environment include safety grab-bars strategically placed in the kitchen and bathroom, kitchen cabinets located within easy reach of the person with restricted reach and mobility, and lighting and textures of furnishings selected to offset the effects of glare or inadequate light. Use of contrasting colors for doorknobs, locks, thermostats, and light switches makes them clearly identifiable for persons with limited vision. Increasing the size of lettering on thermostats, telephones, prescription bottles, and other printed materials gives visually impaired individuals better access to the printed message. Clearly, the environment can be designed to compensate substantially for disabilities of reach, sight, and mobility and therefore to encourage a sense of wellness. Fostering wellness also includes reducing the incidence of illness by managing harmful conditions in the environment and strengthening the ability of people to endure stress and change.[8]

Goffman,[9] in his book *Asylums,* identifies three major forces of institutional life that depersonalize the individual, cause boredom and sameness, and discourage creativity:

1. The residents generally eat, sleep, work, and play in the same environment with the same people under the same set of rules that are promulgated by the institutional staff.
2. Institutional residents are ''batched'' or treated alike or perceived by staff to be alike on the basis of having similar needs. There is no appreciation of the individuality of persons of diverse ages, backgrounds, interests, and capacities.
3. The institutional rules are made by the staff, often for the convenience of the staff, despite the pretense that rules are made for the residents.

Combined, these forces quickly tend to institutionalize the resident and can create the iatrogenic illnesses associated with institutionalization. Such adverse effects can be minimized by persistently emphasizing wellness, rather than illness, and by considering residents as unique individuals. When residents are invited to furnish their living spaces with their own belongings or, in more restrictive settings, to add some personal effects to the institutional furnishings, they feel greater comfort with the environment. When institutional rules are carefully scrutinized to eliminate those that are not required for the welfare of residents, wellness is created. When monotony and boredom are replaced with multiple options for creativity, education, or assumption of responsibility, the negative aspects of illness are replaced by an awareness of wellness.

The concept of wellness also is encouraged when personnel of institutions understand the difference between illness and the aging process and respond accordingly. A good example of this distinction is understanding that hearing loss is a normal change that takes place among all adults; its negative aspects can be offset by understanding personnel. The typical hearing loss of the older person is presbycusis, which is associated with loss of nerve functioning. This may result in confusion of the message heard because of distortion of consonant sounds. The consequent impairment of communication for the older person can cause isolation, loneliness, and withdrawal. An insensitive staff that is unaware of these normal changes, might interpret such behavior as a form of illness. A sensitive and alert staff that properly identifies the problem can help the individual overcome the handicap by using such simple techniques as talking face-to-face so mouth and facial movements can be observed, slowing the speed of the speech pattern, and lowering the pitch of the voice. The alert attendant can reduce the effects of disability through understanding and an affirmative regard for the competencies of the person, thus stressing wellness.

Self-Determination

When the institution becomes a new home, especially for long-term residence, how does the individual relate to the rules and regulations of that home? If an individual can only accept the rules, regulations, and policies of the institution and cannot modify them, then his or her power and control have been transferred to the institutional management. The person may, of course, move to another institution that appears less restrictive, if one can be found. Even then, the individual would merely be submitting to a more compatible authority. Residents enter institutional environments, be they retirement centers, homes for the aged, or nursing homes, to seek assistance that can be provided in those settings. Requiring and obtaining institutional services do not necessarily require as a *quid pro quo* that the residents be denied all opportunities for exercising control over daily living.

In order to encourage greater self-determination by residents, institutions often establish residents' councils, committees, or advisory boards. Yet, generally, the residents' role on councils or committees is advisory, without any obligation on the part of staff to use this advice. Unfortunately, residents' councils often present only a facade of self-determination, permitting residents to advise on such issues as choosing a feature movie, the theme for a party, or a dish for the evening menu. In practice, such an advisory role conveys a clear message to the residents: "You deal with the insignificant issues; staff will deal with important matters, such as personnel, budget, and finances."

One way residents could be involved effectively in a most significant aspect of their environment would be to have them participate in the selection and evaluation of personnel, including the administrator. Evaluating personnel in a formal process would clearly maintain the residents' role as consumers, with power to determine both the nature of services and the level of performance expected. Regardless of their health and need to be in an institutional setting, giving residents the ability to exercise control over their personal environment fosters a sense of wellness. The institution that recognizes and encourages this reality helps its residents perceive themselves as persons, rather than collections of infirmities.

THE COMMUNITY AND PUBLIC POLICY

Probably some of the more pervasive negative forces encouraging the absence of wellness in long-term care are public policies. According to Anne Somers, "Of all the difficult health care problems facing the nation today, none is more complex or urgent than the formulation of a viable policy of long term care for the elderly and the chronically ill and disabled."[10] The real issue is the absence of a national policy that recognizes and pays for the skills that are an essential part of long-term care; namely, the care provided to meet the personal and social needs of the individual.

Somers argues for a new long-term care policy that has the following four characteristics:

1. focus on functional independence for the patient, rather than on "cure"
2. emphasis on prevention at all ages
3. involvement of families in a reasonable way
4. involvement not only of physicians, but of nurses, social workers, aides, and others, and provision of incentives for these workers to master geriatric skills.

The major national health care program in the United States, Medicare, focuses on acute care for the elderly and does not provide any support for the problems related to chronic care. Neither does it offer any assistance to the families of older people, who provide the majority of long-term care services.[11] Rather, both Medicare and Medicaid favor the provision of institutional care programs through their payment and reimbursement policies. The absence of family supports, the rejection of payments for preventive programs, and the emphasis on payments for institutional care demonstrate how present health care policies hamper, or even prevent, the development of appropriate long-term care services to the elderly. If the wellness potential in long-term care is to be realized, the sources of financial payment must support programs that recognize the importance of prevention, education, support for people at home, and maintaining the supportive function of families.

Brody,[12] Somers,[13] and Eisdorfer[14] have described differences between the medical care and the social care models. The medical model is physician-directed, cure-oriented, and dependent on sophisticated medical technology. The social care model responds to the personal and social needs of the individual, who is much more involved in decision making than in the medical model. The social care model has been associated with long-term care, whereas the medical model is used to represent what generally is considered acute care.

Long-term care or chronic care is not solely social care, however. It is social care as part of an overall program that usually includes medical care. What frequently happens is that long-term care is dichotomized into the two care systems, which sometimes may seem to be in opposition or at least in conflict. While long-term care is the appropriate intervention, the medical model is what is delivered.

Wellness in long-term care is dependent on the embodiment of the concept of wellness in the national policies that support that care. It is also necessarily dependent on the interrelationships among the individual, the family, and society. Wellness cannot be implemented in the absence of a whole and integrated system.

NOTES

1. E.M. Brody, *Long Term Care of Older People* (New York: Human Sciences Press, 1977), pp. 14–15.

2. D.L. Featherman, "The Life-Span Perspective in Social Science Research," *SSRC Five Year Outlook,* December, 1981, pp. 621–648.

3. D.A. Hamburg, "Frontiers of Research in Neurobiology," *Science* 222, (December 1983): 4627.

4. P.B. Baltes and M.M. Baltes, "Plasticity and Variability in Psychological Aging: Methodological and Theoretical Issues," in *Determining the Effects of Aging on the Central Nervous System,* ed. G. Guiski (Berlin: Shering, 1980), p. 123.

5. D.L. Featherman, *op. cit.,* pp. 621–648.

6. H. Feifel, *New Meanings of Death* (New York: McGraw-Hill, 1977), p. 181.

7. M.P. Lawton, P.G. Windley, and T.D. Byerts, eds., *Aging and the Environment: Theoretical Approaches,* Gerontological monographs of the Gerontological Society #7 (New York: Springer Publishing Co., 1982), p. 41.

8. S. Nickoley-Colquitt, "Preventive Group Interventions for Elderly Clients: Are They Effective?" in *Aging and Health Promotion,* ed. T. Wells (Rockville, Md.: Aspen Systems, 1982), p. 168.

9. E. Goffman, *Asylums* (New York: Anchor Books, 1961), p. 102.

10. A.R. Somers, "Long Term Care for the Elderly and Disabled," *New England Journal of Medicine,* 307 (July 1982): pp. 221–226.

11. C. Eisdorfer, "Care of the Aged: The Barriers of Traditions," *Annals of Internal Medicine,* 94 (1981): pp. 256–260.

12. S.J. Brody, "The Thirty-to-One Paradox: Health Needs and Medical Solution," in *Aging: Agenda for the Eighties* (National Journal Issues Book, 1980), pp. 17–20.

13. A.R. Somers, *op. cit.,* pp. 221–226.

14. C. Eisdorfer, *op. cit.,* pp. 256–260.

Chapter 9

Growing Old Healthy: Meeting the Emotional Challenges of the Senior Years

James A. Davis, Ed.D.

SENIOR LIFE ADJUSTMENTS

Of all the transitions that Americans face—from moving through the different levels of schooling to marrying, having children, and changing jobs—old age is the one for which there is typically little, if any, formal or informal preparation. This lack of preparation is unfortunate because a potentially rewarding period of life becomes more trying than need be. Yet, it is perhaps most harmful because coping with life adjustments is the greatest challenge the elderly as a group encounter and because how individuals deal with these transitions makes the difference between mental stability and emotional difficulties. The major adjustments of later life include the following.

Change in Role and Status

On retirement, individuals find themselves in a world in which it is more difficult to reflect the traditional work ethic of achievement, productivity, and independence. For an individual who has lived his or her life in pursuit of these goals—and whose very identity has become wrapped up in the status and power these achievements bring—retirement can be particularly difficult. This adjustment difficulty is most prevalent in the professional world and is a major reason why white-collar workers fear retirement more than do blue-collar workers.[1]

Most other social roles in an elderly person's life also change noticeably. The homemaker can face a very serious transition in later life with the loss of the active mother role after her children leave home. A person's role as a friend can drastically change, particularly with friends and associates who continue to work and whose worlds revolve around a different axis than the retiree's. The retiree may suddenly find him or herself in a "senior statesman" role in clubs and professional societies, often eased out of leadership positions to make room for "young blood."

Financial Difficulties

On the average, the elderly's income level is only about one-half of that of adults under age 65.[2] As with individuals of any age, retired persons who have insufficient incomes face a variety of problems. The older person may be unable to pursue a pleasurable hobby, purchase adequate food or health care, retain his or her mobility, or remain in a cherished home.

The problem is multifaceted. Double-digit inflation and high interest rates under the Carter administration have been followed by severe cuts in social service programs under President Reagan. Inadequate health care coverage under Medicare, means that catastrophic illness could easily wipe out an individual's savings in a matter of months.

Yet, the biggest obstacle to financial security is the failure of our system to encourage Americans to plan in advance for their financial needs in retirement. Far too many retirees seem to take their financial security for granted. When they realize that their finances are not secure, it is often too late. It is no wonder that financial problems are a major cause of dissatisfaction and morale problems for retirees.

A New Leisure Life-Style

A retiree's life-style is no longer shaped by work. Instead, every day is like a weekend day, which must be filled with hobbies, volunteer activities, or other outside interests. Rest and relaxation are not arts at which many Americans excel. Most find little time in their workaday world to develop outside interests. When they do play, they "work" very hard at it. Thus, when retirement comes and they have all the time in the world, many individuals quite literally do not know how to relax and enjoy themselves.

Again, a lack of adequate planning comes back to haunt the retiree. Too few people plan for leisure activities in retirement, thinking, "There will be more than enough to keep me busy." However, once retired, the retiree often finds him- or herself at a loss as to how to fill their now extensive leisure time.

Changes in Relationships

Most couples spend their work years going in different directions. Even when they are at home together, they often are occupied with children and other concerns and find little time to work out any problems in their own relationship. When retirement comes, however, suddenly they are with each other 24 hours a day and can no longer avoid these problems. To their surprise, many couples may find they do not know each other as well as they thought and that they must become reacquainted. Whether they can do so may prove a test of stability in the marriage. With proper communication, however, these problems can be dealt with and resolved, resulting in an even stronger marital bond.

Many retirees have used the pressures of a career and outside interests as an excuse to avoid solving emotional problems. When they retire, they inevitably find themselves face-to-face with their problems. Personal difficulties and insecurities can be compounded by the retiree's tendency to see him- or herself as "old" and no longer useful. Such a change in self-concept can isolate an older person.

Loss of Loved Ones

Although most older people realize that they must deal with death as an inevitable part of life, many still cannot help being shocked by the loss of family members, close friends, and associates that accompanies growing older. They may have to face a series of sudden deaths or face a slower, but nonetheless devastating, accumulation of deaths. None of these losses is more stressful than the loss of the spouse. Widowhood means dealing with the tremendous grief encountered by the loss of a partner, lover, and confidant. Lifelong roles are changed overnight, often causing serious problems with identity and self-esteem. One must face the loneliness and isolation that come with severe changes in social circumstances.

Most likely, the wife will outlive her husband. She will likely face many difficult adjustments in widowhood, including serious financial problems and age discrimination in employment. Widows also encounter major social roadblocks. In our couple-oriented society, many friends who socialized in the past as couples begin to lose contact with the widow. Even when she goes out with a couple, she may feel like a "third wheel." Establishing new social contacts is not an easy task and may involve fierce competition for the attention of the few remaining older males.

Experiencing Loneliness and Isolation

Loneliness and social isolation can be caused by living alone, especially if it is not by choice. In addition, social isolation may result from an older person's inability to communicate effectively because of physical defects, such as blindness, deafness, or loss of speech. Poor physical or mental health also can be a major contributor, because of the limitations placed on activities or the reaction of those in contact with the ill individual. In addition, social isolation can be precipitated by the loss of close family members and friends or by changes in familiar surroundings and patterns. Once friendly, close-knit neighborhoods can become built up and highly commercialized. Or the once nice neighborhood may become run down, presenting a greater threat of crime and causing the elderly to become virtual prisoners in their own homes. The situation is no better for the institutionalized elderly, for whom loneliness and isolation can be a constant companion.

Changes in Health and Physical Appearance

Inevitably, older people face changes in health and physical appearance. The vast majority of the elderly suffer from one or more chronic illnesses, the most prevalent of which are heart disease, arthritis, obesity, hernias, cataracts, varicose veins, hemorrhoids, hypertension, and prostate disease. The greatest frustrations are the limitations chronic illnesses can put on daily activities—the difficulty getting around, complete or partial confinement to the home, or the need for assistance. Physical illness shakes one's sense of pride in the reliability of one's body.

Ongoing changes in physical appearance are a constant reminder of the passing years. In our very youth-oriented society, billions of dollars are spent each year to attempt to turn back time with cosmetic surgeries, lotions, hair dyes, and cosmetics. For many, however, decline in their senses is even more disturbing. Failing vision and hearing loss are the most traumatic. The senses of taste, touch, and smell can also be affected.

DEALING WITH EMOTIONAL TURMOIL

Given the tremendous adjustments and transitions faced by older persons, often in shockingly short periods of time, it should come as no surprise that the elderly are at high risk of developing emotional difficulties. The 1978 Presidents' Commission on Mental Health statistics indicate that more than 3 million older Americans need mental health care services.[3] Most experts believe this estimate is conservative.

As a group, the elderly are prone to more frequent occurrences of such common emotional disturbances as depression, sleep disturbance, and hypochondria.

Of those problems, *depression* stands out as the most common and potentially devastating. Trying to cope with a tremendous number of difficult life transitions, often occurring very close in time to each other, can put older persons at high risk of becoming depressed. For those who do become depressed, the result is often a sense of hopelessness and discouragement, which saps their strength and has progressively negative effects on their everyday lives.

Sleep disturbances are also a serious problem for older persons. Some elderly persons have difficulty falling asleep, and others suffer from frequent awakenings and restless sleep. As with depression, the precipitating factors are often the changes and losses that old age brings.

A third common emotional disorder among the elderly is *hypochondria,* or obsessive concern about the functioning of one's body or its parts. Victims of hypochondria either complain about maladies that have no physical basis or exaggerate symptoms for those that do. Often, every possible excuse is used to see a doctor. These reactions are usually a response to unmet emotional needs and may reflect an attraction to the sick role as an answer to perceived failure to meet society's emphasis on success, independence, and financial security. For those who feel neglected, it can be a vehicle for gaining attention. Social isolation, lack of stimulating interests, hostile feelings toward others or oneself, and/or fear of death may also lead older persons to focus excessive attention on their bodies.

Depression, sleep disturbances, hypochondria, and other emotional disorders are problematic for the elderly in and of themselves. Of even greater concern, however, is that, in many such cases, the individual is incorrectly identified as suffering from *organic brain disorder* and thus is considered untreatable when he or she could be helped to overcome these obstacles and regain emotional well-being. For those few who do suffer from organic brain disease, however, the prognosis may be grim.

THE TRUTH ABOUT "SENILITY"

Organic brain disease is perhaps the most debilitating emotional disorder that the elderly face. A victim of the disorder, which is often classified in the catch-all category of "senility" and written off as one of the incurable effects of aging, may experience impairment of intellectual function, comprehension, memory, and judgment. The initial stages often bring confusion about time—hour, day, and year—and later about places and orientation. As the disorder progresses, the individual has increasing difficulty remembering the people actively involved in his or her life, and, finally, the frustration of not remembering his or her own name.

Although one of the prevailing myths about old age is that all the elderly become senile, only about 5 percent of the older population suffers from organic brain syndrome (OBS). There are two distinct categories of OBS, each with vastly different prognoses.

The first type, which represents a surprisingly large percentage of OBS sufferers, is a reversible brain syndrome (RBS) that can be treated. A common cause of RBS is a stroke, after which the individual usually passes through a period of severe confusion before regaining normal capacities. Another cause may be malnutrition caused by isolation, declining appetites, depression, or physical illness. The startlingly high usage of prescription drugs among the elderly population may be still another precipitating factor in RBS, due to unexpected side effects brought on by the drug itself or ill-advised mixtures with other drugs, foods, or alcohol. The lack of intellectual stimulation and meaningful contact with others can also cause disorientation.

The significant number of OBS victims who suffer from the more virulent and irreversible form of the disease are most often victims of Alzheimer's disease or multi–infarct dementia. Alzheimer's disease, found in 50 to 60 percent of all elderly with mental impairment,[4] is caused by changes in the proteins of the nerve cells in the outer layer of the brain, which results in the death of large numbers of brain cells. As the disease progresses, the individual experiences increasing memory loss, confusion, agitation, restlessness, and major personality changes. Finally, the victim becomes helpless and incontinent.

Multi-infarct dementia is a chronic disorder that accounts for 20 percent of all irreversible OBS.[5] It is caused by the hardening or narrowing and closing of blood vessel walls, which restricts the flow of blood—and thus of oxygen and essential nutrients—to the brain and results in permanent brain damage. Decline is erratic and uneven, but irreversible. Among the contributing factors is the traditionally rich diet, high in saturated fats and cholesterol, that many Americans follow.

The greatest tragedy of OBS is that, because their symptoms are quite similar and, in some cases, virtually indistinguishable, reversible disorders are too often mistaken for irreversible impairments. The result can be the denial of needed and valuable treatment, which could help restore the sufferer to good mental health. For the 5 percent of the elderly who suffer from organic brain syndrome, medical treatment is essential either to reverse the symptoms or minimize suffering in the case of an irreversible disorder. Yet, most of the other mental health problems of the later years can be improved by preventive measures that the elderly can take for themselves such as diet, exercise, and stimulating social contact and activities.

SELF-HELP AS A TREATMENT

As with any age group, to a certain extent the elderly are the masters of their own destiny. How they view themselves, how they meet the various challenges of the older years, whether they call into play the coping skills that have allowed them to survive to old age will play a major role in their adjustment to old age. If they see themselves as old, ugly, decrepit, and out-of-the mainstream, this perception may prove to be a self-fulfilling prophecy. If, however, they view old age and all its changes as only another stage of life—a stage that presents new challenges and opportunities, just as growing up, getting married, joining the workforce, and raising a family had their challenges and opportunities—old age will prove to be a much more positive experience.

THE ELDERLY AND THE MENTAL HEALTH SYSTEM

The Youth Orientation of the Mental Health System

Even the most positive attitude cannot cure or forestall all the emotional problems the elderly face. The mental health system must also assist the elderly by providing appropriate services in a timely manner. Unfortunately, the current public and private mental health systems have put priority on their younger and middle-aged clientele.

In the world of private mental health care, the elderly are almost nonexistent. Psychologists and psychiatrists are too often unwilling or hesitant to treat older persons. In fact, research has shown that only 2 to 5 percent of psychiatric services are devoted to the elderly.[6,7]

Instead, mental health professionals tend to treat young, white, and well-educated persons. The American Psychoanalytic Association reported that 98 percent of its members' private patients were white, 82 percent were under 45 years of age, and 78 percent were college-educated.[8] Clearly, private mental health professionals have a bias against treating the elderly.

Money is also a factor in the exclusion of the elderly from private mental health care. Psychiatric care is most frequently utilized by higher-income individuals, who can afford to pay the high cost of private psychoanalytic services, which range from $40 to $80 per hour or more.

Community Mental Health Centers (CMHCs) do no better a job of serving the elderly. A comprehensive study of CMHCs in Oregon showed that they have virtually the same bias against treatment of the elderly as the private mental health system. The Davis study examined the CMHCs' clientele flow from 1976 to 1979. During that period, clients between the ages of 21 and 59 made up more than two-thirds (68.4 percent) of all admissions to CMHCs and 94.5 percent of all adult (21 +) admissions. This compares to 3.7 percent (overall) and 5.5 percent (adult) admission figures for senior clients during those same four years.[9]

Moreover, the Davis study pointed out that the make-up of the senior CMHC clientele (age 60 +) varied widely from that of the nonsenior adult client. The senior clientele were half as likely to refer themselves to CMHCs, but were more likely than the younger clientele to be referred by private physicians, public mental hospitals, and family. The younger client group were more than three times as likely to list problems within their family or marriage or with child guidance as reasons for seeking CMHC assistance. The older clients were widowed more than 10 times as often, yet younger clients were separated or divorced nearly twice as often. As could be expected, nonsenior clientele were significantly more financially secure and received considerably less government assistance. They were also far better educated than their elderly counterparts.

The obvious conclusion that can be drawn from this study is that CMHC service emphasis is on a younger and middle-aged clientele that is strikingly different in its make-up than the elderly clientele. The result is a classic "Catch 22" situation: Because CMHCs see the elderly less often, they are largely unprepared to deal with their special needs. And because they are unprepared to deal with their special needs, they are that much more likely to reach out to the younger group.

Shrinking Funds

A major reason for the private and public mental health sector's lack of attention to the elderly has been money, or the lack thereof. Since the Reagan administration took office, mental health care has been a victim of conservative fiscal policies. The Mental Health Systems Act was effectively dissolved, and most of its progressive programs and funding potential died with it, although some limited sections were picked up in subsequent legislation.

As soon as that act was dissolved, the Reagan administration began consolidating funding for a variety of programs under block grants to the states, which then have the authority to determine how those funds were allocated. Mental health funding was placed in the Alcohol, Drug Abuse, and Mental Health Block Grant, and the overall allotment was reduced.

Public mental health care has suffered significantly as a consequence. For example, CMHCs, which have long been insufficiently funded, have become even more understaffed and overworked and thus less able to reach out to the elderly community.

Medicare continues to offer little to help meet the mental health care needs of its beneficiaries. Since its inception, there has been a $250 ceiling on outpatient treatment of mental health problems per year. Unlike the 80–20 percent co-payment requirement for physical health care services, Medicare pays only 50 percent of mental health care costs. Furthermore, this reimbursement is limited to the services of psychiatrists. In almost all instances, services provided by psychologists, social workers, and psychiatric nurses are not reimbursed. Psychiatric hospitalization coverage is also very limited under Medicare. Unfortunately, private health insurance policies provide equally poor coverage of mental health costs.

It is both tragic and ironic that better mental health care services are not available to the elderly. If mental health care services were strengthened, there would be less need for general medical care. The federal government, however, has yet to acknowledge the value of an improved mental health care system.

Elders' Negative Attitudes toward the Mental Health Field

Another major obstacle to the delivery of adequate mental health care services to the older population is the elderly's own negative attitude toward the mental health field. Having lived through an era when mental health care emphasized institutional alternatives, many elderly still equate mental health care with institutionalization. Because they tend to view such care as being designed for persons who are "senile" or "crazy," they are less likely than younger people to seek assistance for their own emotional problems. As Dr. Robert Patterson found while conducting a survey:

> Normal elderly people outside the centers reacted to questions about mental health problems with anxiety, often expressed by nervous joking. Many thought mental health services were only for "crazy people"; they associated mental problems with long hospitalization. Some described illnesses, but they had not considered it appropriate to take these problems to mental health professionals.[10]

This stigmatization creates a dilemma for the CMHC system. The primary objective of CMHCs is to serve those who seek help. Because the elderly rarely seek mental health care services, they rarely receive them.

Changing and Sensitizing the Present Mental Health System

Given the underutilization of private and public mental health care services by the older population, it is evident that a brighter future for the emotional and psychological well-being of the elderly hinges at least partially on the development of a relatively low-cost continuum of mental health services. Development of such a care continuum would be no easy task, but it can be done. To be successful, it requires the involvement of the CMHCs, agencies that serve the elderly (area agencies on aging, senior services, home health, homemakers, nutrition programs, senior centers), senior groups (Gray Panthers, American Association of Retired Persons, County Senior Councils), and community organizations (churches, advocacy groups). For example, county-wide task forces made up of representatives of these groups can be formed to advocate for improved mental health services to the elderly, incorporate available resources, develop educational programs for service/care providers and the public, and seek out appropriate funding sources.

The following key ingredients are essential to the effort to provide better mental health care for the elderly.

Change the Priorities of CMHC Services

CMHCs need to take a long, hard look at the services they provide and see how they can reshuffle their priorities. It is critical that CMHCs have ongoing contact with the local elderly population and the agencies and programs that serve them. To reach this objective, the following programmatic steps should be taken:

- *Designated staff responsibilities.* Certain CMHC staff should be designated to work with the elderly as a major or at least minor part of their responsibilities.

- *Community contact.* To encourage a change in attitude toward mental health care on the part of the senior community, designated CMHC staff should make themselves available at a certain time each week at locations that are well attended by older persons. Such a program will give the elderly the opportunity to visit and share concerns in a comfortable environment, rather than a mental health facility with its stigmas.

- *Expanded counseling outreach.* Once these initial efforts are underway and a sense of trust is building within the senior community, attempts should be made to expand individual and small group counseling for older persons. Which approach is used depends on the individual and the level of difficulty he or she is experiencing. With budget cutbacks and the limits they place on staff time, however, group work becomes a more attractive alternative to reach more elderly, as well as to provide participants with the opportunity for positive interaction with others who are experiencing similar problems.

- *Self-help/mutual aid groups.* Expanding on the group concept, CMHCs might also attempt to form a network of self-help, mutual aid groups that can deal with common concerns of the elderly, such as role/status changes in retirement, bodily changes, and loss of loved ones. Interested community volunteers or paraprofessionals can be trained to serve as group leaders.

- *Consultation in the community.* CMHCs also should provide consultation to direct service providers—for example, outreach workers, homemakers, home health care employees—who are in daily contact with the elderly to help them respond appropriately when they are confronted by their clients' emotional problems. If individual consultation is unrealistic, a monthly "rap" session would be helpful.

Increased Involvement of Psychologists and Psychiatrists

Private mental health professionals should take advantage of their unique skills to provide psychotherapy and guidance to the older population. Despite the youth orientation of the profession, this objective can be accomplished with some very basic initiatives on the part of psychologists and psychiatrists:

- *Counseling support.* Efforts should be made in conjunction with local psychiatric and/or psychological groups to encourage those in private practice to free up some time to assist elderly person(s) who otherwise could not afford their services. A list of therapists could be compiled and arrangements made for the older person to go to a therapist's office. A more comfortable location may also be selected where possible or appropriate.

- *Consultative support.* The advice and consultation of psychologists and psychiatrists also is extremely valuable to paraprofessionals and volunteers who end up being "counselors" to elderly persons who are experiencing problems and adjustments and who have nowhere else to turn. By setting up "rap" sessions or donating a certain amount of free consultation time to individuals or groups of paraprofessionals/volunteers each month, psychiatrists and psychologists can help these individuals better respond to and refer the problem situations they encounter.

- *Sliding fee scale.* An effort should be made to convince those in private practice to adopt a sliding fee scale that would make private mental health services affordable for the lower- and middle-income elderly. This step could fill some service gaps, especially in more highly populated areas where most psychiatrists and psychologists are located.

Education of Service Providers and the Public

A multifaceted educational program is an important component in any local mental health programming effort aimed at older people. Its objectives would be to (1) provide the proper educational background and knowledge to service/care providers in the closest contact with the elderly, so they can respond to the emotional problems with which they are confronted; (2) help older persons become more comfortable with what mental health care is all about and to demonstrate to them how they can best cope with the adjustment problems they face; and (3) help the general public gain a better understanding of the mental health needs of the elderly and a more honest perspective of growing old. The following are ingredients of a successful education program:

- *Workshop format.* Workshop sessions can be developed on generalized or specific topics, such as senior life adjustments, organic brain disorders, psychiatric problems, response and referral, substance abuse, elderly depression, and exercise and nutrition. The intensity and depth of the training will depend on the educational background and experience of the audience.

- *Electronic media usage.* Television and radio are especially effective educational tools that can reach into thousands of homes at once. If a group is well-prepared, public service programming is easier to obtain than one might imagine. A talk show format—presented as a special series or an ongoing show—can deal effectively with mental health topics—for example, successful retirement, dealing with depression, institutionalization, alcohol and drug use and abuse, the dangers of stereotyping—especially with the winning combination of a solid production, a good host, and interesting guests.

- *Speaker's bureau*. Another logical approach to community education is to utilize knowledgeable mental health professionals and/or gerontologists to speak to groups of seniors or service providers about emotional well-being in the later years. This type of interaction will open up discussion and make all concerned a little more comfortable with a traditionally uncomfortable topic.

Use of Skilled Volunteers

How is it possible to plan an effective approach for reaching older persons in the community with little or no funds?

The answer may be found in the training of skilled volunteers, individuals of all ages and backgrounds who have a sincere interest in older persons and the necessary time to devote to them. Elderly persons themselves, of course, make ideal skilled volunteers as they can best relate to the problems of their peers. The types of services that can be provided by skilled volunteers fall into three main areas:

- *Visitation and referral*. Volunteers can serve as friends for elderly persons in private homes or institutions who are lonely and isolated due to lack of human contact or intellectual stimulation or who are encountering serious adjustment problems or losses and who do not have someone in whom they can confide. Often, simply having someone around who is genuinely concerned can make a big difference.
- *Escort to mental health services*. If an elderly person is referred and agrees to seek counseling or other treatment, skilled volunteers can help relieve anxiety by escorting him or her to and from the counseling site, at least for the initial visit(s). This service will help alleviate some of the initial emotional pressure and allow the older person to discuss his or her experience and reaction.
- *Small group leadership*. Volunteers also can be trained to serve as group leaders for self-help/mutual aid groups. It is preferable that group leaders have personal involvement or experience in the topic area being discussed.

Preretirement Training and Preparation

Traditionally, there has been very little preparation for the retirement years, both because of the strength of the work ethic and the fear of growing old, which have caused our society to virtually ignore the prospect of retirement. As a sad result, adjustment to this phase of life is more difficult than it need be.

To change this, the private and public sectors need to develop comprehensive preretirement programs for their older workers. This effort should begin 5 to

10 years before actual retirement to prepare workers for the effects retirement will have on family relations, leisure time, government benefits, desirable roles and activities in the community, legal affairs, income sources, housing and living arrangements, and physical conditions. Counseling, workshops, and group sessions, preferably with the involvement of the spouse, can provide information, allay apprehensions, and stimulate planning.

CONCLUSION

The elderly face a host of adjustments and losses in the "golden years" of retirement. The result is a population at much higher risk of developing emotional problems, including depression, sleep disturbances, and hypochondria.

To a certain degree, the elderly control their own destiny in later life. Keeping a positive outlook, staying active and involved, maintaining meaningful friendships and associations, eating properly and exercising regularly make adjustments to this stage of life much easier and life satisfaction much greater.

Even the best of self-help approaches, however, cannot solve all the mental health problems of older persons. The mental health system must also play a significant role in meeting the emotional needs of this population. Unfortunately, both the public and private mental health sectors have severely neglected the delivery of needed mental health services to the elderly. Funding shortages have been a major contributing factor to this neglect, particularly for the public mental health system. Federal and state funding has been cut, with particularly damaging effects on the Community Mental Health Centers, which have faced a history of being understaffed and overworked due to inadequate funding levels. Medicare's coverage of mental health care remains startlingly inadequate. Private health insurance policies do equally little to meet this need. If the elderly choose to seek private therapy without appropriate coverage, the cost—ranging from $40 to $80 an hour—would likely be prohibitive. Many older persons also still hold negative attitudes toward mental health care, often equating it with institutionalization or as care designed for the "senile" or "crazy."

A brighter future for the mental health care of the older population, thus, may hinge on the development of low-cost, alternative programming. CMHCs should change their priorities to create a stronger link to the senior community. Private mental health professionals should be encouraged to donate some individual or group counseling time or even to utilize a sliding fee schedule to reach elderly persons who otherwise might not be able to afford their services, as well as to provide consultation to service providers in closest contact with the aged.

A solid base should be built in the community through the use of skilled volunteers and increased training of service providers and the general public to deal more effectively with the emotional concerns of their senior clients or loved ones. In addition, preretirement training should be expanded to prepare people in advance for the stresses and adjustments of the senior years.

In summary, the elderly face special adjustments and transitions in their lives and may need special help in meeting them. Addressing these needs will necessitate a broad-based approach—involving everything from improved self-help techniques to greater participation by the private and public mental health system and development of new, creative alternatives. Given the many contributions older Americans have made to society, meeting these important needs is the least we can do to repay them.

NOTES

1. S. Steury, "The Later Years: A Psychological Perspective," in *Readings in Psychotherapy with Older People,* ed. (Rockville, Md.: National Institute of Mental Health, 1976), p. 4.

2. Bernard Stotsky, "Coping with Advancing Years," in *Quality of Life: The Later Years,* ed. (Acton, Ma.: American Medical Association, Publishing Sciences Group, Inc., 1975), p. 116.

3. President's Commission on Mental Health, *Report to the President from the President's Commission on Mental Health, Volume 1* (Washington, D.C.: U.S. Government Printing Office, 1978), p. 9.

4. National Institute on Aging, "Senility: Myth or Madness ?" in *Age Page* (Washington, D.C.: U.S. Government Printing Office, 1980), p. 1.

5. *Ibid.,* p. 1.

6. R. Butler and M. Lewis, *Aging and Mental Health: Positive Psychosocial and Biomedical Approaches* (St. Louis: C.V. Mosby Company, 1982), p. 183.

7. M. Blank, "Raising the Age Barrier to Psychotherapy," *Geriatrics* (1974): 62.

8. Butler and Lewis, *op. cit.,* p. 183.

9. J. Davis, *An Analysis of Oregon Community Mental Health Program Clientele: Are the Elderly Being Served?* (Salem, Or.: Oregon Mental Health Division, 1981), p. 5.

10. R. Patterson, "Services for the Aged in Community Mental Health Centers," *American Journal of Psychiatry* (1976): 273.

Chapter 10

Worksite Wellness*

Anne K. Kiefhaber
Willis B. Goldbeck

For a variety of reasons, the worksite is a logical setting for wellness programs. Illness results in increased expenditures for health insurance and worker's compensation, reduced productivity, and increased absenteeism and turnover. Statistics clearly demonstrate the costliness of ill health and risk factors for employers. For example:

- Each employee who smokes is estimated to cost employers between $624 and $4,611 dollars annually more than a nonsmoking employee in medical costs, absenteeism, replacement costs, maintenance, property damage, other insurance increases, and lowered productivity.[1,2]
- More than 26 million work days are lost annually due to cardiovascular disease and hypertension.[3]
- Some $19 billion in work-loss days were attributed to excessive drinking in 1979.[4]

Seen more positively, the worksite offers opportunities to facilitate healthy behavior. Most people spend one-third of their time at work. Workplace programs usually have higher participation rates than community programs. For example, New York Telephone achieved 90 percent participation in a multiphasic screening program, whereas a similar community program achieved a 30 percent participation rate, even with extensive publicity. In addition, the corporate culture can contribute positively or negatively to health-related behavior.

Older workers, their spouses, and retired employees are three groups that can be reached through worksite wellness programming. Unfortunately, very little is

---

*Based on article "Work Site Wellness" by Anne K. Kiefhaber and Willis B. Goldbeck as it appeared in *Healthcare Cost Management: Private Sector Initiatives,* published by Health Administration Press, 1984.

known about the effect of worksite wellness programs on the elderly. In this
chapter, worksite wellness programs in general are examined, with a focus on
special applications for the elderly.

PROGRAM INITIATION

In the past few years, there has been a tremendous growth in worksite wellness
programs across the country. The breadth and diversity of these programs stem
from the large variety of individuals who design and conduct them. Most of the
early programs were initiated by very high-level employees within corporations
who believed in the benefits of a corporate culture that promoted wellness.

Other emerging sources of worksite wellness activities are unions, employee
organizations, and employee committees, including the following:

- The Health and Welfare Trust at the Storeworkers Union in the New York
  City area conducts a hypertension screening and treatment program, a breast
  cancer detection program, and weight management courses for members of
  the union.

- Employee associations at companies such as the California sites of Rockwell
  International, Lockheed Corporation, and General Dynamics have focused
  on wellness, in addition to recreation. These associations have a cooperative
  arrangement with the companies. The physical facilities and some staff
  support are provided by the company whereas the operating costs and the
  management of the program are the responsibility of the association.

- Quality of worklife or employee involvement groups established in many
  companies to improve productivity are now developing wellness programs.
  An employee involvement group at the Ford Motor Company, for example,
  has initiated exercise classes, smoking cessation programs, and stress management sessions and has distributed pamphlets on health topics, such as
  weight control and nutrition.

Generally, worksite wellness programs have been developed piecemeal, rather
than as part of an overall strategy. However, although still few in number, some
companies have appointed committees to formulate health enhancement strategies, with representatives from the personnel, safety, medical, benefits, fitness,
employee assistance, and corporate planning departments and from employee
organizations.

ELIGIBILITY

Companies that have wellness programs do not necessarily make them available
to all employees, and dependents or retirees may not be eligible to use them.

Eligibility is determined by the characteristics of the program, the philosophy of the company, and the corporate communications mechanisms. Programs that focus on disseminating information are most frequently extended to dependents and retirees, whereas facility-based programs based on services and activities are often limited to employees only. Examples of the options for eligibility are listed below:

- all employees, retirees, and spouses and at all locations
- all employees at all locations
- all employees, retirees, and spouses, but at selected locations only
- all employees, but at selected locations only
- high-risk employees
- executives only

STAFF AND FACILITIES

The staff and facilities can either be worksite- or community-based. Particularly sites with too few employees to justify the use of extensive internal resources, the trend is toward using community resources. Among the combinations of community and internal resources are the following:

- worksite wellness staff that teach courses on-site
- worksite wellness staff that use community facilities
- community-based instructors (e.g., from private firms and YMCA) that use worksite facilities
- employee volunteers who run the entire program or work in conjunction with wellness program staff

COMPONENTS OF A WELLNESS STRATEGY

Early Detection of Disease and Biological Risk

As more has been learned about the relationship between life-style and illness and as improved diagnostic technology has become available, the worksite has increasingly become the locus for detection and treatment programs. Medical screening programs that are designed to detect disease and/or biological risks include preemployment, periodic, and executive physicals; screens that target a particular risk or disease, such as hypertension or glaucoma; and self-screening programs, such as breast or testicle self-examination. These tests are conducted in a variety of ways, including on-site with company medical personnel and equipment; on-site through mobile screening units, community volunteers, or paid personnel; and off-site but paid for by the company.

The rationale for these physical examinations is that many diseases and biological risk factors can be successfully controlled, if caught early. The wellness concept is incorporated into these examinations when companies screen for risk factors, as well as illness. Increasingly, corporate medical departments seek a balance between illness detection and risk factor identification in their screening programs. By incorporating the latest research on the medical efficacy of conducting each test on particular populations at given time intervals, employers try to determine what tests will have the most significant health effect and be cost-effective. Tests that are often performed at the worksite to detect high-risk populations include hypertension screening, breast cancer detection (often offered in the form of breast self-examination courses), glaucoma screening, sickle cell anemia testing, blood tests, colon cancer screenings (frequently in the form of a self-administered test for blood in the stool), and height and weight measures for recognition of obesity. Most of these tests are inexpensive. Frequently, outside organizations, such as the American Heart Association and the American Cancer Society, as well as insurance carriers, conduct these programs free of charge at the worksite as a community contribution or as a service to their clients.

The potential for risk reduction is great, as the programs of IBM and Pioneer Hi-Bred illustrate. Since 1968, IBM has had a multiphasic screening program that provides all 35-year-old employees with a battery of physical tests, as well as a questionnaire that focuses on medical history and identifiable risk factors. Employees are eligible to repeat the exam every five years or whenever the IBM medical department suggests the tests are necessary. By 1980, approximately 90,000 employees had been screened.[5] The overall findings are striking. Forty-one percent of those screened had an "unknown medical condition" (i.e., of which they were not previously aware); another 33 percent had known conditions of which they were already aware; and 26 percent were "healthy," based on the test results.[6]

Pioneer Hi-Bred in Des Moines, Iowa, is a smaller company, with 2,500 employees, which implemented a health screening and incentive program in 1979 called Health Guard. All employees and their spouses are offered annual health screens, which include vital signs—height, weight, pulse, temperature, and blood pressure—and a urinalysis. They also receive a complete blood chemistry during their first screen. The screens are repeated annually for persons over age 40 and for those with identified problems. Others receive these tests every five years. Participation rates are 97 percent for employees and 70 percent for spouses.

In 1983, the company reported several indicators of success in the first four years of Health Guard's operation. In 1979, serious abnormalities were identified for 6 percent of those screened, compared with less than 1 percent in 1982. Many diabetic individuals identified in the first screen are now being treated through diet and exercise modifications.

Control of Disease and Biological Risk

The workplace, with its regular schedules and economic incentives to help people avoid leaving work to visit the doctor, is an ideal location for treatment or control of diseases that require continual, long-term monitoring that can be performed safely outside a medical care setting. For example, Baltimore Gas & Electric's medical department screens for hypertension, educates hypertensive employees, follows up every three months to ensure compliance with the treatment, and, if necessary, provides the medication. Discussed below are two areas of disease control—hypertension control and employee assistance programs (EAP)—for which the evidence of effectiveness is fairly strong.

Hypertension

The relationship betwen hypertension and mortality is well documented.[7] A recent study has produced results that are highly supportive of hypertension worksite programs. The University of Michigan's Institute for Labor and Industrial Relations, the Ford Motor Company, and the National Heart, Lung, and Blood Institute collaborated on a project to determine the relative effectiveness of the following four methods of hypertension referral and treatment programs.[8]

1. *Site One* served as a control. The program consisted of hypertension screening and referral to the employee's doctor, if appropriate. Except for a courtesy letter to the physician, no follow-up was conducted until the end of the two-year trial period.
2. Employees at *Site Two* were provided minimal follow-up, consisting of referral to the employee's physician with an accompanying letter to the physician and semiannual follow-up sessions.
3. Employees at *Site Three* were provided full follow-up. The main difference between Sites Two and Three was the intensity of follow-up. Although employees at Site Two were contacted only on a semiannual basis, at Site Three follow-up visits were scheduled as needed according to the severity of hypertension.
4. Employees at *Site Four* were offered complete hypertension treatment by the plant physician. Those not electing to accept on-site treatment were followed according to the Site Three protocol.

A correlation between the control of hypertension and absenteeism was found. One year before screening, matched hypertensives were absent more than normotensives at all four sites (30, 28, 12, and 29 percent more for Sites One through

Four, respectively). Hypertensive employees reduced their absenteeism over the two-year period following screening in all three experimental sites. The absence rates of active participants in Sites Two and Four approximated that of normotensives by the second year. In contrast, absenteeism among hypertensive employees increased at the control site.

Employee Assistance Programs (EAPs)

Often an outgrowth of alcoholism programs, EAPs focus on emotional problems of employees that, if left unattended, can be precursors of more significant—and potentially more costly—psychiatric and physical health disorders. According to an unpublished 1982 Washington Business Group on Health survey, more than 75 percent of their membership, which includes predominantly "Fortune 500" size employers, now offer some form of EAP.[9] Some use in-house staff exclusively, others contract out for services, whereas still others use both methods. EAPs often result in referrals to private practitioners for ongoing treatment. Although many insurance plans discriminate against mental health services, particularly outpatient treatment, the basic insurance plan is still the payment mechanism for treatment that exceeds the limitations of the EAP. For example, Standard Oil of California provides full coverage for mental health treatment when it is recommended by the EAP staff.

The primary purpose of most EAPs is to help employees with personal problems (mental, legal, family, or job-related) or illness (substance abuse, emotional illness) that can affect job performance. Employees may enter the program through self-referral or at the request of a supervisor who believes that job performance has declined. Frequently, the alternative to seeking help through the EAP, particularly where the substance abuse problem exists, is disciplinary action or dismissal. Many EAPs have expanded their focus on treatment or crisis intervention to include programs that help individuals effectively manage their time, stress, career, and family relationships to help prevent crises from occurring. Employers have discovered that EAPs reduce accidents, absenteeism, medical utilization, and improve productivity.

Detection of High-Risk Behavior

Many high-risk behaviors are the targets of public service messages provided by voluntary agencies, the government, and health organizations. Employers also provide information through newsletters, posters, audiovisual resources, and materials sent with paychecks. Health Fairs have become a popular community event that combines the resources of many local groups to educate the public about health and risk factors.

The National Health Screening Council for Volunteer Organizations, Inc. (NHSCVO) is the nonprofit organization that has assumed national leadership for developing community Health Fairs. It is the catalyst for media, corporate, volunteer, and public sector financial and in-kind services. In 1983, NHSCVO gained support from more than 120 voluntary organizations that provided health screens across the country. Some employers have held health fairs for their own populations to increase awareness of the dangers of high-risk behaviors and to assist with biological risk and disease detection.

The NHSCVO Health Fair has four components: health education, screening tests, referrals, and follow-up. Specialty programs are now offered to the elderly, minorities, students, the disabled, and local companies as part of a wellness strategy. The program for the elderly now includes a year-round education program. Each month a health message is developed and implemented through classes, printed information, and lectures. This program is conducted at senior citizen centers across the country.

Reduction of High-Risk Behavior

To help employees reduce high-risk behaviors, employers use a variety of approaches, including information dissemination, formal educational programs, behavior modification efforts, and financial incentives.

Information Dissemination

The following information dissemination techniques have been used by employers:

- Many companies provide nutritional information in cafeterias that lists the caloric and cholesterol content of food. Some companies offer a special "heart healthy" menu.
- *Citibank* offers seminars for employees on the appropriate warm-up techniques for exercises, how to buy running shoes, and how to develop an exercise regimen.
- *Ford* posts maps of two of its corporate offices with mileage measurements for employees who wish to walk indoors during breaks.
- *Armco* developed an off-the-job safety program when it discovered that off-the-job accidents caused the loss of 427,457 employee workdays between 1966 and 1977, which was the equivalent of closing a 500-person plant for three years. The program consists of calendars that identify a safety topic for every month, flyers that are sent to employees' homes with safety tips, and a meeting devoted to the safety tip of the month.

154   WELLNESS AND HEALTH PROMOTION FOR THE ELDERLY

Education

Another approach is to conduct educational programs designed to alter personal behavior. In contrast to information dissemination, educational programs attempt to assist the individuals over time by using more elaborate educational methodologies, such as repetition, reinforcement, personal contact, and the tailoring of information to appropriate learning levels. Companies may either employ health educators or contract with community resources to provide this education.

In addition, many employers have found self-help programs to be the most feasible method of providing education on behavior change. These programs are usually cheaper to run than classes, can be conducted at home where family members can participate, and can be offered at all work locations. Instruction methods range from workbooks to audiovisual or computer-taught courses.

One of the most extensive such programs is the *Xerox Health Management Program,* which involves written material, incentives, and peer support. The written material consists of an employee "self-starter" kit, which includes instructions on how to conduct a step-by-step fitness evaluation, begin a personal exercise program, cease smoking, and manage weight; a bi-monthly health management newsletter; posters in the work areas; and a computerized health-risk appraisal. Employees are encouraged to participate and are assisted by worksite-trained volunteer facilitators. In April 1983, a buddy-system incentive program was initiated. Pairs of participants entered into a contract with each other that stated that, by the end of the year, they would not smoke, would be within 10 pounds of ideal weight, and would exercise at least three times per week. Employees who met the contract terms received a T-shirt. In addition, if the pair was still participating in the contract system after a certain number of months, they each received a wallet, and their names were placed in a drawing for items such as home computers and AM/FM stereo systems.

Financial Incentives

A study by Donald Shepherd and Laurie Pearlman, Harvard University School of Public Health, of worksite-based behavioral change incentives identified 25 programs in 19 companies that were operating on or before July 1982.[10] Included were 15 smoking cessation, 5 weight loss, 4 exercise and fitness programs, and 1 stress management program. Some were offered in conjunction with behavioral change assistance, whereas others were independent. Examples of incentives include the following:

- *Analysis and Computer Systems* offers monthly bonuses to those who quit smoking. The bonuses range from $50 for the first 6 months after cessation to $300 for months 7 through 18. Six employees have participated in the program, all of whom successfully stopped smoking.

- In 1967, *City Federal Savings and Loan Association* began paying all nonsmoking employees $20 per month extra. All nonsmokers qualified, regardless of whether they had ever smoked.

- *Coors Industries* provides a $45 rebate for employees who quit smoking for 12 months, $15 reimbursement for a slimness course, and up to $100 if weight loss goals are met during a nine-month period.

- *Intermatic, Inc.* matches up to $100 of smokers' self-placed bets on whether or not they will stop smoking. Successful quitters are also eligible for a trip to Las Vegas. In addition, $4 per pound is paid for those who meet their weight loss target, and $1 per pound is paid for those who do not meet their target but lose at least 15 pounds.

- *Hospital Corporation of America* pays employees to engage in aerobic activities. Twenty-four cents is paid for each "aerobic unit." Examples of units are 1 mile of walking or running, ¼ of a mile of swimming, 4 miles of biking, 15 minutes of aerobic dancing, and 30 minutes of racketball. From June 1982 through June 1983, the company paid a total of $15,000 to the 300 corporate office employees who participated in the program. Twelve hundred employees were eligible to participate.

- *Pioneer Hi-Bred* offers overweight employees and spouses $5 per pound lost until their desired weight is reached. If the desired weight is maintained for one year, the participant has a choice of gifts valued at roughly $75. Of all overweight employees, 60 percent participated in the program, 90 percent of whom lost at least some weight. The company also pays an employee or spouse $150 to quit smoking for one year. A $75 gift is offered to the successful ex-smoker if abstinence is maintained for an additional year. An estimated 37 percent of the workforce smoked at the beginning of the program; 14 percent of these quit for two years as a result of it.

- *Blue Cross of Oregon* offers an insurance plan that integrates a medical expense account with a wellness program. In order to receive the unused portion of the account, the employee must participate in specified wellness activities and be absent from work one day less than the average of days missed for all employees.

- Several companies offer incentives for seat belt usage. *Teletype Corporation* in Little Rock, Arkansas, randomly checks for seat belt usage as employees enter or leave the parking lot and awards wearers with coupons for food at "McDonalds." *General Motors* has given away four cars through a seatbelt incentive program. Employees sign a pledge that they will wear seatbelts. When a certain percentage of employees is found to be wearing seatbelts as determined by a random check, a drawing for a new car is held for all who have signed pledge cards.

- Many companies offer material incentives, such as T-shirts, books, gym shorts, and wristwatches, for achieving a desired health outcome.

Environmental Support

Corporate attitudes, management styles, methods of communication, and the physical environment can all influence healthy behavior. This section discusses two components of an environmental health promotion strategy: the physical environment and the emotional environment.

Physical Environment

The work setting can be altered in many ways to facilitate healthy behavior, including making available facilities that promote physical fitness. Although some employers feel the presence of these facilities is synonymous with wellness programs, they are not essential for a successful wellness program. There is no evidence that fitness facilities stimulate behavioral change, although they clearly are a convenience for employees. Listed below are some options for changing the physical environment:

- nutritious, low-calorie or low cholesterol foods in cafeterias and vending machines
- menus that include nutritional information
- showers to encourage exercise
- bike racks to encourage bicycle commuting
- quiet rooms for meditation and other forms of stress management
- attractive decor
- noise control
- smoking restrictions that protect nonsmokers from exposure to cigarette smoke and reinforce the desirability of not smoking
- refrigeration to allow employees to bring their own food
- fitness facilities providing convenient access to exercise equipment. Some companies offer a full range of exercise options at the worksite, including a swimming pool, a running track, saunas, a whirlpool, and areas for exercise classes and weight training.

One of the most extensive physical facilities is located in Golden, Colorado. A few years ago, a company purchased and renovated a supermarket, making it into their wellness center. Activities at the wellness center include an extensive physical fitness program in which about one-third of employees participate; a stress management program, which includes classroom sessions and one-to-one counseling; a weight reduction program; a smoking cessation program; an extensive alcohol education program; and nutrition counseling. Many of these activities are open to family members. Vending machines have nutritious meals, with calories and cholesterol content marked.

Although this chapter has not focused on occupational safety and health, this important workplace health concern operates synergistically with wellness programs. Optimal health can obviously not be achieved in the presence of toxins and other hazards. Worksite safety and health efforts could be enhanced through wellness programs. In addition, wellness programs are dependent on individuals assuming a greater responsibility for their own health. Little incentive is offered to workers to do this if they perceive the greatest threat to their health to be their work environment over which few workers have much control.

Emotional Environment

The rise in worker's compensation awards for mental illness resulting from job stress is one indicator of the effects that the emotional aspects of a job can have on health. The most frequently cited causes of job stress are lack of control over the job, disrespect and harassment from supervisors, too much work to do in too little time, fear of unemployment, and a lack of opportunity to use one's intelligence.

The pressures of work affect individuals differently. For example, there appears to be a correlation between personality types, the degree of structure in the job, and health. A study at the Lockheed Corporation found that when people with type A personality hold structured jobs that do not permit much autonomy, their blood pressure is much higher than if their work allows a lot of freedom and creativity. The reverse was true for type B people with a more laissez-faire personality. These people experienced lower coronary risk in well-defined jobs with little room for independent action. Their blood pressure rose as job autonomy rose.[11]

There is a growing body of evidence indicating a positive correlation between an individual's ability to receive some degree of personal satisfaction through work and his or her health. Mechanisms that contribute to employee satisfaction include:

- more control over the job through employee participation groups, open lines of communication to management, and the fostering of internal entrepreneurship
- better job fit through job placement programs and opportunities for job shifting or relocating
- opportunities to mesh the job with nonwork responsibilities and desires through flex time, part-time work opportunities, paternity and maternity leave, sabbaticals, and flexible vacation policies

Although these initiatives are not traditional health initiatives, the need to consider these activities as a component of a wellness strategy will become more apparent as the information about their importance to health grows.

EVIDENCE OF EFFECTIVENESS

With the diversity of worksite wellness programs, it is critical to determine which approaches yield the greatest results so that an employer who wishes to make a commitment to wellness can spend limited resources most effectively. Ironically, these limited resources are one reason why more scientifically valid information does not exist; most companies would rather devote funds to programs than to expensive evaluations. However, two companies—Johnson & Johnson and Control Data Corporation—are making the financial commitment to conduct scientifically valid evaluations that will help all companies understand the merits of wellness programs and determine which components produce the desired outcomes. These are discussed below, followed by a summary of some other studies.

Johnson & Johnson—Live for Life

Objectives of the Johnson and Johnson Live for Life program include improvements in nutrition, weight control, stress management, fitness, smoking cessation, and health knowledge. It also encourages the proper utilization of medical interventions such as high blood pressure control and the employee assistance program. Employees are provided with a health risk screen and have the opportunity to participate in health enhancement programs at the worksite. In addition, employee task forces are responsible for creating a work environment that supports positive health practices.

An essential element of the program is the annual health screen, which is available to all employees. The screen includes biometric variables (blood lipids, blood pressure, body fat, weight, and estimated maximum oxygen uptake), behavioral variables (smoking, alcohol use, physical activity, nutritional practices, coronary behavior pattern), and attitudinal measures (general well-being, ability to handle job stress, personal relations, organizational commitment, and job involvement).

Control groups were established for the evaluation. Some 2,100 employees at four Johnson & Johnson facilities with the Live for Life program were compared with 2,000 employees at locations without the program. The evaluation protocol compares the baseline screening results with the findings from two subsequent years. The first report was issued in late 1981.[12]

Significant findings of behavioral changes include a 43 percent increase in aerobic calories burnt measured in kilograms per week in the Live for Life population (the treatment sites) compared with a 6 percent increase in the control group, a 15 percent decrease in smoking at the treatment sites compared to a 4 percent decrease at the control sites, a 1 percent decrease in the percentage of the treatment population that is above ideal weight compared to a 6 percent increase in the control group, and a 32 percent reduction in the percentage of the treatment population with elevated blood pressure compared with a 9 percent decrease at the control site. The evaluation also measured changes in self-reported sick days, with a 9 percent decrease at the treatment sites and a 14 percent increase at the control sites. People at the treatment sites also reported greater satisfaction with working conditions. A preliminary study of the impact of Live for Life program on medical utilization is also underway.

Control Data STAYWELL

STAYWELL was initiated in 1979 and, in 1983, was available to 22,000 Control Data employees and their spouses as a free employee benefit. It is also marketed to other companies as a commercial venture. Participation among Control Data employees ranges between 65 and 95 percent at the various site locations. The program includes a confidential health-risk profile with a workshop to interpret the results, a health screen, one-hour overview courses on life-style and health, and comprehensive sessions given over several weeks to change behavior related to smoking cessation, stress management, weight control, nutrition, and fitness. Control Data also has employee participation groups that attempt to alter the work environment to promote healthy life-styles, as at Johnson & Johnson.

Data for the evaluation are collected primarily through a survey that is administered to a 10 percent sample (approximately 5,000) of all domestic Control Data employees. Employees at STAYWELL locations are compared to those at locations without the program. Respondents in the STAYWELL group are also subdivided based on whether they are:

- not active in the program
- participate only in the health-risk profile
- participate in any other activities beyond health-risk profile, but not in the extensive life-style classes
- participate in the life-style change course

Control Data reported several positive effects of STAYWELL.[13] For example, smokers enrolled in the smoking cessation course smoked an average of 1.6 packs per day at the start of the course. Twelve months after the course, 30.3 percent had stopped smoking, 43.5 percent were smoking less than one pack per day, and 24.2 percent continued to smoke one or more packs per day. The evaluation also determined that people with poor health habits are 86 percent more likely to miss work and 100 percent more likely to limit the amount of work they do. They are also more likely to take prescription drugs. Finally, the Control Data evaluation confirmed the relationship between health habits and health care benefit payments. For example, current smokers and those who quit less than five years ago generated 25 percent more benefit payments and twice the number of hospital days as those who either never smoked or quit more than five years ago. Also, sedentary individuals experienced a claims cost that averaged $436.92 and .57 hospital days as compared with $321.01 and .37 hospital days for the more active people.

Other Studies

There are also less scientifically valid studies that still offer some indication of the benefits of worksite wellness programs. Those studies that are especially convincing relate to hypertension and smoking cessation. According to Jonathan Fielding, M.D., based on a review of available research:

> A voluntary on-site (hypertension) screening, referral and follow-up program at the home office of Massachusetts Mutual Life Insurance Company led to an increase in the percentage under control from 36 percent to 82 percent after one year of operation.
>
> In a three-site industrial hypertension screening, detection, and follow-up program, 92 percent of 120 auto workers, 138 sanitation workers and 106 postal workers referred for high blood pressure saw their physician, and 93 percent of those seeing a physician had treatment initiated. Of those initiating treatment, about 84 percent showed progress towards control. In 28 Chicago-area hypertensive employees who attended a special high blood pressure control clinic near their work place, average diastolic blood pressure fell from 102.6 mm Hg at first screening and 98.8 mm Hg at second screening to 83.1 mm Hg at the end of the first year.[14]

Fielding also reports that smoking cessation programs at the worksite have achieved a 40 to 60 percent abstinence rate over a 6 to 12 month period, as compared to a 15 to 30 percent abstinence rate achieved through community programs.

For many employers, less rigorous evaluation of the positive effect that wellness programs can have on absenteeism, turnover, and on-the-job accidents, and so forth has been sufficient to gain their support. Some of the studies have estimated actual cost savings as a result of wellness strategies. However, the authors are not in a position to judge validity of those results. Furthermore, companies may be more willing to report successes, rather than failures. Examples of results reported by individual companies include the following:

- *New York Telephone,* which has 80,000 employees, estimates an annual savings of $663,000 from its hypertension control program; $1,565,000 from its alcohol control program; $269,000 from its breast cancer screening program; $302,000 from its back treatment program; and $268,000 from its stress management program. [15]
- *The Occidental Life Insurance Company* and *Northern Natural Gas Company* report reduced absenteeism as a result of a fitness program.
- *Canada Life Assurance* found that program participants had a 1.5 percent turnover rate compared to a 15 percent rate for employees who did not participate. Forty-seven percent of fitness program participants reported that they were more alert, enjoyed their work more, and had better rapport with co-workers and supervisors since the program began.
- The *National Aeronautics and Space Administration* and the *New York State Education Department* have reported positive benefits in employee attitude, general sense of well-being, and reduction in absences as the result of fitness programs.
- *Kimberly-Clark* reports a 70 percent reduction in on-the-job accidents among its EAP participants.
- The *General Motors EAP* has been used by 44,000 people in 130 locations. The company reports decreases among program participants of 40 percent in lost time, 60 percent in sickness and accident benefits, 50 percent in grievances, and 50 percent in on-the-job accidents. [16]

WORKSITE WELLNESS AND OLDER WORKERS

Although few programs are designed specifically for older workers, several components of a wellness strategy are frequently tailored to the needs of different age groups. For example, most screening programs are offered more frequently as age increases. The number of tests included in the screenings are also tailored to specific age groups. Therefore, the older the employee, the more frequently the tests are offered and the more procedures are included in the test. Specific screening programs, such as hypertension and glaucoma, although available to all age groups, are more relevant for older workers.

Most corporate fitness programs require a fitness assessment before beginning a program. Many then design a special regimen for each of the participants. This suggests that older employees receive a program that takes their age into account. Moreover, a few companies offer special courses for individuals who have diet-related illnesses that are associated with aging, such as diabetes and hyper-cholesterolemia.

Some of the corporate programs are offered to retirees, and many employers have preretirement programs for employees. Although in the past these courses focused on financial and legal issues, the trend is toward the inclusion of such health issues as nutrition and physical fitness. Some programs also address the coping mechanisms for the stresses associated with retirement.

CONCLUSION

In 1970, only a handful of U.S. employers had initiated any programs that emphasized health promotion and disease prevention. In 1985, a conservative estimate would be that almost all of the larger companies have established at least one element of a wellness strategy. Smaller employers, public sector employers, unions, non-profit sector employers, and hospitals are also offering wellness programs or facilitating access to community services. This phenomenon mirrors the growth in the general public's commitment to healthier life-styles and concern for the escalation of medical care costs.

As programs become more sophisticated, they bring more cultural changes into the workplace. The work setting is becoming more humanistic in nature and is focusing more on self-responsibility. Self-responsibility is the backbone of the wellness programs, but can only be achieved if the environment, particularly the work environment, facilitates the behaviors that achieve optimal health.

NOTES

1. Marvin Kristein, "How Much Can Business Expect to Earn from Smoking Cessation" (Paper presented at the National Interagency Council on Smoking and Health's workshop, "Smoking and the Workplace," Chicago, Illinois, January 9, 1980).

2. William L. Weis, "Can You Afford to Hire Smokers?," *Personnel Administrator*, May 1981.

3. *National Heart Lung and Blood Institute Demonstration Projects in Workplace High Blood Pressure Control*. (Draft paper prepared May 1983), (For further information contact Judith H. LaRosa, NHLBI, Building 31, Room 4A18, Bethesda, MD 20205).

4. Robert M. Cunningham, *Wellness at Work* (Chicago: Blue Cross Association, 1982).

5. Robert N. Beck, "IBM Health Care Strategy" (Presentation made to Council on Wage and Price Stability, April 16, 1980).

6. *Ibid.*

7. Thomas Royle Dawber, *The Framingham Study* (Cambridge: A Commonwealth Fund Book, Harvard University Press, 1980).

8. John C. Erfurt and Andrea Foote, *Final Report: Hypertension Control in the Worksetting—The University of Michigan Ford Motor Company Demonstration Project*, Heart, Lung & Blood Institute NIH, DHHS Contract No. N01-HV-8-2913, 1982.

9. Washington Business Group on Health, unpublished.

10. Donald Shepherd and Laurie Pearlman, *Incentives for Health Promotion at the Workplace: A Review of Programs and Their Results* (Boston: Center for the Analysis of Health Practices, Harvard School of Public Health No. 677, 1982).

11. *USA Today*, 30 November 1983.

12. Curtis Wilbur, Johnson and Johnson, personal communication.

13. M.P. Naditch, "The STAYWELL Program" in *Behavioral Health: A Handbook of Health Enhancement and Disease Prevention,* ed. J.P. Matarezzo et al., (New York: John Wiley and Sons, 1984).

14. Jonathan E. Fielding, "Effectiveness of Employee Health Improvement Programs," *Journal of Occupational Medicine,* (November 1982).

15. Loring Wood, "Lifestyle Management Strategies at New York Telephone" (Paper presented at the Leadership Strategies—Health Conference, Millwood, Virginia, 1980).

16. Charles A. Berry, *Good Health for Employers and Reduced Health Care Costs for Industry* (Washington, D.C.: Health Insurance Institute, 1981).

Chapter 11

Fitness and Exercise for the Elderly

Gregory S. Thomas, M.D., M.P.H.
John H. Rutledge, M.D., J.D., M.P.H.

Hippocrates was one of the first to comment on the possibility that regular exercise might retard the process of aging, noting that "all parts of the body which have a function, if used in moderation and exercised in labors to which each is accustomed, become thereby well-developed and age slowly; but if unused and left idle, they become liable to disease, defective in growth, and age quickly."[1]

Is it possible to postpone or even reverse this process of aging? Wrinkles certainly do not melt away without cosmetic surgery, but short of that, many of the measures of physiological performance that worsen with age, and are indeed regarded as a consequence of old age, can be postponed even a decade or more with regular exercise. Bortz has called attention to the similarities between the physiological changes that occur with aging and those that occur in persons of any age during a period of prolonged bed rest.[2] He has postulated that many of the effects of aging may be related as much to inactivity as to an intrinsic biological aging process. He thus suggests that much of what we regard as aging can be prevented by regular activity.

AEROBIC AND LOW-INTENSITY EXERCISE

Before examining the effect of exercise on the aging process, one must have an understanding of exercise and its effects on persons of all ages.

Research on the effects of exercise has most commonly used young or middle-aged persons as research subjects. Exercise performed by the elderly certainly has many, if not most, of the same effects that it has on a younger population, but one must be cautious not to generalize the findings of research using young persons as research subjects to the elderly. Much of the data on which this discussion is drawn were obtained using young or middle-aged research subjects. The next section, "The Effects of Exercise on the Elderly," focuses specifically on research using only the elderly as research subjects.

Exercise performed by persons of any age can be grouped into two categories: aerobic exercise and low-intensity exercise. Aerobic exercise has come to mean exercise that strengthens the cardiovascular system.[3] Jogging, cycling, skiing, and swimming are all aerobic exercises. Low-intensity exercise has little effect on the cardiovascular system, but is helpful in controlling weight and in halting age-related bone demineralization, as well as in simply staying active and enjoying life.[4] This type of exercise may include walking, bowling, golfing, and fishing. Both types of exercise, aerobic and low-intensity, have obvious benefits for the aged and the young. The type of exercise that one chooses to perform or to recommend that another perform is based on the needs, interest, and medical status of the potential exercise participant.

An aerobic exercise places a moderate stress on the heart. The heart and the rest of the cardiovascular system respond with adaptations to handle this stress. The heart becomes stronger, as manifested by an increase in the volume of blood it expels with each beat, and the rest of the cardiovascular system becomes more efficient. These adaptations enable a person to perform the same amount of physical activity with progressively less effort. Such a stress is produced by exercise that results in a heart rate of 60 to 90 percent of the maximum heart rate.[5] The maximum heart rate can be estimated by subtracting one's age from 220 and multiplying that figure by 60 to 90 percent to obtain the target heart rate. For a 40-year old, the target heart rate would thus be 108 to 162 beats per minute (bpm). For a 65-year old, the range would be only 93 to 135 bpm. However, because little research has been done in the evaluation of the effects of exercise at less than 100 bpm, a floor of 100 bpm should be used in establishing the target heart range for the elderly. Comparing the target heart rates for a 40-year old and a 65-year old—108 to 162 bpm and 100 to 135 bpm, respectively—it is clear that the exercise intensity required to produce a heart rate in the target range is less for the 65-year old than for the 40-year old. For example, walking at an average pace does not result in a heart rate of 108 bpm in the 40-year old, but it may often result in a heart rate of 100 bpm in a 65-year old. The same applies for moderate calisthenics; for the elderly this exercise generally results in a heart rate above 100 bpm and is thus in the aerobic category, but for the middle-aged the minimum heart rate of 108 bpm is usually not reached, and it is thus a low-intensity exercise.

For aerobic exercise to result in beneficial effects on the cardiovascular system, it should be performed at least three times a week for 15 to 60 minutes a session.[6] The minimum session length necessary for the exercise to be aerobic is dependent on the intensity with which it is performed. For exercise near the low end of the target heart range, sessions should last nearly 60 minutes. When exercise is performed with an intensity great enough to produce a heart rate of 90 percent of maximum, a session need only last 15 minutes to be of aerobic benefit. For exercise in the middle of the target range—75 percent of maximum heart rate—sessions should last 30 to 40 minutes.

Aerobic exercise has been reported in epidemiologic and clinical studies to inhibit the development of coronary artery disease. Although this hypothesis has not been proven, the evidence that such an effect probably does occur is substantial.[7,8,9,10,11,12] The mechanism for this effect seems not only to be an effect of exercise per se but also to be the effect of exercise on other risk factors involved in the genesis of coronary disease.

Studies of young and middle-aged subjects have demonstrated that aerobic exercise can lower blood pressure among hypertensive persons, reduce weight among the obese, and improve glucose control among diabetics.[13] In healthy subjects, aerobic exercise has been shown to increase the level of high-density lipoprotein cholesterol (HDL-C),[14,15] which is the type of cholesterol that has been shown to correlate with a lower risk of developing coronary artery disease.[16] There are also indications that aerobic exercise results in the development of a more health conscious life style in the new or continuing exercise participant.[17] Exercise certainly does not totally protect against coronary artery disease, but it does appear to lessen its likelihood.

Low intensity exercise plays a role in maintaining and improving health as well. Maintenance of bone mineralization, joint flexibility, and weight control are among the benefits of low intensity exercise which will be described in more detail in the next section.

If an older person is capable and interested, aerobic exercise has more apparent benefits than low-intensity exercise. For persons not capable or interested in aerobic exercise, the benefits of low-intensity exercise are substantial, and it is preferable to a sedentary life style.

THE EFFECTS OF EXERCISE ON THE ELDERLY

The physiological and psychological effects that exercise has on the elderly have been increasingly examined over the past decade.[18] Because age is measured not only in years but also in the slow decline in the parameters that measure the body's performance, it is these studies of these parameters that have, in effect, examined the effect of exercise on the aging process.

Cardiovascular System

One of the most fundamental measures of a person's physical condition is his or her maximum oxygen consumption ($\dot{V}O_2$ max), which represents the amount of oxygen consumed at the peak of an all-out physical effort. The greater a person's $\dot{V}O_2$ max, the easier it is for that person to cover a given distance by running, swimming, or pedaling.

$\dot{V}O_2$ max diminishes with age;[19,20] Bortz estimates this diminution to be about 1 percent per year.[21] Several studies have shown however, that persons who are physically active—be they young,[22] middle-aged,[23] or elderly[24]—have a higher $\dot{V}O_2$ max than less active persons of the same age. Sidney,[25] deVries,[26] and others have shown that regardless of an elderly person's prior exercise habits, an aerobic exercise program results in an average increase in $\dot{V}O_2$ max of 10 to 30 percent. Sidney found the most significant increases in $\dot{V}O_2$ max to occur among participants in individualized programs who exercised at higher heart rates and for longer session durations than participants in the same program who exercised at lower heart rates for shorter session durations.[27] In general, subjects who had the lowest $\dot{V}O_2$ max on entry had the largest subsequent percent increase in their $\dot{V}O_2$ max. Thus, those who had the poorest fitness on entry into a program gained the most from the program.[28]

The decrease in $\dot{V}O_2$ max seen with age can be regarded as analogous to the decrease in $\dot{V}O_2$ max that occurs with prolonged bed rest. Even well-conditioned athletes have substantial decreases in $\dot{V}O_2$ max following several weeks of bed rest.[29] The similarity between a sedentary life style and bed rest may well be the cause for much of the decrease in $\dot{V}O_2$ max seen with aging.

Another consequence of advancing age is high blood pressure. The gradual increase in peripheral vascular resistance that occurs with age results in a steady increase in blood pressure.[30] Regular exercise, however, often results in a lowering of blood pressure. Such an effect was found by deVries[31] and by Buccola[32] in their studies of exercise in populations of the nonhypertensive elderly. Decreases in both systolic and diastolic blood pressure of about 5 to 10 mm Hg were seen following completion of a multiweek exercise program. Because these study protocols necessarily required that blood pressure be taken frequently during the study, it is possible, however, that part of this decrease in blood pressure may have been due to the possibility that the subjects were less anxious while having their blood pressure taken at the end of the study than they were at the beginning of the study.

Body Composition and Structure

Age affects body composition and structure as well. Lean body mass, a measure of musculature, decreases by 2 to 3 percent for every decade after age 25.[33] Again, exercise can aid in regaining some of this loss. Sidney found a one-year exercise program to result in a 10 percent increase in lean body mass and a similar increase in muscle strength, as measured by hand grip and knee extension.[34] Aniansson found a 12-week exercise program to result in an 8 to 22 percent increase in the strength of knee extension;[35] subjects in another 42-week exercise program realized an increase in arm strength averaging 11.9 percent.[36] Bortz has commented that the decrease in muscularity with age is similar to that which is seen when a cast is removed from a broken leg after six weeks of healing.[37] Although the fracture has mended with time, the muscles around it have weakened and the joints have lost their flexibility. Joint movement is painful and slow. The effect of a lifelong sedentary life style on musculature and joint flexibility is analogous to this effect of a cast on the joint and muscles it surrounds.

One of the principles in the field of physical therapy is that a joint must be put through its range of motion or it will lose that range of motion. In a leg deadened by a stroke, joints and muscles left motionless will develop contractures, and eventually little or no movement is possible. On the other hand, Bassett found a 10-week low-intensity exercise program of light calisthenics to result in an increase in the range of motion of the shoulder, hip, and knee.[38] Buccola found an increase in trunk and leg flexibility during a 14-week walking program.[39]

Bones, too, are involved in the aging process, as manifested by the extraordinarily high incidence of hip, vertebral, and other fractures in the elderly. Skeletal mass begins to decline after age 40 to 50, doing so at a faster rate in women than in men. During the three to four decades after the age of 40, the total loss in skeletal mass may be 30 to 50 percent of that present at an earlier age.[40]

Although the architecture of bone does not change substantially with age, a dramatic decrease in its mineralization causes this loss of mass. This process is termed "osteoporosis."

As occurs with other parameters of the aging process, osteoporosis begins to occur in persons of any age who are subjected to prolonged bed rest.[41] Activity again has a favorable impact; when Huddleston examined 35 competitors in the 1978 United States Tennis Association 70-, 75-, and 80-year old age group Clay Court Championship, he found the competitor's dominant (playing) arms to have a bone mass 12 percent greater than in their nondominant arms.[42] In a group of elderly subjects placed on a three-year low-intensity exercise program, a 4.2 percent increase in bone mineral content was seen in the exercise group, whereas a 2.5 percent decrease was seen in the nonexercising control group.[43] In a similar three-year study, the low-intensity exercise group had an increase in bone mineral content of 2.3 percent, whereas the control group had a 3.3 percent decrease.[44]

Body Weight

Body weight is also affected by age, Shephard estimates that excess weight in the elderly averages 5.1 kg for men and 4.5 kg for women.[45] This excess weight is the result of an increase in both absolute and relative amounts of body fat and a decrease in lean body mass (a measure of musculature),[46] due partly to a decrease in activity. One study found the energy expenditure of middle-aged and elderly mothers to average 165 kcal/day less than the energy expenditure of their daughters; this difference was due mainly to the mothers spending an average of 45 fewer minutes walking per day as compared to their daughters.[47] In regard to body composition, Sidney found that placing a group of elderly persons on a one-year walk-jog program resulted in a 17 percent decrease in skinfold thickness (a measure of body fat).[48,49] Analyzing the subjects' activities following the completion of the program, Sidney found them to spend less time driving a car and more time at active pursuits.[50]

Psychological Status

Because an exercise program increases body strength, joint mobility, and maximum exercise tolerance (as measured by $\dot{V}O_2$ max), one would expect an exercise program to result in elderly participants seeing themselves as stronger, healthier, and more physically fit. Unfortunately, the difficulty in quantifying these feelings has limited the ability of studies to determine accurately the effect of exercise on the mental health of the elderly. Several studies, however, have found an exercise program to produce psychological benefits. Sidney found an exercise program to reduce anxiety and result in a greater regard for activity as a "relief of tension."[51] In his study, favorable changes in body image, mood, and attitudes were most evident in persons who had trained the hardest and who had had the greatest improvement in fitness. An 11-week stationary bicycling study performed by Blumenthal[52] resulted in improved mood and greater feelings of satisfaction, self-confidence, and achievement in 40 to 50 percent of the participants. Worsening of these psychological parameters was seen in 10 to 15 percent of participants, and no change was found in the remainder. Buccola found a 14-week walk-jog program to result in greater feelings of self-sufficiency.[53]

One difficulty in interpreting these results is that psychological changes occurring during an exercise program may have resulted not from the exercise but from the increased personal and medical attention participants received during the testing and training sessions. Moreover, because psychological changes were generally measured by questionnaires, positive results could also have been the result of a desire of the participants to please the investigators.[54] Indications are, however, that exercise is probably of marked psychological benefit in the elderly, despite the methodological problems in study design that have limited the ability of investigators to clearly demonstrate this effect.

MEDICAL EVALUATION PRIOR TO EXERCISE

Elderly persons should consult their physicians before embarking on an exercise program. Such consultation is mandatory before beginning an aerobic exercise program and is preferable before entering a low-intensity exercise program. Although exercise may help prevent coronary heart disease (CAD), it must be performed with caution once an individual has CAD. It has been estimated that by age 70, half of all men have CAD and that half of these persons are asymptomatic.[55] The prevalence of coronary disease among women is only somewhat less dramatic. The high incidence of CAD has been borne out by screening evaluations performed on subjects who initially volunteered to participate in the studies discussed above. For example, of 37 persons who volunteered to participate in Blumenthal's study on the psychological effects of exercise,[56] 10 were found to be medically unsuitable for aerobic exercise following a history, physical examination, and exercise stress test with electrocardiographic monitoring. A medical evaluation of the volunteers for one of Sidney's studies[57] resulted in 21 percent of them being screened out before their entry into an exercise program. In an evaluation of an ongoing low-intensity physical therapy program that did not use medical screening before entry, Gordon randomly selected six subjects whom he subjected to exercise stress testing.[58] Stress tests were positive for a high likelihood of CAD in three of the six. A physician or a nurse practitioner or physician's assistant skilled in the care of the elderly can best determine the likelihood of a person having coronary disease.

In a statement by the American Medical Association (AMA) encouraging physicians to prescribe exercise for their elderly patients, it recommended that a history and physical examination, as well as an exercise stress test when deemed appropriate, be performed before the prescription of exercise.[59] An exercise stress test is not a mandatory segment of this medical evaluation, however, although it can provide a great deal of useful information. For example, a stress test enables one to accurately determine an individual's maximum heart rate and level of fitness; without it, one must estimate maximum heart rate using the formula of 220 minus one's age. It also provides an estimate of the likelihood of a person having either symptomatic or asymptomatic CAD. In many cases, this information alone justifies its expense.

One of the reasons that an exercise stress test is generally not required in young and middle-aged persons prior to the initiation of an exercise program is that it is not as accurate in this age group. The stress test's accuracy is dependent on the prevalence of CAD in the specific population being tested. The lower the likelihood of CAD in a population, the less accurate is the test. Because the risk of having either symptomatic or asymptomatic CAD increases with age, the elderly population has a high prevalence of CAD. Thus, a positive exercise stress test for CAD is more likely to represent true disease in an elderly person than in a young person.

Whether or not participants undergo an exercise stress test, the physician and, if applicable, the leader of a supervised exercise program should warn them of the symptoms of CAD and should instruct them to return to their physician if any of these symptoms develop. A list of these symptoms has been compiled by Fair.[60]

In addition, a list of absolute and relative medical contraindications to participation in an exercise program can be obtained from several sources.[61,62,63,64] The major absolute contraindications include acute myocardial infarction, increasing angina pectoris, severe aortic stenosis, and acute infectious disease. Relative contraindications in which exercise would generally be inadvisable include congestive heart failure, ventricular aneurysm, hypertrophic cardiomyopathy, and moderate aortic stenosis. Conditions that require special consideration or precautions include stable angina pectoris, frequent premature ventricular complexes, severe hypertension, marked obesity, and kidney or liver disease.[65]

THE EXERCISE PROGRAM

The type of exercise program that a person should initiate, either aerobic or low-intensity, is dependent on his or her health, level of fitness, and interests. Once the type of exercise has been established, the specific activity should be determined by the participant's specific interests, as well as climatic, geographic, and economic factors. For example, indoor activities, performed either at home or at a center for the elderly, may be required because of inclement weather or a lack of neighborhood safety.

As discussed above, aerobic exercise is exercise vigorous enough to produce a heart rate of 60 to 90 percent of one's maximum and that is performed for 15 to 60 minutes three or more times a week. For the elderly, walking is generally the most readily available form of aerobic exercise. Because it usually results in a heart rate in the lower half of the target heart range, walking should generally be performed for somewhat more than 30 minutes during each session. Other appropriate aerobic exercises for the elderly include bicycling—either on the road or on a stationary bicycle; swimming; jogging; brisk dancing, such as aerobic dancing; and tennis or other racquet sports.

It is important that a previously sedentary exercise participant begin an exercise program slowly, and because the benefits of exercise appear to remain only as long as one continues to exercise, lifetime exercise participation is the goal. It makes little difference how quickly one advances to a higher level of fitness; what is important is eventually becoming fit and continuing to exercise in order to maintain that fitness. Starting an exercise program with a "slow and easy" attitude is most conducive to avoiding musculoskeletal injury and enhancing the likelihood of long-term participation. This caution is particularly applicable to the older person taking up exercise.

Thus, a walking program could begin with walking two to three blocks each session. The distance would then be gradually increased over several months until the point at which the exercise became aerobic. In the case of walking, for most elderly persons that point would be reached when walking is performed for 30 to 60 minutes at least three times a week.

An aerobic exercise session should also contain a three- to five-minute warm-up and cool-down, performed before and after the activity, respectively. Each is composed of an activity of an intensity that is intermediate between the previous activity and the following one.[4] Slow walking, light calisthenics, and stretching all fit into this category.

As has been discussed, low-intensity exercise can be helpful in weight control, the amelioration of osteoporosis, and the retention of musculature and flexibility. Low-intensity exercises include stretching and light calisthenics. Exercises that are aerobic if performed long enough and frequently enough—for example, walking—are classified as low-intensity exercises when performed for less than the necessary 15 to 60 minutes at least three times a week. The frequency guideline of at least three sessions a week is also a reasonable goal for low-intensity exercise.

Over the past several years there has been a surge of interest in Nautilus and other brands of weight lifting equipment. When performed in the usual fashion, weight lifting is a low-intensity exercise. Although weight lifting certainly places stress on several different muscle groups, the stress it places on the entire body is generally not enough to maintain the heart rate within the target heart range needed for the exercise to be aerobic. Circuit training, however, is an aerobic exercise. Circuit training consists of 20 to 40 minutes of lifting relatively light weights for 10 to 20 repetitions at each different exercise station. Only a short time—usually 15 to 30 seconds—is allowed between each station. The short duration of the rest period ensures that the heart rate does not fall below the target heart range. Compared to circuit training, traditional weight lifting uses heavier weights that are necessarily lifted fewer times at each exercise station. Rest periods between stations are also longer, generally lasting several minutes. Circuit training is thus much closer to a continuous exercise than is traditional weight lifting.

Studies of the effects of circuit training in young and middle-aged men and women have found an increase in $\dot{V}O_2$ max of 5 to 8 percent following the completion of a 12- to 20-week program.[66,67] This is considerably less than the approximate 25 percent increase in $\dot{V}O_2$ max generally seen among the young and middle-aged during a traditional aerobic exercise program, such as jogging.[68]

Although studies have not been published examining the effects of circuit training on the elderly, a similar aerobic benefit would be expected in this population. A number of health clubs throughout the country have initiated individually supervised circuit training programs for the elderly. Because of the risks of this form of exercise, including potential muscle damage caused by improper technique and inadequate supervision, any circuit training program for the elderly should be supervised by a trained instructor. Further, because circuit training produces only a modest increase in $\dot{V}O_2$ max, its role as an aerobic exercise for the elderly is limited to those highly motivated to increase their upper body strength and for those who are particularly interested in this form of exercise.

The elderly can participate in an aerobic or low-intensity exercise program either alone or in a group. However, because studies among the middle-aged population have found that the dropout rate is lower in a group program than in an individually performed program,[69,70] group exercise is preferable. An exercise class at an elderly center would be ideal for many persons. Participants in a group exercise program have the benefit of a group leader, who can prod them and encourage their continued participation. The presence of other participants makes the session a social event.

Although certainly not yet at an optimal level, the availability of exercise classes for the elderly is steadily increasing. Centers for the elderly, either free-standing or within a residential community for the elderly, the local YMCA, neighborhood parks, and health clubs, may all offer such classes. An aerobic or low-intensity exercise program designed within the guidelines presented above can meet the needs of most elderly exercise participants. Other sources are available that describe specific aerobic[4,71] and low-intensity[4,72] exercise programs for the elderly. The exercise program chosen for an exercise class should be as enjoyable as possible because exercise programs, including those for the elderly, are known to have excessively high dropout rates.

Every incentive to continued participation should be considered in designing a group exercise program for the elderly. A time should be selected when transportation to and from the program is most readily available.[73] If the program is being held at an elderly center where meals are also being provided, exercise sessions held immediately before a meal can encourage continued compliance. A prominently posted attendance chart and a secluded area in which to exercise are ideal.[74] Even group T-shirts may spur continued enthusiasm. The maintenance of an individual exercise diary in which the details of each session and of one's physical and mental reactions to it can be recorded may encourage continued participation as well.

CONCLUSION

In sum, many of the physiological changes seen with aging are due as much to prolonged inactivity as to an intrinsic biological aging process. The initiation of a regular exercise program, following the completion of a careful medical examination, can allow an elder to regain some of the physical characteristics of his or her more youthful years. A low-intensity exercise program offers improvements in muscle and bone strength, flexibility, weight control, and psychological well-being. An aerobic exercise program offers these same benefits, as well as improvements in cardiovascular fitness and blood pressure control.

NOTES

1. Kayleen Sager, "Senior Fitness—For the Health of It," *The Physician and Sports Medicine* 11 (1983): 3–36.

2. Walter M. Bortz, "Disuse and Aging," *Journal of the American Medical Association* 248 (1982): 1203–1208.

3. Gregory S. Thomas et al., *Exercise and Health: The Evidence and the Implications* (Cambridge, Ma.: Oelgeschlager, Gunn and Hain, 1981), p. 17.

4. American Medical Association Council on Scientific Affairs Advisory Panel on Exercise and Fitness, *Physical Activity . . . for Fitness and Health* (Monroe, Wi.: American Medical Association, 1981).

5. American College of Sports Medicine, *Guidelines for Graded Exercise Testing and Exercise Prescription,* 2nd ed. (Philadelphia: Lea and Febiger, 1980), pp. 12–15.

6. *Ibid.,* pp. 12–15.

7. Victor F. Froelicher and P. Brown, "Exercise and Coronary Heart Disease," *Journal of Cardiac Rehabilitation* 1 (1981): 277–288.

8. Victor Froelicher, *Exercise Testing and Training* (Chicago: Year Book Medical Publishers, 1983), pp. 179–263.

9. Nancy A. Rigott, Gregory S. Thomas, and Alexander Leaf, "Exercise and Coronary Heart Disease," *Annual Review of Medicine* 34 (1983): 391–412.

10. Gregory S. Thomas, "Physical Activity and Health: Epidemiologic and Clinical Evidence and Policy Implications," *Preventive Medicine* 8 (1979): 89–103.

11. Gregory S. Thomas et al., "Exercise and Health" (Discussion paper, Health Policy Program, University of California, San Francisco, 1979), pp. 7–19.

12. Thomas S. Gregory et al., *Exercise and Health: The Evidence and the Implications, op. cit.,* pp. 23–54.

13. *Ibid.,* pp. 55–74.

14. K.D. Brownell, P.S. Bachorik, and R.S. Ayerle, "Changes in Plasma Lipid and Lipoprotein Levels in Men and Women After a Program of Moderate Exercise," *Circulation* 65 (1982): 477–483.

15. A. Lopez et al., "Effects of Exercise and Physical Fitness on Serum Lipids and Lipoproteins," *Atherosclerosis* 20 (1974): 1–9.

16. T. Gordon et al., "High Density Lipoprotein as a Protective Factor against Coronary Heart Disease: The Framingham Study," *American Journal of Medicine* 62 (1977): 704–714.

17. J.V.G.A. Durin, E.C. Blake, and J.M. Brockaway, "The Energy Expenditure and Food Intake of Middle-aged Glasgow Housewives and their Adult Daughters," *British Journal of Nutrition* 11 (1960): 85–94.

18. Pat Franks, Phillip R. Lee, and Jane E. Fullarton, *Lifetime Fitness and Exercise for Older People* (Policy Paper No. 4, Aging Health Policy Center, University of California, San Francisco, 1983), pp. 26–43.

19. J.L. Hodgson and E.R. Buskirk, "Physical Fitness and Age, with Emphasis on Cardiovascular Function in the Elderly," *Journal of the American Geriatrics Society* 25 (1977): 385–392.

20. Roy J. Shephard, "World Standards of Cardiorespiratory Performance," *Archives of Environmental Health* 13 (1966): 664–672.

21. Walter Bortz, *op. cit.,* pp. 1203–1208.

22. Roy J. Shephard, *op. cit.,* pp. 664–672.

23. *Ibid.,* pp. 664–672.

24. Nanette K. Wenger, "Rehabilitation of the Elderly Cardiac Patient," in *Geriatric Cardiology,* ed. R. Joe Noble and Donald A. Rothbaum (Philadelphia: F.A. Davis, 1981), 221–230.

25. Kenneth H. Sidney, Roy J. Shephard, and Joan E. Harrison, "Endurance Training and Body Composition of the Elderly," *The American Journal of Clinical Nutrition* 30 (1977): 326–333.

26. Herbert A. deVries, "Physiological Effects of an Exercise Training Regimen upon Men Aged 52 to 88," *Journal of Gerontology* 25 (1970): 325–336.

27. Kenneth H. Sidney and Roy J. Shephard, "Activity Patterns of Elderly Men and Women," *Journal of Gerontology* 32 (1977): 25–32.

28. Albert Oberman, "Rehabilitation of Patients with Coronary Artery Diseases," in *Heart Disease: A Textbook of Cardiovascular Medicine,* ed. Eugene Braunwald (Philadelphia: W.B. Saunders, 1984), 1384–1398.

29. Bengt Saltin et al., "Response to Exercise after Bed Rest and after Training," *Circulation* 38 (1968) Supplement 7:1–78.

30. Stevo Julius et al., "Influence of Age on the Hemodynamic Response to Exercise," *Circulation* 26 (1967): 220–230.

31. Herbert A. deVries, *op. cit., pp.* 325–336.

32. Victor A. Buccola and William J. Stone, "Effect of Jogging and Cycling Programs on Physiological and Personality Variables in Aged Men," *The Research Quarterly* 46 (1975): 134–139.

33. D.H. Calloway and Eline Zannie, "Energy Requirements of Elderly Men," *The American Journal of Clinical Nutrition* 33 (1980): 2088–2092.

34. Kenneth H. Sidney, Roy J. Shephard, and Joan E. Harrison, *op. cit., pp.* 326–333.

35. Amelie Aniansson et al., "Physical Training in Old Age," *Age and Aging* 9 (1980): 186–187.

36. Herbert A. deVries, *op. cit., pp.* 325–336.

37. Walter M. Bortz, *op. cit., pp.* 1203–1208.

38. Christine Bassett, Elizabeth McClamrock, and Marilee Schmelzer, "A 10-Week Exercise Program for Senior Citizens," *Geriatric Nursing,* March/April 1982, pp. 103–105.

39. Victor A. Buccola and William J. Stone, *op. cit., pp.* 134–139.

40. Stephen W. Krane and Michale F. Holick, "Metabolic Bone Disease," in *Harrison's Principles of Internal Medicine,* ed. Robert G. Petersdorf et al. (New York: McGraw-Hill, 1983), 1949–1960.

41. Everett L. Smith, "Exercise for Prevention of Osteoporosis: A Review," *The Physician and Sportsmedicine* 10 (March 1982): 72–83.

42. Alan L. Huddleston et al., "Bone Mass in Lifetime Athletes," *Journal of the American Medical Association* 244 (1980): 1107–1109.

43. Everett L. Smith and William Redden, "Physical Activity: A Modality for Bone Accretion in the Aged," *American Journal of Roentgenology* 126 (1976): 1297.

44. Everett L. Smith, William Redden, and Patricia E. Smith, "Physical Activity and Calcium Modalities for Bone Mineral Increases in Aged Women," *Medicine and Science in Sports and Exercise* 13 (1981): 80–84.

45. Roy J. Shephard and Kenneth H. Sidney, "Exercise and Aging," *Exercise and Sport Sciences Review* 6 (1978): 157.

46. *Ibid.,* p. 157.

47. J.V.G.A. Durin, E.C. Blake, and J.M. Brockaway, *op. cit., pp.* 85–94.

48. Kenneth H. Sidney and Roy J. Shephard, "Activity Patterns of Elderly Men and Women, *op. cit.,* pp. 25–32.

49. Kenneth H. Sidney, Roy J. Shephard, and Joan E. Harrison, *op. cit., pp.* 326–333.

50. *Ibid.,* pp. 326–333.

51. Kenneth H. Sidney and Roy J. Shephard, "Attitudes towards Health and Physical Training in the Elderly: Effects of a Physical Training Program," *Medicine and Science in Sports* 8 (1976): 246–252.

52. James A. Blumenthal et al., "Psychological and Physiological Effects of Physical Conditioning on the Elderly," *Journal of Psychosomatic Research* 26 (1982): 505–510.

53. Victor A. Buccola and William J. Stone, *op. cit.*, pp. 134–139.

54. Gregory S. Thomas, *op. cit.*, pp. 89–103.

55. Richard J. Radeheffer, "Exercise Cardiac Output Is Maintained with Advancing Age in Healthy Human Subjects: Cardiac Dilation and Increased Stroke Volume Compensate for a Diminished Heart Rate," *Circulation* 69 (1984): 203–213.

56. James A. Blumenthal, *op. cit.*, pp. 505–510.

57. Kenneth H. Sidney and Roy J. Shephard, "Maximum and Submaximum Exercise Tests in Men and Women in the Seventh, Eighth, and Ninth Decades of Life," *Journal of Applied Physiology: Respiratory, Environmental, and Exercise Physiology* 43 (1977): 280–287.

58. N.E. Gordon, et al., "Assessment of a Geriatric Exercise Programme Using Ambulatory Electrocardiography," *South African Medical Journal* 64 (1983): 169–172.

59. American Medical Association Council on Scientific Affairs, *Exercise Programs for the Elderly* (Chicago: American Medical Association, 1983).

60. J. Fair, J. Rosenaur, and E. Thurston, "Exercise Management," *Nurse Practitioner* 4 (1969): 13–15, 17–18.

61. American College of Sports Medicine, *op. cit.*, pp. 12–15.

62. American Medical Association Council on Scientific Affairs, "Indications and Contraindications for Exercise Training," *Journal of the American Medical Association* 246 (1981): 1015–1018.

63. Stephen M. Krane and Michael F. Holick, *op. cit.*, pp. 1949–1960.

64. Gregory S. Thomas et al., *Exercise and Health: The Evidence and the Implications, op. cit.*, pp. 75–95.

65. *Ibid.*, p. 94.

66. Larry R. Gettman et al., "Physiologic Effects on Adult Men of Circuit Training and Jogging," *Archives of Physical Medicine and Rehabilitation* 60 (1979): 115–120.

67. Larry R. Gettman and Michael Pollack, "Circuit Weight Training: A Critical Review of its Physiological Benefits," *The Physician and Sportsmedicine* 9 (January 1981): 44–60.

68. Gregory S. Thomas et al., *Exercise and Health: The Evidence and the Implications, op. cit.*, pp. 17–20.

69. American Heart Association Committee on Exercise, *Exercise Testing and Training of Apparently Healthy Individuals: A Handbook for Physicians* (New York: American Heart Association, 1972), p. 26.

70. M. Guidry, "Programming for Physical Fitness," *Parts Recreation,* August 1976, p. 48.

71. Kenneth H. Cooper, *The Aerobics Way* (New York: Bantam Books, 1970).

72. Pat Franks, Phillip R. Lee, and Jane E. Fullarton, *op. cit.*, p. 44.

73. James H. Price and Stephen L. Luther, "Physical Fitness: Its Role in Health for the Elderly," *Journal of Gerontological Nursing* 6 (1980): 517–523.

74. *Ibid.*, pp. 517–523.

Chapter 12

Dietary Recommendations for Older Americans

Nathan Pritikin
Nan Cisney

Inconclusive studies of nutrition, particularly of the contemporary American diet's effect on older people, make complete certainty regarding nutritional recommendations impossible. However, from the available research, we can infer that, when the elderly are in good health, are not alcoholic, are drug-free, have been eating a well-balanced diet, and remain physically active, their nutritional needs are the same as those of younger adults, with the exception of an increased need for calories and iron by women before menopause. Unfortunately, aging is frequently accompanied by the onset of diet-related degenerative diseases, borderline deficiency states from long-term or recent changes in dietary habits, the excessive use of alcohol, or a decrease in physical activity. These factors can cause an increased or decreased need for nutrients.

The discussion that follows and the dietary guidelines in Appendix 12–A pertain to the entire cross-section of the older population from the age of menopause to the age of death of both men and women. Although there are profound differences between persons at the age of 65 and 95, their nutritional needs do not change significantly if they are in good health. Frequently, as people get older, however, they are not encouraged to venture outdoors; lack the motivation to prepare proper meals and rely heavily on commercially processed foods that are of low-nutrient density but are high in fats, cholesterol, sugar, and salt; and are heavily medicated. These factors all contribute to the tendency of the elderly to be marginally deficient in certain nutrients, although their requirements are not intrinsically higher than those of younger people.

NUTRITIONAL REQUIREMENTS

Energy

Older persons' caloric intake must be sufficient to prevent them from being excessively underweight. A major cause of calorie malnutrition in the elderly is the poor condition of their teeth and gums. Half of Americans at age 60 and 66 percent at age 75 have lost all their teeth. As people age and gum tissues shrink, dentures can become more difficult to fit. As a result, too many elderly people subsist on soft, refined, ready-to-eat foods that are low in nutrient density. Because they are unable or unmotivated to prepare more nutritious foods in a manner that makes them easier to chew, their diet may contain little variety, provide marginal levels of many nutrients, and be deficient in calories.

Loss of the sense of taste can also be responsible for a lack of appetite, which results in inadequate calorie intake. The taste buds in the front of the tongue and palate that are responsible for identifying sweet and salty tastes atrophy first. This condition may be exacerbated by the loss of sensitivity to taste caused by smoking and/or the excessive intake of salt, sugar, and medication.

Being over- rather than underweight is more frequently a problem among the elderly.[1,2] As people age, the proportion of muscle tissue is gradually reduced, although to a large extent, the process can be halted by exercise.[3] The loss of muscle mass results in a decrease in metabolism rate and therefore a decrease in the number of calories needed to maintain body weight. Because maintenance of body weight in the elderly could actually indicate fat accumulation, a gradual loss of weight after age 60 may be desirable in the sedentary older person. Caloric intake should be reduced if energy expenditure decreases because obesity is considered a risk factor in many diseases and conditions to which the elderly are particularly susceptible.

Older people often eat alone and are therefore not motivated to spend time in meal preparation. Instead, they may subsist on prepared foods lacking in fiber. These foods can be extremely high in calories, and because of their lack of bulk, people consume more of such foods more often.

The older person should be taught to eat lightly cooked vegetables, especially leafy greens, in the first part of the meal. These harder-to-chew foods that take longer to eat are lower in calories and higher in calcium, iron, and in vitamin C, which facilitates the absorption of these minerals. They are also higher in folacin and carotene; both of these vitamins tend to be consumed in inadequate amounts by the older population. These foods lack cholesterol and are lower in calories, fat, and salt than other foods. It is better to serve vegetables to people not used to eating them as a first course when their appetite is greater. Otherwise, they are apt to cater to their desire for foods higher in calories but lower in other nutrients. If they are accustomed to highly adulterated foods, simply prepared vegetables might be considered somewhat uninteresting and bland due to lack of salt. It has been demonstrated, however, that the desire for salt falls, over time, to meet the amount consumed.[4] Salt can be replaced as a flavor enhancer by lemon juice, spices, and herbs. Many herb blends containing no salt are presently on the market.

Protein

It was thought by some nutritionists that protein was utilized less efficiently by the elderly and that their protein requirements were therefore substantially higher.

However, recent data indicate that protein requirement is not affected by the aging process.[5,6]

The RDA (recommended dietary allowance) for protein is 12 percent of calories. It would be difficult to devise even a vegan diet—a vegetarian diet with no dairy foods or eggs—containing less than this amount. Diets higher than the RDA in protein are implicated as causative factors in osteoporosis[7] and kidney disease.[8] Evidence from some laboratory studies suggests that high-protein intake may be associated with an increased risk of cancers at certain sites.[9]

Dietary surveys show that protein is one of two nutrients—the other is niacin—found most frequently in adequate amounts in the diet of elderly people.[10] Because of this fact and the possible ill effects of a diet in which protein is more than 14 percent of total calories, it would be ill-advised to attempt to increase the proportion of protein in the diet of the elderly as long as their caloric intake is adequate.

Neither is it necessary to be concerned with the outmoded idea of complementing proteins. This is the term used when foods low in one essential amino acid are eaten at the same meal with foods high in that amino acid. For example, grains are relatively low in the amino acid lysine, whereas beans, peas, and dairy products are high in lysine. Some people eat these foods in the same meal to provide "complete" proteins in the diet. However, protein and the amino acids from which it is comprised are contained in foods in varying amounts. Some foods are somewhat higher in certain amino acids and lower in others. If the diet is at all varied and contains sufficient calories, all the essential amino acids are provided in amounts several times the RDA. Therefore, complementing proteins is entirely unnecessary for those eating enough to maintain their weight.

Carbohydrate

The highest priority among nutritional requirements is sufficient nutrient to provide energy, and the most efficient source of energy is carbohydrate. Without a constant source of energy, life itself cannot be sustained. Most nutrients are needed because they play a role in the conversion of carbohydrate to energy, and without carbohydrate, the other nutrients provide little benefit, regardless of age. Healthy older people still require most of their calories to be derived from this efficient fuel source.

Carbohydrates have been much maligned, and it is necessary to bear in mind that there are two kinds: complex carbohydrates, or starches and fiber, and simple carbohydrates, or sugars. Starches and sugars can be parts of whole or lightly processed plant foods, or they can be highly refined. White bread, white spaghetti, and white rice, for instance, remain complex carbohydrate foods, but the fiber and many of the nutrients have been lost. Most of our calories should be derived from unrefined, complex carbohydrate foods.

White sugar is so highly refined that it is an almost chemically pure substance. It is rapidly absorbed and has a powerful effect on body chemistry. It contributes only calories and no nutrients, and because it has no lasting satiety value, it is conducive to consuming far more calories than desirable. Refined sugar should be kept to a minimum, especially in the diet of the elderly who need to obtain the necessary nutrients spiced with as few calories as possible.

Dairy foods, eggs, and meat are devoid of fiber and, except for dairy products that contain a type of sugar called lactose, contain no carbohydrates. Most of the carbohydrate and calories in the diet should come from unrefined grains and grain products, potatoes, vegetables, fruit, beans, and peas.

The diet should be comprised mostly or entirely of these foods, so that it will provide the macronutrients in the optimal proportions, calculated as percent of total calories: protein, 12–14 percent; carbohydrate, approximately 80 percent; fat, 8–10 percent. It will also contain 50 or more grams of dietary fiber per day. These recommendations are based on epidemiologic studies of native populations and the relationship between their diet and state of health and on studies of the effect of dietary intervention in persons with degenerative diseases, such as cardiovascular disease and diabetes.

Fat

Except for the essential fatty acids, there is no requirement for dietary fat. Because almost all foods contain fat, it is not necessary to eat such visible fats as margarine or oil in order to have fat in the diet. If one eats a variety of plant foods and includes no visible fat in the diet, about 10 percent of calories would still be derived from fat. Any excess of energy in the body—whether derived from dietary carbohydrate, fat, protein, or alcohol—is converted to fat. A diet based on the guidelines at the end of the chapter provides 8 to 10 percent of total calories as fat and meets the requirements for essential fatty acids.

It is extremely difficult to obtain too little fat in the diet, as fatty acids occur in optimal amounts and ratios in plant foods that have not been overprocessed. It is, however, all too easy to obtain an *overabundance* of dietary fat. In fact, it is difficult *not* to obtain far more than the optimal amount of approximately 10 percent of total calories when foods from animal sources, extracted vegetable oils, and oil products comprise a significant part of the diet.

The Senate Select Committee on Nutrition and Human Needs, in its *Dietary Goals* (1977), admonished Americans to curtail their fat consumption.[11] Fat seems to be an important factor associated with the early advent of cardiovascular disease and other degenerative conditions, such as cancer and disturbed carbohydrate metabolism. There is a positive relationship between hypertension and dietary fat.[12,13] Fat and cholesterol also appear to have an inhibitory effect on the immune response in both animals and humans.[14]

Fats can be saturated, monounsaturated, or polyunsaturated. Saturated fats occur predominantly in foods of animal origin and tend to be solid at room temperature. Unsaturated fats occur mostly in plant foods, especially in oil seeds, and tend to be fluid at room temperature. To harden them into margarine, they are partially hydrogenated or rendered less unsaturated.

Twenty-five years ago, researchers believed that replacing the saturated fats in the diet with unsaturated fats would afford protection from heart disease and they became preoccupied with the P/S ratio—ratio of polyunsaturated to saturated fats in the diet. Data gathered within the past ten years, however, imply that unsaturated fats are also harmful and that a healthful diet is low in total fat. Because most foods contain fat, care must be taken to avoid concentrated sources, such as extracted oils and high-fat animal products.

Dietary Cholesterol

Dietary cholesterol, a waxy substance found in foods of animal sources, has been demonstrated to increase the amount of cholesterol in the blood and to increase the risk of developing heart disease.[15,16,17]

The American Heart Association (AHA) diet of 30 percent fat, 300 mg cholesterol per day was demonstrated in the multimillion dollar MRFIT (Multiple Risk Factor Intervention Trial) report to achieve an insignificant 4 percent reduction in serum cholesterol. The National Institutes of Health were not satisfied with this result. Therefore, they recommended the cholesterol-lowering drug, cholestyramine, be used in conjunction with the AHA diet. This drug, however, is prohibitively expensive, is not only bulky but must be taken six times a day, and has many serious side effects, some of which are life threatening. And it only lowers cholesterol an additional 8 percent!

The most effective diet to reduce the risk of heart disease is a 10 percent fat diet permitting 100 mg cholesterol per day. This diet achieves a 25 percent drop in cholesterol in 3 weeks and, if followed, could almost eliminate heart disease in the United States. In 1958, the 10-year Framingham Study and other studies reported data that would have justified the recommendation of such a diet.

The AHA is slowly revising its dietary guidelines in the direction of reduced fat and cholesterol intake. Since 1961, the AHA has been trying to determine how little the American diet can be improved and still decrease the incidence of heart disease. That effort is similar to recommending that Americans smoke one cigarette less each year until the incidence of lung cancer starts to decline. Based on past revisions, the AHA will not recommend the optimal diet until the year 2025!

Cholesterol can only be lowered enough to eliminate the risk of heart disease almost completely by limiting its intake to 100 mg a day and fat to 10 percent of total calories. This lowered intake can be achieved by limiting meat, fish or poultry to 3 to 4 ounces a day; not eating egg yolks; using only nonfat dairy products; and preparing foods without oils or fats.

Minerals and Vitamins

Certain conditions, such as loss of blood due to trauma, gastrointestinal disease, or parasitic infestation, naturally demand replacement of various nutrients. However, normal persons of any age, without metabolic abnormalities and who are in good health, will meet their need for all nutrients with the exception of vitamin B_{12} by following the guidelines outlined in this chapter. For people who have eaten no dairy or other animal products for a number of years, vitamin B_{12} nutriture could be compromised, and they should consult with their physician.

DIET-RELATED DISEASES

Diet-related diseases associated with middle and old age are diabetes, cancer, cardiovascular disease, and osteoporosis. In addition, diet can contribute to kidney disease and anemia, and it can exacerbate arthritic degeneration.

Cardiovascular Disease

Atherosclerotic heart disease is not uncommon in middle-aged men and becomes increasingly prevalent among both the male and female elderly population. About 1,500,000 Americans are expected to have a heart attack this year, and half of them will die.[18]

The amounts of fat and cholesterol in the diet and in the blood affect the prevalence of atherosclerosis. In most populations where the average serum cholesterol is high, a high incidence of heart disease exists,[19,20,21] and where serum cholesterol is maintained below 180 mg/dL over the lifetime of people, heart disease is uncommon.[22] Both dietary cholesterol[23] and dietary fat[24] are major factors causing the elevation of serum cholesterol. Almost without exception, populations with a low incidence of heart disease consume diets containing approximately 10 to 15 percent of calories from fat and less than 100 mg of cholesterol per day.

In the past, some investigators argued that only low serum cholesterol levels due to heredity, and not low levels due to diet, were related to the incidence of atherosclerotic heart disease. However, in 1981, data obtained from a 19-year evaluation of diet, serum cholesterol, and other variables in 1,900 middle-aged men were published.[15] The findings support the conclusion that dietary fat and cholesterol affect serum cholesterol *and* risk of death due to heart disease in middle-aged

American men. It was further found that *eating large amounts of foods rich in cholesterol can result in heart disease even if a person's serum cholesterol is low.*

Keeping the cholesterol content of the diet low can not only help prevent atherosclerosis but also can cause its regression.[25,26,27] A diet of 10 percent protein, 10 percent fat, 80 percent complex carbohydrate, and less than 100 mg cholesterol a day has also been demonstrated to be useful in the treatment of patients with peripheral vascular disease.[28]

Cancer

The Committee on Diet, Nutrition and Cancer of the National Research Council concluded that the differences in the rates at which various cancers occur in different human populations are often correlated with differences in diet. The prevailing research suggests that most cancer is caused by nutritional excesses, mainly of fats and especially of those that are polyunsaturated. A positive correlation exists between fat intake and the incidence of colon, breast, uterine, ovarian, and prostate cancer.[29]

The risk of cancer is decreased to the greatest degree when the diet is low in fat.[30] However, other dietary factors play a role in altering this risk. For example, the consumption of salt-cured, salt-pickled, and smoked foods correlates with stomach and esophageal cancer, and the ingestion of tannins, found in tea and some foods, correlates with oral and esophageal cancer.

On the other hand, the risk of cancer tends to be *decreased* when diets are consumed that are high in vegetables containing beta-carotene or certain substances that tend to protect against cancer. Beta-carotene can be obtained from orange vegetables, such as carrots, sweet potatoes, or winter squash, or from leafy greens. Other naturally occurring substances in certain vegetables, especially of the cruciferous family that includes cabbage, Brussels sprouts, turnips, kohlrabi, cauliflower, and broccoli, have also been shown to inhibit the development of cancer.[31]

Bone and Joint Disease

Osteoporosis is becoming one of the most important health problems in our population. The resulting fractures are a major cause of disability in middle-aged and elderly persons in Western countries, most of whom suffer a progressive decrease in bone density as they age. About 25 percent of Caucasian women 65 years and older have osteoporosis.[32] However, increasing age does not appear to be associated with any change in the absorption of calcium,[33] and the excretion of calcium has been shown to diminish with age, rather than to increase.[34]

Although the elderly frequently take drugs, such as laxatives and antacids containing aluminum and/or magnesium that compromise mineral nutriture and contribute to bone loss,[35,36] the most important factor contributing to fragile bones in old people appears to be the nature of the diet consumed during their entire lifetime. As a result, osteoporosis is occurring in an ever increasing number of the elderly population—especially thin, postmenopausal women—and the age of onset seems to be decreasing.[37] The problem, however, is not a result of an increased requirement of the elderly for calcium. Rather, older people tend to eat fewer vegetables that are rich sources of calcium and vitamin C than when they were younger. This decreases both the amount of calcium in the diet and the amount that is absorbed, as vitamin C enhances the absorption of calcium.

However, although the calcium content of the diet plays a role, it does not appear to be the most important factor relating to bone density. The most significant dietary characteristics relating to osteoporosis appear to be those that cause bone-forming minerals to leave the bones: the high protein content and excessive amounts of acid-forming minerals due to predominance in the diet of foods of animal origin.[38] Other dietary factors that decrease the amount of calcium absorbed from food include:

- excessive oxalates due to consumption of vegetables with high oxalate content, such as spinach, chard, beets, and beet greens
- excessive dietary fats causing formation of insoluble calcium soaps and acidic ketone bodies
- excessive consumption of alcoholic beverages that drastically reduces the absorption of calcium

The most effective way to halt the loss of minerals from aging bones is to lower the amount of foods from animal sources in the diet of persons between the middle and late years. Of special concern should be postmenopausal women. A secondary measure would be to include generous amounts of calcium in the diet.

All too often, dairy products are seen as the "magic" source of calcium. Even the government Women, Infants and Children's (WIC) program for pregnant women and young children subsidizes only dairy food sources of calcium. Unfortunately, this program does not help the increasing number of Asians in our population, a large percentage of whom are young children and people in their early childbearing years. Asians, as some other peoples, not only have a psychological aversion to milk and dairy products but also have the physiological problem of lactose intolerance, which causes diarrhea.

Even among Caucasians, the incidence of lactose intolerance increases among the elderly. In addition, some older people may be vegans or consume few dairy foods because of their religious beliefs.

Many vegetables are good sources of calcium. Table 12–1 shows the calcium content of selected vegetable and dairy foods that are rich sources of calcium.

Table 12–1 Dietary Sources of Calcium and Iron

FOOD	AMOUNT	CALCIUM mg	IRON mg	CALORIES
Collards	1 cup cooked	357	1.5	63
Turnip greens	1 cup cooked	267	1.6	29
Kale	1 cup cooked	206	1.8	43
Mustard greens	1 cup cooked	193	2.5	32
Nonfat milk	1 cup	296	0.1	88
Nonfat yogurt	1 cup	296	0.1	88
Nonfat cottage cheese	2 ounces	52	0.2	48

Source: Adapted from *Nutritive Value of American Foods in Common Units* by Catherine F. Adams, Agriculture Handbook No. 456. (Washington, D.C., United States Department of Agriculture, 1975)

Calcium absorption is also affected by vitamin D, the main source of which is the skin where its synthesis is dependent on ultraviolet radiation and is not affected by any known nutritional factors. Suboptimal vitamin D nutrition develops in some elderly persons in the United States as a result of diminished sun exposure. In old age homes, a small increase of ultraviolet exposure from specially designed bulbs was found to increase calcium absorption.[39] It would be highly commendable if the elderly, even those institutionalized and confined to wheelchairs or bedridden, were provided with some time outdoors on a regular basis. However, self-medication by the elderly with vitamin D should be strongly discouraged as the margin of safety is low.

Fat is suspected as a causative factor in various joint diseases, including osteo-arthritis.[40,41] The large number of elderly who already suffer with some degree of arthritis would do well to avoid high-fat foods to halt progression of the degenerative joint changes and to help keep their weight down, minimizing the stress to the already damaged joints. In gouty arthritis, yeast, sardines, and organ foods, such as sweetbreads, pancreas, liver, and spleen, that are high in nucleic acids or purines should be avoided because, even in healthy persons, they can raise uric acid levels to levels within the gout range.[42] At these levels, the uric acid can crystallize, precipitating an acute attack of gout. For persons with the metabolic disorder that causes this type of arthritis, drugs do not cure the disorder, but adherence to a diet low in fat, nucleic acids, purines, and alcohol can prevent both the recurring attacks and the crippling formerly associated with gout.

Many factors play a role in causing rheumatoid arthritis, including emotional stress, disturbed carbohydrate metabolism, or a fatty diet[43] that can create high amounts of fats in the blood, resulting in the inability to deliver optimal amounts of oxygen to the tissues. Arthritic persons have very little oxygen in their joints;[44]

this condition can cause white cells to increase and rupture, discharging their corrosive digestive enzymes into the joints.

Anemia

The main blood-building nutrients are iron, folic acid, and vitamin B_{12}, and in most cases, anemia is due to deficiency in one or more of these nutrients.

Iron deficiency anemia in the elderly can easily be prevented as the body's iron requirements are lowest in old age, and the average iron intake is adequate in older Americans.[45] The RDA of 10 mg iron daily can be satisfied by a diet moderate in calories that includes fruits and vegetables containing vitamin C, which causes the iron in these foods to be more readily absorbed. Only 66 mg of vitamin C, the amount in one orange, can increase the absorption of iron fivefold.[46] Iron deficiency anemia in the older person is often related to internal bleeding caused by cancer or the intake of a large amount of salicylates.[47]

The small segment of the population receiving insufficient dietary iron is comprised of isolated individuals consuming very low-calorie diets that contain marginal levels of a broad spectrum of nutrients.[48] The diet of elderly people, especially those who live alone, tends to contain a smaller variety of foods than when they are part of a larger family group. They also tend to drink more tea, as coffee and other acid beverages are apt to cause indigestion in older people. Not only does a diet limited in variety tend to provide little iron but also tea, which contains tannins that bind many nutrients, is the most potent inhibitor of iron absorption known.[49] Coffee also has this effect, but to a lesser extent. The inhibitory effect is greatest when these beverages are drunk with or immediately after meals. Milk taken with tea binds the tannins responsible for the inhibitory effect, but coffee with milk was found to inhibit iron absorption to a much greater degree than when it was taken black.

Despite the lowered requirement of the elderly for iron, many take large quantities of iron supplements. This could present a danger for the significant proportion of the population with abnormal regulatory mechanisms for the absorption and excretion of iron, which result in iron overload. Occasionally, iron supplementation can even harm normal people.[50] It could also compromise zinc nutriture. Because of the interrelationship among zinc, copper, and selenium, self-medication of any of these minerals should not be undertaken, as homeostasis can easily be disturbed. Only if iron deficiency is substantiated by a physician should iron supplementation be undertaken. It should be discontinued after menopause unless a woman's physician recommends otherwise.

Folic acid requirements can readily be met by most older people who are not alcoholic. Folic acid is found in nearly all foods, although it tends to be low in foods of animal origin. The highest amounts are found in fruits and vegetables that are rich sources of vitamin C. For instance, one broccoli spear contains a quarter of the RDA of 400 μg and half the recommendations of the Food and Agricultural Organization and the World Health Organization.[51]

Vitamin B_{12} deficiency can occur in older persons whose stomachs no longer secrete a substance that permits its absorption. For older people who do not have this rare problem, requirements can be met by only occasionally including small amounts of foods of animal origin in the diet. Half a cup of skim milk each day provides ample amounts of the vitamin B_{12}.

Disorders of the Gastrointestinal Tract

Approximately a quarter of all elderly people who visit physicians complain of constipation and spend huge sums of money on laxatives. A large and increasing body of evidence seems to point to our fiber-depleted diet as the main causative factor not only of constipation but also of various conditions and diseases of the gastrointestinal tract. Fiber retains large amounts of water in the intestines, giving bulk to the fecal mass and allowing it to move more rapidly through the colon. When there is not sufficient bulk in the diet, the muscles of the colon have to work harder to propel the contents forward. The resulting increase in pressure can cause a ballooning out of little pouches along the wall of the colon. This condition is called diverticulosis. Food particles that become lodged in the pouches allow the multiplication of bacteria, resulting in diverticulitis.

High fiber diets are now being used to treat diverticular disease.[52,53] Although fiber might not effect a cure, it usually controls the disease unless it is very advanced. People with digestive tract disorders should be, however, under the supervision of a physician. During acute episodes, it may be necessary to take certain precautions, such as abstaining from uncooked foods.

People with a low intake of fiber have a greater risk of developing colorectal cancer.[54,55] A high fiber diet causes a significant decrease in the intestinal bacteria that break down bile acids into powerful cancer-causing substances. Fiber, however, is broken down by other intestinal bacteria that play an important role in the normal metabolism of cholesterol.

Fiber exerts its most important effects in the large bowel or colon. The richest source of this fiber is wheat, but it is found in all plant foods from which it has not been extracted. A varied diet of whole, unrefined foods supplies all the fiber needed.

Kidney Disease

As people in industrialized countries age, kidney function often declines due to progressive hardening of tiny vessels in the kidneys. By the age of 75, function can have declined by as much as 50 percent, and those with diabetes, hypertension, or heart disease are at great risk of total kidney failure.

The large amounts of protein in the Western diet may be one of the main causative factors responsible for this degeneration.[56,57] Increasing protein in the diet causes the filtering system of the kidneys to work overtime, resulting in thickening of the capillaries leading to the tiny filter units. This thickening makes the capillary lumen smaller and reduces or cuts off the blood supply to the filters. Kidney failure can result.

Because kidney function so often deteriorates with age, it is best to keep the protein intake of the elderly at a maximum of 12 percent of the caloric total to prevent the necessity of eliminating excessive amounts of toxic nitrogenous protein waste products.

Senility

Deterioration of the mental faculties can occur as a result of hardening of the arteries that supply the brain. A diet low in cholesterol and fat is the nutritional approach to both the prevention and the treatment of senility. Symptoms of senility can also be the result of Alzheimer's disease, which produces intellectual impairment in as many as 2 million people in the United States over age 65, and possibly 1 million who are under age 65. Evidence is mounting that the aluminum in antacids, such as Amphojel and many others, may be a causative agent of Alzheimer's disease in patients undergoing kidney dialysis.[58,59,60,61,62,63] More recent research indicates that, although the body absorbs ingested aluminum poorly, it may be an important toxicant for normal people, as well as for those with kidney disease.[64] It now appears that the excessive use of aluminum-containing antacids may impair the absorption and utilization of essential minerals, causing anemia and softening of the bones, as well as Alzheimer's disease. It is therefore advisable to avoid the habitual use of aluminum-containing antacids or other aluminum compounds.[65] It is also prudent to store cooked foods, especially those that are salty or highly acid, in glass, stainless steel or plastic, rather than in aluminum containers.

Abnormal Carbohydrate Metabolism

Frequent high complex carbohydrate, high fiber meals have been found to be beneficial both for people with hypoglycemia[66,67] and for those with diabetes.[68,69] Blood sugar approaches normal levels after just a short time on this diet, and most adult-onset diabetics taking insulin can become drug-free on it. Those who do not become drug-free can substantially reduce their insulin dosage, thus decreasing the risk of developing the crippling complications associated with diabetes.

FOOD, NUTRIENT, AND DRUG INTERACTIONS

The effects that foods and drugs have on each other can determine whether medications do their job and whether the body gets the nutrients it needs. Natural substances in foods can render some drugs almost useless or cause them to be dangerous or even lethal.

It is safer to take medicinal tablets with water than with acidic fruit, vegetable juices, or carbonated beverages. These beverages could cause some drugs to be dissolved rapidly in the stomach, instead of the intestines, and be absorbed too quickly.

One of the most hazardous food-drug reactions occurs between the monoamine oxidase inhibitors prescribed for depression or high blood pressure and tyramine-containing foods, such as aged cheese, pickled herring, salami or pepperoni, bananas, avocados, soy sauce, and Chianti wine, sherry, or beer. Combining the drug with these foods and possibly also with cola drinks, coffee, chocolate, and raisins could result in dangerously high blood pressure.

Drugs do not always mix well with vitamins; some can prevent absorption and utilization of many vitamins and lead to certain deficiencies. Some prevent the synthesis of vitamins in the body as well. Mineral oil, sometimes used as a laxative, prevents the absorption of two fat-soluble vitamins—A and D. Many drugs, including aspirin and barbiturates, increase the requirements for vitamin C. Prolonged use of most antacids depletes the body of thiamin. The antacid, aluminum hydroxide, interferes with the absorption of vitamin D. Diuretics cause the body to lose water-soluble vitamins. Anticonvulsants inhibit the absorption of folacin and vitamin B_{12}. Sugar and alcohol, both of which would technically be considered drugs, cause the body to be depleted of B vitamins. Sometimes vitamin E lowers the insulin requirement of diabetics. Finally, detoxification of drugs in the body may cause an increased need for certain nutrients.

Barbiturates are frequently prescribed for elderly people to help them sleep. Because many older people do not eat balanced diets, they tend to suffer from marginal nutritional deficiencies. In addition, most older people suffer from osteoporosis, the softening and shrinking of bone tissue. Barbiturates make less calcium available for bone maintenance because they adversely affect metabolism of the vitamin D that is necessary for the absorption and utilization of calcium. Phenobarbitol has also been found to increase the rate at which vitamin C is excreted from the body. The glucocorticoids—antiinflammatory drugs used in the treatment of arthritis—have similar effects.

If vitamin supplements are taken, they should be discontinued at least a week before blood tests are taken. Supplements can cause false results on some tests, thereby making diagnosis more difficult. When going for a medical examination, a patient should tell the doctor exactly what supplements are being taken and in what quantities.

Drugs can also affect mineral nutriture. Diuretics (water pills) cause the body to lose potassium and are especially dangerous if the patient is also taking digitalis. Aluminum-containing antacids can inhibit the absorption of phosphorus and fluoride and increase the excretion of calcium. If drugs are to be taken for a prolonged period of time, supplementation of one or more nutrients may have to be considered.

A physician or pharmacist should be asked about possible food-drug reactions. In addition, people on drug therapy or their caretakers should have a reliable reference book describing all known food-drug reactions. One of the better ones is *Interactions of Selected Drugs and Nutrients*,[70] by Daphne Roe, published in 1982 by the American Dietetic Association.

Labels on nonprescription drugs and the inserts that come with prescription drugs should always be read carefully. A few drugs come with a warning against taking them and alcohol at the same time. Indeed, alcohol does not mix well with a wide variety of drugs, such as antibiotics; anticoagulants; antidiabetic drugs, including insulin; antihistamines; blood pressure drugs; and sedatives. It is best to avoid alcohol when taking drugs of any kind.

Other forms of medical intervention besides drug therapy can influence the need for many nutrients. Nutrition should be considered before and after surgical procedures and radiotherapy.

ALCOHOL

Immoderate drinking contributes to malnutrition in several ways. Alcohol is devoid of carbohydrates, fats, protein, fiber, vitamins, or minerals, but it does contain many calories and often replaces nutritional foods in the diet. It causes inflammation of the stomach, intestines, and pancreas, which results in the malabsorption of many vitamins, as well as calcium and iron. It causes the rapid excretion of magnesium, zinc, calcium, and potassium, and it impairs the body's ability to utilize nutrients properly once they have been absorbed. Both alcohol and its breakdown product, acetaldehyde, interfere with the activation of vitamins by liver cells. This is especially true of thiamin. Exacerbating this problem is the fact that the metabolism of acetaldehyde requires large quantities of thiamin, further depleting the body stores.

Thiamin deficiency is often responsible for the tremors, psychosis, and amnesia of alcoholics. Beriberi—the thiamin deficiency disease causing nerve and heart damage—is almost never seen in this country except in alcoholics. Although generally vitamin supplements are not needed, it is recommended that heavy drinkers consult their physician in this regard. A vitamin B complex formula would prevent some of the damage caused by alcohol.

CONCLUSION

The low-income elderly constitute one of the groups in American society particularly vulnerable to malnutrition. Yet, they are at risk neither because their nutritional needs are any greater nor because they cannot afford nutritious food. The foods that constitute a healthful diet are often less expensive than the highly processed foods that comprise the diet of a great proportion of elderly Americans.

Instead, malnutrition among the vast majority of our elderly is the result of a dearth of constructive nutritional information and a wealth of misinformation, lack of motivation, and insufficient human resources to provide for their care. To ensure that elderly Americans are fed properly is more within the domain of social than nutritional science. However, elaborate nutrition programs set up in the past have often done more harm than good. The nutritional problems of the elderly can best be solved by educational programs aimed at the elderly themselves and those directly or indirectly responsible for their care.

NOTES

1. Mary Bess Kohrs et al., "Nutritional Status of Elderly Residents in Missouri," *The American Journal of Clinical Nutrition* 31 (1978): 2186–2197.

2. Sharon Fisher et al., "Nutritional Assessment of Senior Rural Utahns by Biochemical and Physical Measurements," *The American Journal of Clinical Nutrition* 31 (1978): 667–672.

3. Gilbert B. Forbes and Julio C. Reina, "Adult Lean Body Mass Declines with Age: Some Longitudinal Observations," *Metabolism* 19 (1970): 653–663.

4. Mary Bertino et al., "Long-term Reduction in Dietary Sodium Alters the Taste of Salt," *The American Journal of Clinical Nutrition* 36 (1982): 1134–1144.

5. Ricardo Uauy et al., "Human Protein Requirements: Obligatory Urinary and Fecal Nitrogen Losses and the Factorial Estimation of Protein Needs in Elderly Males," *The Journal of Nutrition* 108 (1978): 97–103.

6. Anthony H.R. Cheng et al., "Comparative Nitrogen Balance Study between Young and Aged Adults Using Three Levels of Protein Intake from a Combination Wheat-Soy-Milk Mixture," *The American Journal of Clinical Nutrition* 31 (1978): 12–22.

7. Hellen M. Linkswiler et al., "Calcium Retention of Young Adult Males as Affected by Level of Protein and of Calcium Intake," *Transactions of the New York Academy of Sciences*, Ser. II, 36 (1974): 333–340.

8. Barry M. Brenner et al., "Dietary Protein Intake and the Progressive Nature of Kidney Disease: The Role of Hemodynamically Mediated Glomerular Injury in the Pathogenesis of Progressive Glomerular Sclerosis in Aging, Renal Ablation, and Intrinsic Renal Disease," *The New England Journal of Medicine* 307 (1982): 652–669.

9. National Academy of Sciences, National Research Council, Committee on Diet, Nutrition, and Cancer, *Diet, Nutrition and Cancer* (Washington, DC: National Academy Press, 1982), pp. 6-1–6-11.

10. Pauline O'Hanlon and Mary Bess Kohrs, "Dietary Studies of Older Americans," *The American Journal of Clinical Nutrition* 31 (1978): 1257–1269.

11. U.S. Senate, Select Committee on Nutrition and Human Needs, *Dietary Goals for the United States*, 2nd ed. (Washington, DC: U.S. Government Printing Office, February 1977), p. 12.

12. James M. Iacono et al., "Effect of Dietary Fat on Blood Pressure in a Rural Finnish Population," *The American Journal of Clinical Nutrition* 38 (1983): 860–869.

13. R. James Barnard et al., "Effects of a High-Complex Carbohydrate Diet and Daily Walking on Blood Pressure and Medication Status of Hypertensive Patients," *Journal of Cardiac Rehabilitation* 3 (1983): 839–846.

14. William R. Beisel et al., "Single-Nutrient Effects on Immunologic Functions: Report of a Workshop Sponsored by the Department of Food and Nutrition and Its Nutrition Advisory Group of the American Medical Association," *The Journal of the American Medical Association* 245 (1981): 53–58.

15. Richard B. Shekelle et al., "Diet, Serum Cholesterol, and Death From Coronary Heart Disease: The Western Electric Study," *The New England Journal of Medicine* 304 (1981): 65–70.

16. Lipid Research Clinics Program, "The Lipid Research Clinics Coronary Primary Prevention Trial Results: I. Reduction in Incidence of Coronary Heart Disease," *The Journal of the American Medical Association* 251 (1984): 351–364.

17. Lipid Research Clinics Program, "The Lipid Research Clinics Coronary Primary Prevention Trial Results: II. The Relationship of Reduction in Incidence of Coronary Heart Disease to Cholesterol Lowering," *The Journal of the American Medical Association* 251 (1984): 365–374.

18. *Heart Facts 1983* (Dallas, TX: American Heart Association, 1982), 25pp.

19. W.B. Kannel et al., "Serum Cholesterol, Lipoproteins, and the Risk of Coronary Heart Disease: The Framingham Study," *Annals of Internal Medicine* 74 (1971): 1.

20. Ancel Keys, "Coronary Heart Disease—The Global Picture," *Atherosclerosis* 22 (1975): 149.

21. Ancel Keys, *Seven Countries* (Cambridge: Harvard University Press, 1980), p. 135.

22. W.E. Connor and S.I. Connor, "The Key Role of Nutritional Factors in the Prevention of Coronary Heart Disease," *Preventive Medicine* 1 (1972): 49.

23. F.H. Mattson et al., "Effect of Dietary Cholesterol on Serum Cholesterol in Man," *The American Journal of Clinical Nutrition* 25 (1972): 589.

24. Ancel Keys et al., "Lessons from Serum Cholesterol Studies in Japan, Hawaii and Los Angeles," *Annals of Internal Medicine* 48 (1958): 83.

25. M.I. Armstrong and M.B. Megan, "Lipid Depletion in Atheromatous Coronary Arteries in Rhesus Monkeys after Regression Diets," *Circulation Research* 30 (1972): 675.

26. R.G. DePalma et al., "Animal Models for the Study of Progression and Regression of Atherosclerosis," *Surgery* 72 (1972): 268.

27. R.W. Wissler and D. Vesselinovitch, "Regression of Atherosclerosis in Experimental Animals and Man," *Modern Concepts of Cardiovascular Disease* 46 (1977): 27.

28. Nathan Pritikin et al., "Diet and Exercise as a Total Therapeutic Regime for the Rehabilitation of Patients with Severe Peripheral Vascular Disease," (Abstract) *Archives of Physical Medicine and Rehabilitation* 56 (1975): 558.

29. National Academy of Sciences, *op. cit.*, pp. 17-6–17-11, 17-19–17-21.

30. *Ibid.*, p. 5–21.

31. Saxon Graham and Curtis Mettlin, "Diet and Colon Cancer," *American Journal of Epidemiology* 109 (1979): 1–20.

32. E. Seeman and B.L. Riggs, "Dietary Prevention of Bone Loss in the Elderly," *Geriatrics* 36 (1981): 71–79.

33. H.H. Draper, "Physiological Aspects of Aging. V. Calcium and Magnesium Metabolism in Senescent Mice," *The Journal of Nutrition* 83 (1964): 65–72.

34. Leo Lutwak, "Nutritional Aspects of Osteoporosis," *Journal of the American Geriatrics Society* 17 (1969): 115.

35. "Antacids: Small Doses Damage Bones," *Medical World News*, June 6, 1975, p. 6.

36. Karl L. Insogna et al., "Osteomalacia and Weakness from Excessive Antacid Ingestion," *The Journal of the American Medical Association* 244 (1980): 2544–2546.

37. G. Alan Rose, "Study of the Treatment of Osteoporosis with Fluoride Therapy and High Calcium Intake," *Proceedings of the Royal Society of Medicine* 58 (1965): 436–444.

38. Ammon Wachman and Daniel S. Bernstein, "Diet and Osteoporosis," *The Lancet* 1 (1968): 958–959.

39. R.M. Neer et al., "Stimulation by Artificial Lighting of Calcium Absorption in Elderly Human Subjects," *Nature* 229 (1971): 255–257.

40. M. Silberberg and R. Silberberg, "Studies Concerning the Specificity of the Skeletal Effects of Enriched Diets in Aging Mice," *Laboratory Investigation* 6 (1957): 372.

41. Leon Sokoloff et al., "Experimental Obesity and Osteoarthritis," *The American Journal of Physiology* 198 (1960): 765.

42. Carol I. Waslien et al., "Uric Acid Production of Men Fed Graded Amounts of Egg Protein and Yeast Nucleic Acid," *The American Journal of Clinical Nutrition* 21 (1968): 892–897.

43. Charles P. Lucas and Lawrence Power, "Dietary Fat Aggravates Active Rheumatoid Arthritis," (Abstract) *Clinical Research* 29 (1981): 754A.

44. Knud Lund-Oleson, "Oxygen Tension in Synovial Fluids," *Arthritis and Rheumatism* 13 (1970): 769–776.

45. Sean R. Lynch et al., "Iron Status of Elderly Americans," *The American Journal of Clinical Nutrition* 36 (1982): 1032–1045.

46. M. Layrisse et al., "Measurement of the Total Daily Dietary Iron Absorption by the Extrinsic Tag Model," *The American Journal of Clinical Nutrition* 27 (1974): 152–162.

47. W.J. McLennan et al., "Anaemia in the Elderly," *Quarterly Journal of Medicine* 42 (1973): 1–13.

48. G. Clifford, "Hematological Problems in the Elderly," In *Clinical Geriatrics*, ed. I. Rossman (Philadelphia: J.B. Lippincott, 1971), 253–266.

49. Timothy A. Morck et al., "Inhibition of Food Iron Absorption by Coffee," *The American Journal of Clinical Nutrition* 37 (1983): 416–420.

50. L.A. Turnberg, "Excessive Oral Iron Therapy Causing Haemochromatosis," *British Medical Journal* 1 (1965): 1360.

51. American Dietetic Association, *Handbook of Clinical Dietetics* (New Haven, CT: Yale University Press, 1981), pp. 171–180.

52. A.J.M. Brodribb and Daphne M. Humphreys, "Diverticular Disease: Three Studies. Part I—Relation to Other Disorders and Fibre Intake. Part II—Treatment with Bran. Part III—Metabolic Effect of Bran in Patients with Diverticular Disease," *British Medical Journal* 1 (1976): 424–430.

53. Gene A. Spiller and Hugh J. Freeman, "Recent Advances in Dietary Fiber and Colorectal Diseases," *The American Journal of Clinical Nutrition* 34 (1981): 1145–1152.

54. M.J. Hill, "Bacteria and Aetiology of Cancer of the Large Bowel," *The Lancet* 1 (1971): 95–100.

55. Susan H. Brammer and Robert L. DeFelice, "Dietary Advice in Regard to Risk for Colon and Breast Cancer," *Preventive Medicine* 9 (1980): 544–549.

56. B.M. Brenner et al., *op. cit.*, pp. 652–669.

57. E.M. Darmady, J. Offer, and M.A. Woodhouse, "The Parameters of the Aging Kidney," *The Journal of Pathology* 109 (1973): 195–207.

58. Jay E. Gorsky and Albert A. Dietz, "Aluminum Concentrations in Serum of Hemodialysis Patients," *Clinical Chemistry* 27 (1981): 932–935.

59. Allen C. Alfrey et al., "The Dialysis Encephalopathy Syndrome: Possible Aluminum Intoxication," *The New England Journal of Medicine* 294 (1976): 184–188.

60. George Dunea et al., "Role of Aluminum in Dialysis Dementia," *Annals of Internal Medicine* 88 (1978): 502–504.

61. M.K. Ward et al., "Dialysis Encephalopathy Syndrome," *Proceedings of the European Dialysis and Transplant Association* 13 (1976): 347–354.

62. "Dialysis Dementia," (Editorial) *British Medical Journal* 2 (1976): 1213.

63. William A. Banks and Abba J. Kastin, "Aluminum Increases permeability of the Blood-Brain Barrier to Labelled DSIP and -Endorphin: Possible Implications for Senile and Dialysis Dementia," *The Lancet* 2 (1983): 1227–1229.

64. G.H. Mayor and M.A. Burnatowska-Hledin, "Impaired Renal Function and Aluminum Metabolism," *Federation Proceedings* 42 (1983): 2979–2983.

65. Gilbert H. Major et al., "Aluminum Absorption and Distribution: Effect of Parathyroid Hormone," *Science* 197 (1977): 1187–1189.

66. James W. Anderson and Robert H. Herman, "Effects of Carbohydrate Restriction on Glucose Tolerance of Normal Men and Reactive Hypoglycemic Patients," *The American Journal of Clinical Nutrition* 28 (1975): 748–755.

67. Steven B. Leichter, "Alimentary Hypoglycemia: A New Appraisal," *The American Journal of Clinical Nutrition* 32 (1979): 2104–2114.

68. James W. Anderson and Kyleen Ward, "Long-Term Effects of High-Carbohydrate, High-Fiber Diets on Glucose and Lipid Metabolisms: A Preliminary Report on Patients with Diabetes," *Diabetes Care* 2 (1978): 77–82.

69. R. James Barnard et al., "Long-Term Use of a High-Complex Carbohydrate, High-Fiber, Low-Fat Diet and Exercise in the Treatment of NIDDM Patients," *Diabetes Care* 6 (1983): 268–273.

70. Daphne Roe, *Interactions of Selected Drugs and Nutrients* (New York: American Dietetic Association, 1982), p. 142.

Appendix 12–A Pritikin Dietary Guidelines

Category	Foods to Use	Quantity Permitted	Foods to Avoid
Fats, Oils	None.		All fats and oils, including butter, margarine, shortening, lard, meat fat, all oils, lecithin (as in vegetable spray).
Sugars	None.		All extracted sugars, including syrups, molasses, fructose, dextrose, sucrose, and honey.
Poultry, Fish, Shellfish, Meat, and Soybeans	Chicken, turkey, Cornish game hen, game birds (white meat preferred; remove skin before cooking).	Limit acceptable poultry, fish, and meat to 3 to 4 oz per day, maximum 1½ lb per week.	Fatty poultry such as duck, goose.
	Lean fish, lobster, squid, and other shellfish.	Lobster, oysters, clams, scallops, or squid; 3½ oz/day (replaces entire daily allotment of poultry, fish or meat).[1]	Fatty fish such as sardines, fish canned in oil, mackerel.
	Lean meat.	Shrimp or crab, 1¾ oz/day (replaces entire daily allotment of poultry, fish, or meat).[1]	Fatty meats such as marbled steaks and pork.
	Soybeans and tofu (soybean curd).	Soybeans and tofu: 3½ oz/day (replaces entire daily allotment of poultry, fish or meat).	Processed meats such as frankfurters and luncheon meats.
			Organ meats: liver, kidneys, hearts, sweetbreads.
			Smoked, charbroiled, or barbecued foods.
Eggs	Egg whites.	7/week max. (Raw: 2/week max.)	Egg yolks. Fish eggs, such as caviar, shad roe.
Dairy Foods	Nonfat (skim) milk, nonfat buttermilk (up to 1% fat by weight). (8 oz = 1 serving)		Cream, half-and-half, whole milk, and low-fat milk or products containing or made from them, such as sour cream, lowfat yogurt.
	Nonfat yogurt. (6 oz = 1 serving)	2 servings/day (on vegetarian days);	
	Nonfat (skim) dry milk. (5T = 1 serving)		Nondairy substitutes such as creamers, whipped toppings.

	Evaporated skim milk. (4 oz = 1 serving)	1 serving/day (on other days)	Cheeses containing over 1% fat by weight.
	100% skim-milk cheese, primarily un-creamed cottage cheese such as hoop cheese or dry curd cottage cheese, or cheeses up to 1% fat by weight. (2 oz = 1 serving)		
	Sapsago (Green) cheese.	1–2 oz/week max.	
Beans, Peas	All beans and peas (except soybeans).	Limit to 8 oz cooked beans on days when fish, poultry, or meat is not eaten. Avoid on other days except for small amounts in salads, or other dishes.	Soybeans and tofu (soybean curd) unless substituted: 3½ oz soybeans or tofu = the poultry, fish, or meat allotment.
Nuts, Seeds	Chestnuts.	Not limited.	All nuts (except chestnuts). All seeds (except in small quantities for seasoning as with spices).
Vegetables	All vegetables except avocados and olives.	Limit vegetables high in oxalic acid such as spinach, beet leaves, rhubarb, and Swiss chard.	Avocados. Olives.
Fruits[2]	All fresh fruits.	5 servings/day max.	Cooked, canned, or frozen fruit with added sugars.
	Unsweetened cooked, canned, pureed, or frozen fruit.	24 oz/week max.	Jams, jellies, fruit butters, fruit syrups with added sugars.
	Dried fruit.	1 oz/day max.	
	Unsweetened fruit juices.	4 oz/day max. (28 oz/week). or	Fruit juices with added sugars.
	Frozen concentrates, unsweetened.	1 oz/day max. (7 oz/week).	

Category	Foods to Use	Quantity Permitted	Foods to Avoid
Grains	All whole or lightly milled grains; rice, barley, buckwheat, millet, etc. Breads, cereals, crackers, pasta, tortillas, baked goods, and other grain products without added fats, oils, sugars, or egg yolks.	Unlimited. Limit refined grains and grain products (i.e., with bran and germ removed) such as white flour, white rice, white pasta, etc.	Extracted wheat germ. Grain products made with added fats, oils, sugars, or egg yolks. Bleached white flour; soy flour.
Salt	Salt.[3]	Limit salt intake to 3–4 gms/day by eliminating table salt and restricting use of high salt or sodium (Na) foods such as soy sauce, pickles, most condiments, prepared sauces, dressings, canned vegetables, and MSG (monosodium glutamate).	Salt from all sources in excess of permitted amount.
Condiments, Salad Dressings, Sauces, Gravies, and Spreads	Wines for cooking. Natural flavoring extracts. Products without fats, oils, sugars, or egg yolks.	Dry white wine preferable. Moderate use.	Products containing fats, oils, sugars, or egg yolks such as: mayonnaise, prepared sandwich spreads, prepared gravies and sauces and most seasoning mixes, salad dressings, catsups, pickle relish, chutney.
Desserts or Snacks	Dessert and snack items without fats, oils, sugars, or egg yolks.	Plain gelatin (unflavored): 1 oz/week max.	Desserts and snack items containing fats, oils, sugars, or egg yolks such as: most bakery goods, package gelatin desserts and puddings, candy, chocolate, and gum.
Beverages[4]	Mineral water, carbonated water. Nonfat (skim) milk or nonfat buttermilk.	Limit varieties with added sodium. See restrictions under DAIRY FOODS above.	Alcoholic beverages. Beverages with caffeine such as coffee, tea, cola drinks, cocoa.

Unsweetened fruit juices.	See restrictions under FRUITS above.	Decaffeinated coffee.
Vegetable juices.	Not limited.	Beverages with added sweetners such as soft drinks.
Red bush or chamomile tea preferred.	2 cups per day.	Diet and other soft drinks with artificial sweetener.

[1] Our revised recommendations are based on a conservative interpretation of the newest data concerning cholesterol and other possibly atherogenic sterols in shellfish.

[2] If triglycerides are above 125 mg percent, eat only fresh fruit in the permitted amount.

[3] Normal salt (sodium) needs are provided by food in its natural state, and additional intake should be kept to a minimum.

[4] Recommendations on herb tea (other than those given) and coffee substitutes are under study.

Source: Reprinted from *The Pritikin Promise: 28 Days to a Longer, Healthier Life* by Nathan Pritikin, pp. 162–164, with permission of Pritikin International, Inc. and Simon & Schuster, Inc., © 1983.

Chapter 13

Longevity: What Can Centenarians Teach Us?

Kenneth R. Pelletier, Ph.D.

A CENTURY OF LIFE

To date studies have been undertaken of several major centenarian communities and individuals throughout the world, including the Vilcabamba in the Ecuadorian Andes, the Hunza who live deep in the Karakoram Range of the western Himalayas in northern Pakistan, the Abkhazians in the Caucasus Mountains of Georgia in the Soviet Union, the Mabaans of Sudan, and the Tarahumara Indians of the Sierra Madre Occidental mountains in the north central state of Chihuahua in Mexico. There has also been limited research with centenarian individuals in the United States and extensive case studies of individuals with extended longevity. Most of this research has been conducted by Alexander Leaf of Harvard and is clearly of an "observational" nature, according to Leaf's own criteria.[1] Despite the cautions clearly stated by many researchers, there has been a tendency for public and professional journals to overstate the conclusions of such findings.

World attention focused on centenarian communities in 1973 when *National Geographic,*[2] *Scientific American,*[3] and *Hospital Practice,*[4] all published reports by Alexander Leaf on three communities of individuals who apparently were living well beyond 100 years of age in extremely good health. His interest had been prompted by earlier research by the Ecuadorian physician, Miguel Salvador,[5] and reports of a research team of scientists and physicians studying the Vilcabamba. At the same time, researchers pointed out a small but significant body of data indicating the common phenomenon of "age exaggeration" by the extremely elderly people of populations throughout the world.[6] Exaggeration of age had been studied in the United States,[7,8] as well as in the Soviet Union.[9,10,11] Overall these studies indicated consistent excesses in the self-reporting of age by elderly people and cast doubt on subsequent reports of extreme longevity.

However, although extreme ages of 150 are unlikely, instances of age 110 are thoroughly documented. Leaf did not rely on subjective reports alone, but used baptismal and marriage records, church documents, notations in family Bibles, letters, passports, "the person's memory of outstanding events," and "even carvings on walls and doors that record the birth of a new member of the family."[12] Due to the obscure and unwritten Hunza language, Leaf generally accepted the verbal reports of age in that community, which may mean that age exaggeration influenced those reports. Other researchers, such as Miguel Salvador in Ecuador, Professor G.Z. Pitskhelaurt in the Soviet Union, and S. Magsood Ali of Pakistan, have independently verified the ages of the three centenarian communities observed by Leaf. Professor Pitskhelaurt assessed the self-report ages versus documented ages of 704 Georgian centenarians and reported, "Almost 95% had given correct ages; the rest were within 5% of the correct age. In no case was the stated age more than 10 years above or below the documented age."[13] Age exaggeration is a potentially confounding variable, but because subjective reports were not the only indicator of longevity in any of the previous studies, it is not adequate grounds to dismiss their results.

The research generally cited to disprove claims of longevity in centenarian communities was conducted by Richard B. Mazess of the Department of Radiology at the University of Wisconsin and Sylvia H. Forman of the Department of Anthropology at the University of Massachusetts. They found that the rate of bone aging in Vilcabamba was almost identical to the rate in the United States. However, osteoporosis did not occur among elderly Vilcabambas, leading Mazess to speculate that factors other than decreased bone mass can affect the development of osteoporosis. The study cast doubt on the claims of extreme longevity among the Vilcabambas while documenting that there was a large population of relatively healthy older people free from osteoporosis.[14]

After reviewing this research, Alexander Leaf himself concluded, "Thus, though I think the health message that I was trying to promote is still correct, the evidence of unusual longevity in the populations that I visited is certainly not correct."[15] Leaf's emphasis on health is important. Interest in extended life expectancy can take attention away from the quality of life. The older people in these communities teach us that individuals can remain optimally healthy and actively involved in the entire psychosocial matrix of their culture far beyond the point considered possible at the present time.

Although a person of 96 may not seem so impressive as one of 140 or 150, that is an impressive age by any standards, at any time, in any geographic location. Another 30 to 40 years of healthy life is similar to another full lifetime. The health of the Vilcabamba elders remains highly significant and thoroughly documented.

More accurate physiological measures of age are clearly needed. Jeffrey L. Bada and Patricia M. Masters of the Scripps Institution of Oceanography in San Diego have adapted methods used in dating the antiquity of fossils. "By examining proteins in the teeth or lenses of the eyes . . . it is possible to calculate the year of birth with only a 10 percent margin of error."[16] When Russian gerontologists gave the researchers a tooth from a Soviet Georgian, the researchers estimated her age at 91 when her documented age was known to be 96 years old. Such biologically based approaches are promising, although they clearly require further development. Even if the results of such inquiries demonstrate 120-year life spans as opposed to the reported 150-year life spans, that discovery would be highly significant.

Actually there is a great deal more evidence to suggest the possibility of an extended life expectancy than there is to support a built-in limit at the present average life expectancy. There are sufficient basic and observational data to leave open the question of whether there are living populations that demonstrate the biological potential of the human species.

Although clearly there are no universal factors underlying increased longevity, it is possible to identify certain common denominators and their variants that are characteristic of centenarian populations. These influences are of equal importance, although any one or any subgroup may assume greater emphasis in a given person or culture for a given time and circumstances. Among the common denominators of longevity in individuals and cultures throughout the world and in the United States are (1) hereditary or genetic influences; (2) dietary and nutritional factors; (3) consumption of moderate amounts of alcohol; (4) physical activity throughout life; (5) sexual activity prolonged into advanced years; (6) environmental influences; and (7) psychological factors, including continued productive involvement in family and community affairs.

This list is of course not exhaustive, no one variable is mutually exclusive of the others, and future research may yet indicate that all of these are the superficial aspects of a yet undiscovered factor of paramount importance. Yet, even before such final answers are discovered, research in centenarian communities may have many benefits. By studying people who attain extended longevity in optimum health, it may be possible to learn how to enhance these conditions in our own population.

GENETIC FACTORS

In all discussions of longevity, genetic or hereditary influences are probably cited more often than any other explanation. There is a tendency to attribute any unknown influence to genetic endowment. However, the influences that determine whether a genetic predisposition is expressed can occur at any time in an organism's development and are probably as important as the infinitesimal event of the sperm fertilizing an egg. Addressing the issue of heredity, Alexander Leaf has concluded:

> Heredity is generally thought to be a significant factor in long life, as indeed it is. Several studies of life expectancy of offspring of long-lived

parents indicated a significant advantage over that for offspring of short-lived parents. The advantage, however, is a modest one. One study of the inheritance of longevity based upon life insurance records indicated that offspring of long-lived parents had a life expectancy at age 20 that probably does not exceed by three years the life expectancy of a smiliar aged group whose parents were short-lived. This was the maximal statistical advantage that could be attributed to heredity according to this study.[17]

Genetic variables were of particular importance in Leaf's observations because the Vilcabambas are primarily of European-Spanish, rather than Indian, descent and appear to be highly inbred and isolated. In the Hunza these conditions of inbreeding were also evident and could indicate a genetic expression of longevity. The centenarians of the Caucasus region, however, do not exhibit a limited gene pool. A 1970 census listed ten different ethnic groups in that region. Among the 4,500 to 5,000 centenarians noted in that census, there were Russians, Georgians, Armenians, Turks, and others "suggesting that no single isolated genetic factor is involved in longevity."[18]

A possible indication of how genetic influences interact with life-style variables is that people of the centenarian communities have a marked absence of cardiovascular and coronary heart disease. Several recent studies have a bearing on this issue. Research by E. Cuyler Hammond and his colleagues from the Department of Epidemiology of the American Cancer Society examined the longevity of parents and grandparents in relation to coronary heart disease and associated variables in their offspring. After examining the records of over 15,000 men and 50,000 women over a period of six years, the researchers concluded, "Death rates from coronary heart disease, hypertensive heart disease, and stroke were found to be considerably higher among subjects with short-lived parents than among subjects with long-lived parents."[19] Because this conclusion is often cited, it is important to acknowledge several contributing influences that make the genetic factor more equivocal. First, the actual mortality age differences were rather small, although statistically significant. Second, the researchers acknowledged that, although some risk factors, such as hypertension and lack of exercise, were considered, others, such as glucose tolerance and serum lipid, were not. The researchers themselves acknowledged, "However, we cannot rule out the possibility that nongenetic transmittal of some factor or set of factors might have accounted for the findings."[20] Although the inextricable interaction among genetic, environmental, and life-style variables is consistently acknowledged throughout such research, the myth of genetic causation persists, particularly with regard to centenarian cultures.

It appears certain from research with long-lived individuals both within and outside centenarian communities that genetic influences on longevity are a contributing but highly limited factor. Data from a 12-year study of the Abkhazians by

Georgian cardiologist David Kakiashvili show how life-style influences can affect possible genetic factors. From a series of electrocardiogram studies Kakiashvili found that these elderly people

> "do have the usual range of cardiovascular disease. [However,] contin-uous physical activity develops and maintains an extensive collateral blood supply to the heart, and . . . if one artery gets pinched off because of localized arteriosclerosis, the collateral circulation is suffi-cient to prevent atrophy of the affected heart muscles."[21]

Such influences that enhance or suppress genetic predispositions are most often referred to, in a derogatory manner, as confounding variables because they inconveniently contaminate or obscure reductionistic models of cause and effect. Every attempt is made to eliminate or control such variables. In a similar manner, most researchers dismiss the contaminating influences of placebo, consciousness and belief systems, spontaneous remission, regenerative psychosis, and a host of phenomena that may be more significant than the effects being researched. Rather than viewing such influences as contaminating and extraneous and attempting to eliminate them, a more wholistic approach emphasizes the necessity of multiple variables and their interactions. It is possible to recognize and acknowledge genetic, medical, psychosocial, environmental, and other influences and to deter-mine the ratio of each given factor's effect on a given individual or culture. Although such approaches are considerably more difficult to design and imple-ment, they are not only possible but mandatory in the study of longevity.

From the point of view of people already born, concern with genetic endowment is, of course, academic. The other six factors in longevity discussed here are within the control of individuals.

NUTRITION

After genetic endowment, the second common denominator found in observa-tions of centenarians that is conducive to longevity is nutritional and dietary practice. The Vilcabambas are a totally agricultural community where people raise their own vegetables and grain. Their diet is almost exclusively vegetarian, with small amounts of protein and fat derived from vegetable sources. According to physician Guillermo Vela of Quito, the daily caloric intake is very low at 1,200 calories. The Hunza are also an agricultural community with diets similar to that of the Vilcabambas. In a survey of 55 adult male Hunzakuts, Pakistani nutritionist Magsood Ali determined their average daily caloric intake at 1,923 calories, comprising 50 grams of protein, 32 grams of fat, and 354 grams of unrefined carbohydrate.[22] Animal protein and fat constituted less than 1 percent of the daily caloric intake. Oil extracted from apricot seeds is used in cooking. Grains, leafy green vegetables, root vegetables, dried legumes, fresh milk and buttermilk, clarified butter and cheese, fresh and sun-dried apricots, mulberries, and grape wine make up the usual diet. Portions consumed are quite frugal. In summer, a typical meal consists of a "soup made from grain, corn, yuka (a kind of root), beans and potatoes. This mainstay is augmented with oranges, bananas, and a little unrefined sugar. A considerable quantity of vegetables is eaten. . . . In winter less fruit is available."[23] Many of the dietary practices and actual recipes of the Hunza have been adapted to ingredients readily available in the United States by Renee Taylor in *Hunza Health Secrets for Long Life and Happiness*.[24]

Among the Hunza, crops of vegetables, grains, fruits, and nuts are often inadequate to last through the severe winters. As a result, "before the new greens come through in the spring, the people have gone through a period of semistarvation."[25] This is a very important observation, consistent with all the research concerning the longevity-enhancing effects of prolonged caloric restriction. These conditions are of course imposed by circumstance, rather than voluntarily undertaken. Examination of early dietary patterns is of great importance because diet during the critical stages of early development appears to be at least as important as, if not more so than, dietary habits during the rest of life. Moreover, it would be important to examine the components of centenarian diets in infancy, because these imposed restrictions may have inadvertently created the particular caloric, protein, and tryptophan moderate deficiencies noted to double the life expectancy of laboratory animals.[26,27]

However, the diet of the Georgians of the Soviet Union is quite different from that of the Vilcabambas and Hunzakuts:

> Theirs is a mixed agriculture-dairy economy and they consume animal products almost daily. The people live not only by their vegetables and fruits but also by their herds of cows, goats, and sheep. They drink milk, eat cheese and yogurt three times a day and often have meat.[28]

Despite these animal products in the diet, the caloric consumption for people over age 50 remains low—1,800 calories—as opposed to an average of 3,300 calories in the United States. Their diet is high in roughage and in unrefined carbohydrates and low in salt, refined carbohydrates, and refined sugar consumption. This is in contrast to the average diet in the United States with its intake of high levels of fat, salt, and sugar and low roughage content. Some aspects of the Georgian diet fall short of the nutritional recommendations of the National Academy of Sciences, yet virtually none of the inhabitants have been found to be either malnourished or obese. Although the dairy product intake is higher than might be expected, it is still considerably lower than in the average American diet.

The Abkhazian consumption of dairy and animal products raises the question of serum cholesterol levels. In two journal articles, Alexander Leaf reported the results of research by Miguel Salvador, who noted a low level of 219 ± 10 mg per 100 ml of serum for 49 Vilcabambas aged 60 and over. Reported levels for the Abkhazians were at an astounding 91.8 ± 4.2 mg per 100 ml of plasma for males and females.[29,30] For males in the United States there is a normal increase in serum cholesterol from ages 18 to 32, where it tends to level off at 250 mg per 100 ml. For women, this same trend begins approximately 13 years later and peaks at age 50. Leaf challenges the normality of such trends by citing data from primitive inhabitants of the Solomon Islands where "there is no tendency for plasma cholesterol to rise with age. Thus even our notions of the 'normal' or average values for the cholesterol may be biased by the prevalence of atherogenic diets in our own culture."[31] The Abkhazian diet demonstrates that dietary influences cannot be divorced from lifelong physical activity and other factors known to modify nutrition and diet.

Although the protein intake of the vegetarian Vilcabambas and Hunzakut is low at 35 to 38 grams and 50 grams, respectively, this intake is not necessarily dictated by their vegetarian diet. The vegetarian diet of corn and beans of the Tarahumara Indians provides a high level of 79 to 96 grams per day. These communities are not undernourished in any dimension of diet, but are living examples of the advice of the American Heart Association: "for long life, maintain a moderate caloric intake that generally avoids obesity, and a diet low in animal and saturated fats."[32]

Although there is a considerable amount of data concerning diet and nutrition among these three centenarian communities, there are many questions that have not been addressed. For example, Leaf notes that no one has yet studied the intake of magnesium or cobalt or other essential substances in the three areas.[33] Another variable may be the quality of the water. Many of the centenarians attribute their long life to "various herb teas they drink," according to David Davies[34] in the Unit of Gerontology of University College, London. Mo Siegel, of Celestial Seasonings Tea in Boulder, Colorado, noted, "They never heat their teas above 140 degree Fahrenheit."[35] Actual methods of food preparation are another variable worth studying, because preparation can enhance or nullify nutritional constituents.

Even with all these questions still unresolved, the influence of nutrition on health, life expectancy, and longevity must still be recognized as of major importance.

ALCOHOL CONSUMPTION

A third common factor, which is related to nutrition, in each of these communities is the consumption of alcohol. Each had its own alcoholic drink, yet there is no evidence of alcoholism in these communities. The Vilcabambas imbibe a potent liquor made from sugar cane, and the Abkhazian people drink two or three glasses of wine at each meal, in addition to a moderate amount of vodka and brandy.[36] David Davies made this observation of the Vilcabambas:

> One particularly remarkable feature is that the inhabitants drink two to four cups of rum a day, and smoke anything from 40 to 60 cigarettes each day. But the rum is unrefined and the cigarettes are home-made, usually from tobacco grown in their gardens, and wrapped in maize leaves (though toilet paper is preferred if available).[37]

Similar observations have been noted for the Hunza, who liberally enjoy a red wine called "Hunzapana," and the Abkhazians, who make a wine as well as a strong vodka from their own grapes. To date, there are no actual measures of the alcohol content of these drinks, the actual amount consumed, or consumption patterns, although drinking alcohol before or with breakfast is not uncommon.

Because there is no evidence of alcoholism, this consumption of alcohol needs to be explored in the context of other variables, such as adequate diet, physical activity, and lack of social stigma surrounding the appropriate use of alcohol. When residents of the centenarian communities cite reasons for their long lives, they often mention the local alcoholic beverage, their vigorous sexual activity, or both.

PHYSICAL ACTIVITY

Physical activity is the fourth and perhaps the most important factor in the longevity and optimum health exhibited in these centenarian communities. Associated with it is the fifth factor—active sexuality—which is also consistently noted. Alexander Leaf observed, "The level of physical activity and fitness among the aged was very striking in all three areas . . . the expenditure of physical energy probably is a better explanation of exceptional longevity than any other apparent influence."[38] Further, "in all three cultures the people are physically active throughout life since they are primarily farmers who labor by hand and walk a great deal in mountainous terrain or ride horses."[39] If hard physical labor seems a dour prescription for longevity, it is also important to note that there are numerous festivals among these people and a great deal of toasting with alcohol, as well as "native dances which are performed for us with such vigor in the mid-day heat."[40]

The benefits of physical activity that is well-integrated into a person's entire life, rather than confined to mandatory exercise periods, is clear from two classic studies undertaken in Great Britain and the United States. J.N. Norris compared the incidence of heart attacks among postal workers in London who delivered mail versus those who had desk positions. Only 51 of 171 mail carriers suffered myocardial infarctions, whereas nearly half, or 70 of 143 office workers, had heart attacks. Norris also conducted extensive postmortem studies indicating that:

> men in physically active jobs have less coronary heart disease during middle age, what disease they have is less severe, and they develop it later than men in physically inactive jobs. The hearts of sedentary workers showed the pathology of the hearts of heavy workers ten to fifteen years older.[41]

The other study was initiated by Curtis Harnes, an astute general physician in Evans County, Georgia. Harnes had observed a high incidence of coronary heart disease among his white male patients, but few cases of heart attacks among black male patients. A detailed survey of this observation was conducted by J.C. Cassel, who studied all adults over age 40 and half of the males between the ages of 15 and 39 in Evans County between 1960 and 1962. From 1967 to 1968, 91 percent of this population was reexamined. Three groups of white sharecroppers were identified, and it was found that two of these groups and the black men had less than half the incidence of coronary heart disease of the third group, who were white non-farmers.

> Analysis of the data revealed that it was the level of physical activity required by the blacks and white sharecroppers which largely protected these two groups from coronary artery disease. Most known risk factors were measured—namely, blood pressure, serum cholesterol level, cigarette smoking, body weight, and diet—and could not account for the differences.[42]

These studies make it clear that physical activity helps burn excess calories and dispose of undigested fats and thus appears to be a significant factor in preventing cardiovascular disease. Exercise may well prove to be the most significant factor mediating nutrition and may help account for the great individual differences in tolerance for high-risk diets.

After extensive physical examinations of the people of the Caucasian village of Duripshi, Alexander Leaf concluded that physical activity was a potent preventive measure not only against cardiovascular disease, such as myocardial infarction and atherosclerosis, but also against other disorders, such as osteoporosis. This latter condition, an increased porosity of the bones, is common among the elderly of the United States. When this condition is present, the calcium and salts that harden bones, as well as the collagen and cartilage matrix for these components, begin to deteriorate, and bones become thin, less dense, and fragile. Among the people of the centenarian communities Leaf saw no evidence of osteoporosis and found them to be strong and active.

For the people of long-lived regions of the world, regular exercise derives largely from activities essential to survival: extensive walking, climbing in rugged terrain, farming, and folk dancing. Exercise needs to be regular, frequent, and continued throughout life to be of benefit for any individual.

SEXUAL ACTIVITY

Sexual activity prolonged into later life is the fifth major common denominator noted by researchers in the centenarian communities. Aging is generally associated with a gradual decrease in the number of cells in certain organs, including the male testes. Cells that produce sperm are the first to be affected, but later the number of cells producing testosterone may also diminish. For females the ovaries gradually cease functioning during their late forties or early fifties. Despite these tendencies, sexual potency in the male and sexual interest in the female continue into advanced age. Sexual interest is more evident in females of advanced age than in males.

Although there is no systematic research concerning sexual activity in the centenarian communities, there is anecdotal evidence. Healthy sperm specimens have been obtained from a supposedly 119-year-old Abkhazian man; Vilcabamba women bear children in their late fifties and are usually observed to assume the initiating role, especially in advanced age. By contrast, our present attitudes reflect a "sexual inhibition in intimacy as a heritage of Victorian attitudes and repressive religious thinking."[43] Vestiges of Victorian censures persist for the elderly, despite a relative sexual revolution among younger people. Colloquialisms, such as "out to pasture, fogy, geezer, over the hill, and dirty old man,"[44] reveal a great deal about attitudes toward sexuality and the elderly. The elderly are also objects of sexist attitudes. An older man with a younger woman is clearly more socially acceptable than an older women with a younger man, even though there is no rational reason for such a judgment. Freedom from these censures and anachronistic attitudes will portend freedom for both sexes. In Vilcabamba there are no comparable stigmatizing terms for the elderly, who are respected. *Los viejos* (the elders) is the name for those approaching or beyond the century mark.

Sexuality is not limited to sexual intercourse, but has infinite expressions. A variety of forms of physical sexual contact can be clearly noted among the centenarians. Extramarital relationships and out-of-wedlock children are not taken as an indication of promiscuity in these cultures. However, Leaf has noted, "Strong taboos against sex outside of marriage and equally strong traditions about the sanctity of the family probably limit extramarital sex in all three areas, . . . everywhere I saw couples who had been married for 80 years or more."[45] Among the Caucasians, Professor Pitskhelaurt believes that a happy marriage and a prolonged, active sex life clearly contribute to their unusual longevity. The Abkhazians themselves concur most heartily. Unmarried individuals are the exception, with 44 percent of the families having 4 to 6 children and 5 percent with 10 to 15 children. Some families have over 20 children. Even in our culture it has been observed that married individuals tend to live longer and often remarry soon after the death of a spouse.

As with any single factor in the dynamic process of longevity, it is important not to overemphasize the factor of sexual activity among centenarian people. Certainly no direct causation has been proved nor advocated by any of the centenarians. All too often the small amount of information concerning long-lived individuals is presented in a sensationalist manner, or they are relegated to the status of a curiosity; certainly their sexual attitudes and habits are subject to such exploitation. Rather than seeing these magnificent people as curiosities, it is more rewarding to look for the wisdom in their life styles. Whatever the relationship between longevity and continued sexual activity, both indicate a life of activity and fulfillment.

SOCIAL ENVIRONMENT

The single most important and most frequently overlooked factor in longevity is the psychological dimensions. These include the prolonged and productive involvement in family and community affairs, an acquired status of dignity and wisdom, and an enduring sense of the meaning and purpose of life itself. The role of human consciousness in determining longevity is the reason that any search for a simple formula, recipe, or secret is doomed to failure. This dimension is generally relegated to minor status in research with centenarians because it is impossible to quantify consciousness or dissect it under a microscope.

An intact and stable social system may play a more important part in longevity than any nutritional, exercise, environmental, or other factor. Alexander Leaf has noted, ''It is characteristic of each of the areas I visited that the old people continue to be contributing, productive members of their society . . . people who no longer have a necessary role to play in the social and economic life of their society generally deteriorate rapidly.''[46] In these communities, increased age is accompanied by increased social status, such as presiding over community councils. Meanwhile, the elders remain active in the chores of farming and other natural labor. Retirement is unknown, and daily hikes, swims, and horseback rides are common. None of the Vilcabamba live alone, and unproductive idleness is unknown. Sula Benet has pointed out that the Abkhazian elderly are:

a life loving optimistic people. . . . Unlike so many very old dependent people in the United States who feel they are a burden to themselves and to their families (the Abkhazians) enjoy the prospect of continued life . . . in a culture which so highly values continuity in its traditions. The old are indispensable in their transmission. The elders preside at important ceremonial occasions, they mediate disputes and their knowledge of farming is sought. They feel needed because they are.[47]

When these factors of involvement are considered, the parallels independently observed among the Ecuadorians, the Abkhazians, and the populations of Roseto, Pennsylvania, and of Brunei, Borneo, by Stewart Wolf[48] are very striking. Active participation and community involvement have been demonstrated to be of major significance in determining an elderly person's level of functioning in later years.

The attribution of dignity and wisdom to the aged of the centenarian communities is perhaps the pivotal point between health and illness, life and death. In carefully considering the effect of such intangibles as the prestige of the elderly, Alexander Leaf has concluded:

I am now convinced that when the social environment encourages one to feel socially useful and needed in the economy, and to be looked up to and revered as a wise figure, the extremely elderly keep their mental faculties and physical abilities so that they can respond appropriately. This is quite contrary to prevailing trends in modern industrialized societies, which tend to emphasize youth and to regard old people as useless and standing in the way of progress.[49]

Evidence of the strength of such an influence on both health and longevity has been provided by two kinds of research from outside these communities: (1) studies of the health effects of ongoing, purposive activity into advanced age and (2) studies showing a direct relationship between prominence and recognition late in life and extended longevity.

Physician Leslie S. Libow, of the Mount Sinai Hospital Center in New York, conducted an 11-year longitudinal study of 27 "optimally healthy" men compared to 20 men of "average" health, with the mean age being 70 years old. The most significant finding was "the role of psychosocial factors in contributing to mortality, for example, the increased mortality related to environmental losses. . . . "[50] Among the optimally healthy elderly people, it was evident that "upward mobility and striving in midlife were related to better adaptation in late life . . . highly organized, purposeful, complex and variable daily behavior together with the absence of cigarette smoking were highly correlated with survival for these healthy elderly men."[51]

Other studies have confirmed a high level of "life satisfaction" as a precondition of extended longevity.[52,53] Research data also indicate that an active life style allows "development, change and growth to continue through the later years of the lifespan in spite of the decrement of social, psychological and physiological functioning which typically accompanies the aging process."[54] Such observations throw into question the appalling practice of relegating elderly people to geriatric centers or the enforcement of an arbitrary retirement age. Only in a youth- and performance-fixated culture would the normal decrease in peak performance be viewed as pathological or as a way of rationalizing neglect of the elderly. Advanced age is not inherently a period of physical or psychological impairment in any sense. However, the expectation of decline can result in a self-fulfilling prophecy.

In the centenarian communities it is evident that the *viejos* remain active at a level of participation suited to their mental and physical abilities. Although they remain highly active, they also have the wisdom to recognize futile, stress-inducing striving and "have learned to accept things as they are, if they cannot change them."[55] Perhaps that philosophy is at the heart of the prolonged health and longevity sustained by these people.

PHYSICAL ENVIRONMENT

Environmental factors among the centenarian communities are the seventh and last major influence on longevity. They are also the least researched. In a few instances, the quality of the water and the mountainous terrain in these geographic areas have been described, but not systematically. Of the three major communities observed by Alexander Leaf, Vilcabamba in the Andes is located at an elevation of 4,500 feet; Hunza communities are spread over a mountainous area ranging from 3,500 to 7,000 feet at the palace of Mir; and in the Caucasus region the elevations were lower, with most centenarians living between 3,000 and 5,000 feet. "In none of these areas is the altitude high enough above sea level for the atmosphere to be rarefied. Rather, the significant factor seems to be the mountainside existence and the incredible amount of physical exertion necessary just to attend to the daily business of living."[56] Again this indicates an interaction between life-style factors and environment, rather than a cause-and-effect relationship between the physical environment per se and longevity.

There is some preliminary evidence from the research of Marian C. Diamond of the University of California at Berkeley that environmental stimulation, including physical, as well as mental stimuli, can result in an increase in nerve cell branching on the cerebral cortex even in advanced age. Although the research has been conducted with laboratory animals, this "increase in mammalian cerebral cortex"[57] could indicate a regenerative potential in the human nervous system and in the areas of the brain involved in higher-order thinking. At present, Diamond's research is being extended to consider the precise nature of the environmental stimulation that would enhance such nerve growth in advanced age.

Purely environmental determinants in these communities, including trace-element concentrations in the water and soil, relative concentration of negative ions that are in greater abundance in proximity to water or at high altitudes, presence or absence of carcinogenic agents, presence or absence of naturally occurring antioxidants, and the absence of electromagnetic activity generated from power lines and media stations, need further study. Numerous other variables will undoubtedly be found that make these environments different from those of postindustrial nations.

These isolated communities are all threatened by modernization and the pollution it can bring. Dramatic negative effects on both health and mortality can be seen when outside influences begin to permeate these societies. Guillermo del Pozo, physician for the Vilcabambas, has stated that 25 of the oldest residents have died during this period of modernization, and "I don't think it's a coincidence."[58] If the delicate balance and harmony of these societies are upset, the health and longevity of their members may be severely affected. For the dignity and integrity of these centenarian people, researchers and reporters should be aware of the effects of modernization they may inadvertently cause.

THE HUMAN BIOLOGICAL POTENTIAL

Extended human longevity is a biological reality. Evidence for it comes from basic biochemical research, laboratory experimental studies, single case reports, and observations of centenarian communities. Although this extensive body of research and data clearly predicts and supports the possibility of extended human longevity, there is virtually no research proving that it is impossible. There is actually far more evidence to support the possibility of longevity than there is to explain the present rates of life expectancy. Although centenarians are relatively rare, the fact of their existence could indicate an inherent but latent biological capacity.

Centenarians are not exclusively isolated in remote geographic regions, with questionable birth certification, but are increasingly evident in Europe and in the United States. In 1969, only 3,200 Americans lived past age 100; in 1978, that figure rose to 13,000.[59] The reported health of many individuals at extreme ages is of far greater importance than the absolute number of years, even according to the centenarians themselves. These people, it must be emphasized, are not located in relatively inaccessible regions of the world. Longevity has been observed in a great diversity of places throughout history. It is not a restricted greenhouse phenomenon but is manifest under a wide range of circumstances. One of the oldest documented centenarians was Charlie Smith, who died at age 138 in 1979 at a veterans' hospital in the United States. Longevity is a reality here and now.

In any new area of research, caution needs to be exercised, but that is not an adequate reason to retard the dissemination and implementation of current knowledge concerning longevity. In his excellent book, *The American Way of Life Need Not be Hazardous to Your Health,* John Farquhar urges:

> Thus we should continue to support basic research while simultaneously implementing our best efforts for appropriate preventive measures, rather than sit passively and wait for basic research to yield conclusive findings on *all* facets of the complex puzzle. The combination of a normal lag and 'let's wait' attitude can erect impressive barriers to preventive action.[60]

Measures conducive to the enhancement of the quality and quantity of human life are noninvasive, with a low risk factor and an extremely positive potential. Virtually all the measures conducive to longevity adhere to the most fundamental tenet of the Hippocratic oath: *Primum nil nocere,* or "do no harm." The reason such measures continue to be overlooked is due to economics and politics.

More important than the incidence of longevity in isolated geographic regions is its incidence throughout history in all regions and, increasingly, in the United States at the present time. This pervasive incidence indicates a biological potential of the human species. Centenarian individuals represent a living prototype that is both predicted and supported by laboratory and observational research. The instances of longevity evident in every region of the world and throughout history show a latent biological potential that may become manifest in the next evolutionary stage of the human species.

NOTES

1. Alexander Leaf, 1978: personal communication.

2. Alexander Leaf, "Every Day Is a Gift When You Are Over 100," *National Geographic* 143, no. 1 (1973): 93–119.

3. Alexander Leaf, "Getting Old," *Scientific American,* September 1973, pp. 45–52.

4. Alexander Leaf, "Unusual Longevity: The Common Denominators," *Hospital Practice,* October 1973, pp. 75–68.

5. M. Salvador, *Vilcabamba: Tierra de longevos* (Quito, Ecuador: Casa de la Cultura, 1972).

6. R.B. Mazess and S.H. Forman, "Longevity and Age Exaggeration in Vilcabamba, Equador," *Journal of Gerontology,* 34, no. 1 (1979): 94–98.

7. R.J. Myers, "Overstatement of Census Age," *Demography* 3, no. 2 (1966).

8. I. Rosenwaike, "On Measuring the Extreme Aged in the Population," *Journal of the Statistical Association* 63 (1968): 29–40.

9. W.C. McKain, "Are They Really That Old?" *Gerontologist* 7 (1967): 70–80.

10. Z.A. Medvedev, "Caucasus and Altay Longevity: A Biological or Social Problem," *Gerontologist* 14, no. 5 (1974): 381–387.

11. R.J. Myers, "Analysis of Mortality in the Soviet Union According to 1958–59 Life Tables," *Transaction of Society of Actuaries* 16 (1965): 309–317.

12. Alexander Leaf, "Unusual Longevity: The Common Denominators," *op. cit.*, pp. 75–68.

13. *Ibid.*, pp. 75–68.

14. R.B. Mazess, "Bone Mineral in Vilcabamba, Ecuador," *American Journal of Roentgenology* 130 (April 1978): 671–674.

15. Alexander Leaf, 1980: personal communication.

16. D. Sobel, "Proof of Age," *OMNI,* October 1979, p. 53.

17. Alexander Leaf, "Unusual Longevity: The Common Denominators," *op. cit.*, pp. 75–68.

18. *Ibid.*, pp. 75–68.

19. E. Hammond, L. Garfinkel, and H. Seidman, "Longevity of Parents and Grandparents in Relation to Coronary Heart Disease and Associated Variables," *Circulation* 43, no. 1 (January 1971): 31–44.

20. *Ibid.*, pp. 31–44.

21. *Ibid.*, pp. 31–44.

22. Alexander Leaf, "Observations of a Peripatetic Gerontologist," *Nutrition Today,* September–October 1973, pp. 4–12.

23. D. Davies, "A Shangri-la in Ecuador," *New Scientist,* February 1, 1973, pp. 104–106.

24. Renee Taylor, *Hunza Health Secrets for Long Life and Happiness,* (Dallas, Tx: Keats Publishing Co., 1964).

25. Alexander Leaf, "Unusual Longevity: The Common Denominators," *op. cit.*, pp. 75–68.

26. P.E. Segall, H. Ooka, K. Rose, and P.S. Timiras, "Neural and Endocrine Development after Chronic Tryptophan Deficiency in Rats: Brain Monoamine and Pituitary Responses," *Mechanisms of Aging and Development* 7 (1978): 1–17.

27. P.E. Segall, "Interrelations of Dietary and Hormonal Effects in Aging," *Mechanisms of Ageing and Development* 9, no. 5–6 (1979): 515–525.

28. Alexander Leaf, "Unusual Longevity: The Common Denominators," *op. cit.*, pp. 75–68.

29. *Ibid.*, pp. 75–68.

30. Alexander Leaf, "Observations of a Peripatetic Gerontologist," *op. cit.*, pp. 4–12.

31. *Ibid.*, pp. 4–12.

32. Alexander Leaf, "Unusual Longevity: The Common Denominators," *op. cit.*, pp. 75–68.

33. *Ibid.*, pp. 75–68.

34. D. Davies, *op. cit.*, pp. 104–106.

35. M. Woodfin, "Want to See 140? Don't Boil the Tea," *The Denver Post,* 3 December 1978.

36. A.R. Favassa, "The Day of Our Years," *M.D.,* October 1977, pp. 19–101.

37. D. Davies, *op. cit.*, pp. 104–106.

38. Alexander Leaf, "Unusual Longevity: The Common Denominators," *op. cit.*, pp. 75–68.

39. N.K. Witte, W.W. Kryshanowskaja, and E.I. Steshenskaya, "The Process of Aging in the Light of Work Physiology," *Zeitschrift fur Alternsforshung* 20, no. 2 (1967): 91–98.

40. Alexander Leaf, "Observations of a Peripatetic Gerontologist," *op. cit.*, pp. 4–12.

41. Alexander Leaf, "On the Physical Fitness of Men who Live to a Great Age," *Executive Health* 13, no. II (August 1977).

42. *Ibid.*

43. R.N. Butler, *Why Survive? Being Old in America* (New York: Harper and Row, 1975).

44. *Ibid.*

45. Alexander Leaf, "Unusual Longevity: The Common Denominators," *op. cit.*, pp. 75–68.

46. Alexander Leaf, "Every Day is a Gift When You are Over 100," *op. cit.*, pp. 93–119.

47. S. Benet, *Abkhasians: The Long Living People of the Caucasus* (New York: HREW: 1965).

48. S. Wolf, "Presidential Address: Social Anthropology in Medicine. The Climate You and I Create," *Trans-American Clinical and Climatological Association* 88 (1977): 1–17.

49. Alexander Leaf, "Unusual Longevity: The Common Denominators," *op. cit.*, pp. 75–68.

50. L.S. Libow, "Interaction of Medical, Biologic, and Behavioral Factors on Aging, Adaptation, and Survival: An 11-year Longitudinal Study," *Geriatrics,* November 1974, pp. 75–88.

51. *Ibid.,* pp. 75–88.

52. E.B. Palmore and W. Cleveland, "Aging, Terminal Decline, and Terminal Drop," *Journal of Gerontology* 31, no. 1 (1976): 76–81.

53. B.D. Bell, "Cognitive Dissonance and the Life Satisfaction of Older Adults," *Journal of Gerontology* 29, no. 5 (1974): 564–571.

54. G.L. Maddox and E.B. Douglass, "Aging and Individual Differences: A Longitudinal Analysis of Social, Psychological and Physiological Indicators," *Journal of Gerontology* 29, no. 5 (1974): 555–563.

55. M. Stanyan, "Secrets of Long Life from the Andes," *San Francisco Examiner and Chronicle,* 26 September 1976: 3.

56. Alexander Leaf, "Unusual Longevity: The Common Denominators," *op. cit.*, pp. 75–68.

57. M.C. Diamond, "Using Your Brains," *The Independent and Gazette,* Berkeley, California, 13 February 1980: 3.

58. A. Goodman, "Secret of the Old Ones," *The Berkeley Barb,* September 20–October 3, 1979, p. 4.

59. "176 Year-Old Woman with Baby Teeth," *San Francisco Chronicle,* 23 November 1978: 12.

60. J.W. Farquhar, "Stress and How to Cope with It," *The Stanford Alumni Magazine,* Fall/Winter, 1977.

Chapter 14

Designing Health Promotion Programs for Elders*

Stephanie FallCreek, D.S.W.
Anne Warner-Reitz, B.A.
Molly H. Mettler, M.S.W.

In this chapter, the practical question of how to develop health promotion services is addressed. Three important steps in the development process—building a base of operations, program design, and program evaluation—are highlighted in this discussion, which is based primarily on the authors' experiences with several health promotion projects:

- the Healthy Lifestyles for Seniors project—Santa Monica, California
- the Wallingford Wellness Project—Seattle, Washington
- the Santa Monica City Senior Nutrition and Recreation Program—Santa Monica, California
- the state-wide Health Promotion with Elders project—New Mexico

The authors also incorporate, wherever possible, knowledge gained from the experiences of others who have developed and delivered successful health promotion programs in other locations. Every health promotion program must respond to the unique context within which it is developed. Consequently, the strategy that best utilizes available resources to meet the needs of the target population and the goals of the sponsoring organization(s) is somewhat different in each setting.

BUILDING A BASE OF OPERATIONS

The first phase of planning a health promotion program includes the following steps: identifying the resources of the sponsoring organization(s), identifying the

*This chapter was based on material that appeared in *Healthy Lifestyle for Seniors: An Interdisciplinary Approach to Healthy Aging* by Anne Warner-Reitz and Carolyn Grothe, Meals for Millions/ Freedom from Hunger Foundation, New York, © 1981; and *A Healthy Old Age* by Stephanie FallCreek and Molly H. Mettler, Haworth Press, © 1984.

target population(s), and locating additional needed resources in the community. In theory, these steps occur sequentially; however, the constraints of time, staff commitment level, and available resources for the planning phase often dictate that they occur simultaneously. Each is important, however, if planner and sponsors are to obtain the information needed to develop a practical program that responds to consumers' needs and interests. The planning process also begins to establish the links between existing aging network and health network services that will eventually secure a place for ongoing and growing health promotion activities.

Defining the Sponsor's Resources

The goals and resources of the program's sponsors, as well as the expertise of the staff, determine the degree to which program planners can respond to the community's needs. If the sponsor's mandate is a limited one—to improve nutrition among the elderly, for example—program planners need to concentrate on nutrition education, even when other health education needs have been identified. The greater the sponsor's expertise, resources, and openness to various kinds of intervention, the greater will be the ability of program planners to respond to the community's needs.

The inception of the Healthy Lifestyles for Seniors (HLS) program as an integral part of the Meals for Millions/Freedom from Hunger Foundation (MFM/FFH), its sponsoring organization, is an example of a skillful linkage of health promotion to the sponsoring organization's purpose and resources. MFM/FFH is dedicated to strengthening the capabilities of communities to solve their own food and nutrition problems, thereby advancing the self-help approach to achieve lasting behavioral change. Emphasis is placed on the health and nutritional needs of special at-risk groups: elders, infants, children, and pregnant and lactating women.

In 1977, the MFM/FFH Foundation initiated a survey of the health and nutrition needs of elders in its home community of Santa Monica, California. Program planners quickly located Community Chest and United Way studies of the aged living in the west side of Los Angeles documenting health and nutrition as top priority needs. Local providers, including the staff of a health screening clinic for elders, supported these findings. However, the clinic staff and the MFM/FFH program planners agreed that nutrition education alone would not be sufficient to affect nutritional status and the other nutrition-related chronic health problems common to this age group, such as heart disease and diabetes. Instead, it was agreed that an intensive interdisciplinary program was needed to break the circular pattern of unhappy and unhealthy aging that resulted in and from poor nutritional intake, lack of physical and social activity, depression, and chronic disease. Based on these findings, program planners proposed the HLS program, an intensive interdisciplinary health promotion approach to meeting the health and nutrition needs of elders. The acceptance of the proposal marked a new direction for the foundation, as HLS was the first project it had undertaken with elders.

The Santa Monica Senior Nutrition and Recreation Program, sponsored by the City of Santa Monica and funded in part through Title III of the Older Americans Act, provides hot noon meals for elders, as well as a range of recreational and ˙ educational activities. The introduction of health promotion programming to the Santa Monica Senior Nutrition and Recreation Program was a less complex task than proposing Healthy Lifestyles for Seniors to the Meals for Millions/Freedom from Hunger Foundation. Health promotion activities were seen as a welcome addition by the city's administrative staff and the program's participants. The challenge of the nutrition program was to provide educational and recreational services without any additional funds. As is discussed below, this challenge was met by a creative use of community resources.

In contrast, the Wallingford Wellness Project (WWP) was sponsored by a grant from the Administration on Aging. Its program planners were specifically mandated to develop and evaluate a multifaceted health promotion program, which addressed physical fitness, nutrition, stress management, and communication skills for elders living independently in the community. The joint university-community-based organizational auspices of the project not only provided great flexibility for program design—reinforcing its innovative approach—but also a valuable pool of expertise on which to draw. Program planners were relatively free to design the program of their choice, within the limits of time and money. The planning and implementing staff chose to emphasize self-determination and personal empowerment. One of the challenges presented by this form of sponsorship was the requirement that a significant portion of available resources—approximately 30 to 40 percent—be expended on evaluation.

The New Mexico Health Promotion with Elders project is sponsored by the state agency on aging with a legislative appropriation from the state. It is a two-pronged program that focuses both on directly promoting fitness of elders and on training elders as "health promotion specialists." These elder health promotion specialists are recruited from low-income elders over 55 years of age. Because the ultimate objective is to develop in the elder health promotion specialists the skills and confidence needed to implement fitness programs in their own communities, the content of the training program and the intervention method were already set, at least in part. The resources available from the sponsoring agency, in addition to financial resources, include a state-wide network of staff in the field of aging, contacts with representatives of a variety of agencies and organizations, the considerable social and political influence that may be exercised by a state agency, and available data about the needs and interests of the target populations.

Identifying the Target Population

A successful health promotion program must be designed to meet the unique needs of its target population; for example, the hypertensive elderly, poor rural elders, those living independently, or some combination of the above. Recruitment tactics, promotional materials, curriculum, and evaluation are influenced by the target population's age range, health status and needs, ethnic heritage, religion, socioeconomic status, and educational sophistication. The target population's relationship to the existing health care delivery system, as well as their receptivity to new ideas and to program participation, should also be taken into account. For example, when developing a program in a community that historically has had a hostile relationship with publicly funded health care service, it may be unwise to locate the program in the public health department offices or to rely heavily on public health staff to provide initial educational programs. Or if one's target population includes elders who have been isolated from the mainstream of human services due to sociocultural discrimination, intensive outreach efforts and a curriculum that incorporates their traditions, beliefs, and values may be needed. Utilizing traditional health care providers—for example, an herbalist or a *curandera*—as recruiters may prove effective.

At the same time, if relatively healthy, independent, socially active elders are one's target, their interests, abilities, and gathering places also must be identified. It is important to recognize that members of any target group—however disabled, poor, isolated, well-educated or healthy they may be—have unique contributions to make in terms of experience, skills, and knowledge. The program design must take into account these aspects of the target population as well.

The Healthy Lifestyles for Seniors (HLS) program was originally targeted for high-risk, motivated elders. Consequently, an intensive, multifaceted approach that sought behavioral changes leading to health status changes was a viable one. The participants in the program met twice weekly for 3½ hours each for a six-month period. During the first hour of each session, individual health monitoring interviews were scheduled with the nurse practitioner. The remaining 2½ hours consisted of group nutrition or stress management sessions and yoga and aerobic exercise sessions.

As the target population of the HLS program was expanded to include less motivated individuals, the intensity of the schedule and the goals were modified to meet these individuals' level of interest and commitment.

The health promotion program sponsored by the Santa Monica Senior Nutrition and Recreation Program was targeted for a group of individuals who came to the nutrition program primarily for a hot meal and for socialization. Although these individuals were keenly aware of their health problems, most were not interested in devoting much time to self-help activities. This lack of interest was evidenced when they bypassed the opportunity to participate in the HLS program and by the fact that they rarely joined in the other educational and recreational opportunities available through the city's recreation and parks department and through the local college for elders. To stimulate their interest in health-related programming, a survey was conducted that asked them to identify their foremost health concerns.

Based on these findings, six hour-long sessions, held either directly before or after the meal, were planned for a six-month period. The purpose of each presentation was to provide information about the subject—be it memory loss, eye care or arthritis—to suggest two or three self-help activities that could improve or prevent the problem, and to provide information on where to obtain more intensive help if needed. The intensive schedule of the HLS program represents one end of the spectrum of health promotion programming, and the Senior Nutrition Program represents the other. However, the design of each program was appropriate to the level of interest of each target group.

The original target population of the Wallingford Wellness Project (WWP) was the high-risk, over-75 age group of elders. As with the HLS program, the WWP approach to this population was intensive and broad, meeting over a four- to six-month period for one to three hours per week. Participants recruited in the first three cohorts differed from the target group as originally identified. Their median age was 71, and their health status ranged from excellent to extremely disabled. These results of recruitment efforts suggest the following possibilities: Planners may not have recruited appropriately for the target age group; the program may have been designed to attract younger, rather than older, elders; or the over-75 group may simply be slower to enter such an innovative program as the WWP. Interestingly, as the program trained new groups, the health status at entry was significantly lower with each group although the target population defined by staff did not change.

The New Mexico Health Promotion with Elders project is directed toward a diverse target population. In order to reach the multicultural, geographically dispersed older population of the state, a "shot gun" strategy is employed. Older people, including paid staff, volunteers, and consumers, as well as some non-elderly service providers, take part in the training sessions. The emphasis is on training older people to establish local health promotion activities for their peers. Because many of these peer trainers are unfamiliar with the concept of health promotion, speak limited English, and have culturally distinct health values, beliefs and practices, the training program must be very flexible and staff must be sensitive to cultural differences and able to think and respond very quickly "on their feet."

Surveying Community Resources

Surveying local services, such as community clinics, the visiting nurse service, senior centers, and day care facilities, provides valuable information about the health needs and concerns of the community's elders and their use of existing services. Providers can also help identify gaps in the existing services that might be addressed by a health promotion program, as well as potential community resources, such as funders, providers, and volunteers. Input from a health screening clinic for elders, for example, played a significant role in shaping the HLS program. The screening revealed that a majority of elders were suffering from chronic degenerative diseases, many of which were exacerbated, if not caused, by life-style factors, such as a poor adaptation to change. Clinic staff recognized the need for an intensive and integrated program—one that would provide training and support in these individual but interrelated life-style areas—but were unable to provide such a program at the time. The clinic was therefore pleased to work out a collaborative agreement with the HLS staff. The HLS program agreed to accept clinic-referred participants into their program, and the clinic agreed to provide free health screening examinations to HLS participants. In addition, when participants completed the HLS program, they were referred to the clinic for follow-up examinations and activities.

As mentioned previously, the challenge of the Santa Monica Nutrition and Recreation Program was to provide health promotion activities without the use of additional funds. Program staff were able to accomplish this by linking the needs of the nutrition program to the mandates of several provider organizations in the community: two local (and competitive) hospitals, a county medicine education program, professional nurses bureau, and a health screening clinic. After conducting a survey of participants' health concerns, the project director contacted the patient and community education department of the two hospitals. One of the hospital departments, which was coincidentally staffed by two health promotion enthusiasts, was recently mandated by its board to provide community health education for elders. The hospital was currently conducting forums at the hospital in the afternoons and evenings, but attendance was low. The hospital staff quickly saw the advantages of offering forums at the nutrition sites. Based on their interest and resources, the hospital selected two of the health concerns identified in the nutrition program survey and agreed to arrange for hospital physicians to present hour-long presentations at each of the four sites. Everyone benefited from these programs; the participants felt that the information presented was interesting and useful, the hospital received recognition for its contribution, and the physicians distributed their business cards to several participants who requested them. The hospital was so pleased with the outcome that, after their presentations on eye care, they offered to return to the sites for free glaucoma testing. Likewise, the other service providers mentioned above selected one or two of the health problems identified in the survey and gave presentations at the sites. Thus, 24 hours of health education programs were provided at no additional cost to the sponsoring agency. It should be noted, however, that the project director spent a considerable amount of time coordinating and publicizing the programs.

Although the Wallingford Wellness Project (WWP) core staff had the expertise and time available to lead the basic class in the program, outside resources enriched and strengthened the program offerings. Other social and health service providers were informed of the WWP and brought "on board" through at least three strategies. First, staff interviewed many service providers in the Seattle target area before designing the program. Face-to-face or telephone interviews were conducted to share information about WWP plans with providers, to solicit assistance from them with recruitment, to invite them to attend the program themselves, and to identify possible resources for future activities. Second, a public informational meeting about the WWP was presented specifically for service providers in the target area. Third, information provided by program participants and colleagues at the University of Washington brought staff together with service providers, such as dental hygienists, public health department staff, and community health practitioners who had not previously been contacted. The service providers served as valuable resources in many ways: They offered guest lectures to the classes in their area of special expertise, they recruited participants for the program, they provided service to program participants who needed assistance not offered by the program, and they improved the program's public image through both formal and informal (personal) communications.

Another very important community resource for the WWP was the university. Both graduate and undergraduate students did practicum or intern placements with the program. These students provided time, energy, enthusiasm, and their own special brand of expertise to the program. Their services enabled the WWP to provide much more individualized attention than otherwise would have been possible. They also "co-facilitated" classes with core staff, contributing to the participatory teaching-learning philosophy that provided the foundation for the project's classes. Student participation varied from cohort to cohort, with two to six students involved at different points in the project.

The New Mexico Health Promotion with Elders project also relies on outside resources to enhance program activities. In many respects, New Mexico faces unique challenges—a very low-income elder population, tremendous ethnic and cultural diversity, a rapid rural-to-urban transition in several areas, and a widely dispersed rural elderly population in most of the state. In combination with a scarcity of community resources for social and health services generally, these factors force health promoters to be creative, flexible, and diligent in their identification and utilization of community resources, particularly the use of volunteers.

Because training is short-term—(two 2-day workshops with telephone follow-ups for most participants—and is conducted by outside staff, elder health promotion specialists must depend on the resources of the home communities to implement programs. The elder trainers focus on physical fitness and utilize other local resources for different aspects of health promotion. Because every community and every community's elders are different, the resources available and those utilized also vary tremendously. Most trainers have secured space and some minimal program support from local senior centers. Nursing homes, churches, tribal community centers, or public schools also provide sites. Because local financial support is extremely limited, these programs function with the barest essentials, perhaps not even a telephone or phonograph at some of the more remote sites. Public health nurses are a resource for several aspects of the programs, providing blood pressure screening, weight control, and smoking cessation classes, for example. Cooperative extension specialists or home economists provide nutrition education or assistance with menu planning or food budgeting concerns.

As can be seen in the examples above, an initial survey of the community's resources is ideal; it lays the basis for future collaborative efforts and for mutual referrals, and it helps establish a niche for the program within the network of respected community health delivery services. It is also important to consider some of the nontraditional health services in a resource identification effort. Health clubs, adult education programs, preretirement program providers, cable intensive stations, and public libraries are among the many possible sites and sources of support.

If resources are not available to conduct an organized survey of available resources, health promotion planners and providers simply must make a conscious and ongoing effort to identify and involve those other individuals and organizations in the area that contribute time, fiscal support, and personal expertise to health promotion activities. As the program grows and becomes visible, new resources for support and assistance will become known and available.

PROGRAM DESIGN

The program's design should be based, at least in part, on the information gathered during the needs and resources assessment. Components of program design include budget, time frame, philosophy, goals and objectives, curriculum, schedule and educational approach, staffing, site selection, recruitment and screening, and insurance and release forms.

Budget

Funds may be obtained through government grants, private foundations, churches, individual donors, clients paying for services, and fund-raising events. However, care must be taken when generating cash by charging participants a fee for service. Usually, the elders most in need of preventive health services live on limited incomes. When funding is limited, program planners need to rely almost entirely on already existing community resources, such as the hospital; local colleges; the city's department of recreation and parks; voluntary organizations, such as the heart and lung associations, and by training volunteers. By coordinating these resources, a health promotion program can be offered at minimal cost, as was illustrated in the example of the Santa Monica Senior Nutrition and Recreation Program.

In-kind contributions can also be very important. Although cash support may not be forthcoming, local businesses, service clubs, and special interest organizations often provide valuable program support. For example, the local newspaper can cover activities, thus assisting with recruiting. Or they could "publicize" the program's need for supplies, equipment, or volunteer time, thereby reaching an audience not typically accessible to solicitation. Service clubs often provide support related to their unique organizational objectives, if the program planner is specific in making requests. For example, approaching the "Lion's Club" for support for classes that address visual impairment remedies and prevention strategies is likely to meet with success, whereas a request for general nutrition education support may be less well received. Special interest organizations, such as the Heart Association or the American Cancer Society, are sources both for materials (handouts, posters, etc.) and expertise (volunteer presentations on a variety of topics). In sum, when seeking support for program activities, it is best to tailor requests to the needs, interests and available resources of the potential sponsoring source.

Time Frame

The three major phases of a program are planning, implementation, and evaluation. Once a program is underway, these three phases may take place simultaneously. The first time a program is implemented, however, it is important to set aside two to four months for planning. Tasks during this initial planning stage typically include conducting a needs assessment, recruiting staff, defining the program philosophy, setting goals, developing the curriculum and evaluation methodology, fund raising, budgeting, site selection, participant recruitment, and screening.

Sometimes a small successful program—one that begins with 5 or 10 participants and achieves its realistic educational and behavioral objectives—can help inspire local enthusiasm and build the community support that is needed to secure resources for a more extensive program. Developing community advocates is a critical aspect of building the program into a solid community-based service. Starting small also provides the opportunity to refine and improve the program design before involving large numbers of participants.

Philosophy

The evolution of both the HLS and the WWP's philosophies, and the consequent development of their program approaches, was a professionally exciting and personally rewarding experience for the staff. Rather than working on their individual components in an isolated way, staff became a team working together toward a common goal. In the HLS project, for example, each staff member was responsible for developing and implementing the curriculum of a particular program component. In both programs, a considerable amount of time was spent sharing experiences, giving feedback, and brainstorming new activities and approaches. The teamwork that grew out of these frequent meetings resulted in the staff's increased awareness of the content, characteristics, and special problems of each of the program components. As staff members saw how their individual components fit into the whole and how component activities could be mutually supportive, they were better able to assess and respond to participants' needs. As they shared their perceptions of individual participants, behavior patterns became apparent that might otherwise have gone unnoticed. The staff even applied this understanding of behavior patterns to their own actions. In the HLS project, for example, as the nurse practitioner learned more about diet and the physiological and psychological consequences of too much stress, she not only was able to offer participants a more complete understanding of the risk factors associated with heart disease but she also began to lose weight and to cut out some of the activities in her life that were causing headaches and excess irritability.

Participants also benefited from this integrated and evolving philosophy and approach. Just as staff did not view the program components as isolated units, so participants came to understand and experience the individual components of the program as various dimensions of one movement toward better health. As they sensed the unifying purpose behind activities, participants were more willing to try new ideas and behaviors and to benefit from their synergistic health-promoting effect.

Goals and Objectives

Program goals and objectives should reflect health improvements that participants can realistically achieve, given their health status and motivation to change. Although staff can establish overall program goals, it is preferable that participants set individual objectives for themselves. The more that participants take responsibility for deciding the changes that they wish to make, the greater will be their motivation and commitment to making those changes. For example, as part of the WWP nutrition curriculum, participants fill out contracts with individual goals for dietary change. Contracts specify the goals about salt, fat, sugar, and complex carbohydrate intake and how participants will reward themselves for achieving their goals.

Regular monitoring of progress is an important part of helping participants achieve their goals.

Curriculum, Schedule, and Educational Approach

Ideally, health promotion programs are comprehensive, addressing more than one issue or focusing on more than one area of health. Program components that are often included successfully in a health promotion program are nutrition, physical fitness, stress management, health monitoring, communication skills, environmental awareness and action, and a variety of special interest health topics, such as accident protection, foot care, hypertension, substance abuse, and common health concerns. Such programs speak to the individual in his or her wholeness as an integrated body, mind, and spirit. This integration facilitates a synergism that increases participants' motivation, strengthens the effectiveness of each component, and results in more rapid and greater improvements in health.

The duration and intensity of a program are determined by the resources of the sponsors, the receptivity of the target population, and the range and depth of the program goals. When participants are motivated to make life-style changes and sufficient funds are available, an intensive multifaceted course, such as the HLS program or WWP, is appropriate. When, as is more typical, the target population is less motivated, it is wise to design a shorter, more limited course, perhaps lasting three or four sessions. Building on the success of a low-key program, planners might then design an intermediate-level course for those individuals who are ready to make a greater commitment. For example, an intermediate-level follow-up to a senior nutrition course might be a four-week course on how diet and exercise can alleviate arthritis, heart disease, and depression.

Regardless of the program's structure and intensity, it is most effective to use a combination of didactic and experiential educational strategies. Short lectures, perhaps 10 to 20 minutes in length, followed by discussion provide participants with a base of health information and the rationale behind proposed attitudinal and behavioral changes. Group discussions encourage participants to learn from and support one another, thereby promoting socialization. Experiential exercises provide participants with an opportunity to try out new behaviors. Positive experiences in the classroom are an important component of helping participants integrate these behaviors into their lives.

For example, the HLS sessions on assertion—part of the stress management component—illustrate this educational approach. The leader opens the session by introducing the concept of assertion, the benefits of assertive behavior, and the personal and health problems associated with nonassertive behavior. Participants formulate a group definition of assertiveness and give examples of assertive and nonassertive behavior. Leaders may need to help the group distinguish between assertion and aggression. A brief pencil-and-paper exercise follows that helps participants identify whether, when, and with whom they are assertive. Another exercise helps them identify and evaluate lifelong beliefs that may block assertive behavior, such as "it is selfish to put your needs before others' needs." Group discussions in which participants share personal experiences are encouraged after each exercise. Such discussions may become very emotionally charged, as participants recount situations in which they were assertive (or aggressive) or in which they felt taken advantage of. Leaders must guide the group in a way to support these individuals without letting them monopolize the discussion. To end the session, participants are given an outline that summarizes the day's discussion: a definition of assertion, getting in touch with one's feelings, exploring options for expressing one's self, the benefits of assertion, and situations in which assertive behavior is appropriate. For homework, participants are asked to note when they do and do not assert themselves effectively. They are asked to practice asserting themselves in low-risk situations and to say "no" when they would normally say "yes," even if they wanted to say the opposite.

A New York-based HLS program—modeled after the Santa Monica HLS program and sponsored by the State University of New York at Binghamton— conducted a research study comparing a solely didactic approach with one that included both didactic and experiential sessions. Participants of the group that received both the experiential and didactic sessions demonstrated greater behavioral and physiological changes and reported greater satisfaction with the program.

Staffing

Health promotion programs are staffed in a variety of ways. Staffing patterns are influenced by available funds, by the expertise required to accomplish program goals and to administer specific program components, and by the target populations' attitudes toward service providers. Training community members to administer the program, for example, may reduce service delivery barriers in a program targeted for minority elders and may also be less costly than employing a paid professional staff.

The WWP successfully trained enthusiastic program graduates to facilitate alumni groups, as well as to teach courses on their own. The HLS staff helped train a group of senior peer health advocates to provide individual and group instruction in nutrition, exercise, and stress management at the local health screening clinic.

Staff members should possess the following abilities and characteristics (1) expertise, or the ability to gain expertise in their content areas; (2) sensitivity to older people; (3) the ability to work as team members; (4) involvement in their personal health processes; and (5) friendliness, compassion, and respect toward all people involved in the program.

Site Selection

Health promotion programs can easily and successfully take place in a large variety of sites. Potential sites include locations where seniors already congregate—senior centers, senior nutrition sites, residential facilities—as well as locations where seniors can be brought together, such as the YMCA, the YWCA, and community rooms in banks, malls, or churches.

The staff of the HLS and WWP programs found that the managers at senior residential projects and senior recreation centers were receptive to providing the space for health promotion programs. Health promotion adds something special to the facility's existing program at little or no cost. Frequently, the managers publicized the program through their monthly newsletters. Often, janitorial services were provided.

Factors that should be taken into consideration in selecting a site include its size, accessibility, safety, physical layout, opportunity for privacy and for quiet, and availability of equipment and support personnel.

Recruitment and Screening

A comprehensive recruitment plan uses tactics that quickly and easily arouse the interests of the target group and help build community support for the program.

The most effective outreach efforts in the HLS and WWP programs included brief presentations to senior groups, contacts with local providers, and articles in local newspapers and senior bulletins. Person-to-person contact with seniors is the easiest way to build enthusiasm and interest, especially in groups that might otherwise not be interested in health programs. Personal contact with providers helps them better understand the scope of the program's services and also helps dissolve turf issues before they grow out of proportion. Newspaper articles are the easiest way to reach those elders who are currently not involved in the mainstream senior activities and services.

Once the target population parameters have been identified, a one-page newsletter should be developed, outlining the program goals and philosophy, the needs and attributes of the desired participants, program sponsorship, and location and schedule. These flyers should be distributed at recruitment talks, posted at key locations, and mailed to agencies and individuals. Once the program is underway, participants and local providers become enthusiastic referral sources, and recruitment becomes increasingly easy and less time-consuming.

It is often necessary to develop screening procedures to determine candidates' suitability for the program. Selection criteria may be based on such factors as age, health status, readiness and motivation to change, commitment, income, and ability to provide necessary personal and physician release forms. Candidates may be asked, for example, to fill out a screening questionnaire and be notified as to their eligibility by phone or by mail. A more personal procedure would be to interview them by phone or in person.

Insurance and Release Forms

The purpose of carrying insurance is to protect the assets of the sponsoring organization and to protect the employees and the participants of the program. The sponsoring organization can insure itself in two ways: by taking preventive measures that minimize its exposure to liability ("lessening exposure") and by carrying appropriate insurance policies, some of which are mandatory by law.

Lessening exposure can be accomplished through participant screening procedures and appropriate release forms. In the HLS model, each participant has a preprogram health screening examination. All participants are required to sign a program release-from-liability form; physician release forms are obtained when possible. Although such measures are not always legally binding, they demonstrate that care and precaution have been taken to provide for participants' safety.

To further protect the employees, participants, and the sponsoring organization, four types of insurance should be considered: worker's compensation, health and welfare, general liability, and malpractice. It is good practice to have an independent insurance broker, rather than a single company agent, help secure the most appropriate coverage.

PROGRAM EVALUATION

There are several reasons to evaluate a program, the primary one being to improve it. A successful evaluation assesses the degree to which the program is accomplishing its objectives and points to weaknesses that can be modified to improve it. A second reason for evaluating a program is to ensure participants' safety. This is especially important when working with a high-risk group, such as elders. Information obtained from a preprogram health screening examination, for example, serves the dual purpose of providing baseline data and alerting staff to health problems that need immediate attention or ongoing monitoring. Finally, an evaluation demonstrates the program's effectiveness to funding agencies. Although this is not always necessary, it is often an asset when submitting future proposals.

The range and sophistication of an evaluation depend on several factors: funding, staff expertise, program goals, the target population, the setting, and the needs of the sponsoring organization. A community-based program with limited funding, for example, might focus on easy-to-measure parameters, such as changes in health knowledge, physiology (e.g., weight and blood pressure), and behavior (e.g., time spent exercising). A university-based research project might evaluate more elusive parameters, including attitudinal change or long-term variables, such as the program's effect on the number of doctor visits and medical expenditures.

A variety of instruments and procedures, such as blood pressure and weight measures, health risk assessments, knowledge questionnaires, attitude scales, and exercise logs, can be used to assess participants' changes. Pre- and postprogram self-report questionnaires and interviews can supplement such data. Whenever possible, evaluation tools should serve an educational function. Keeping a food journal and setting goals for nutritional change at the beginning of the program, for example, can provide participants with an opportunity to take a critical look at their diets.

Administering evaluation instruments calls for flexibility. Participants with limited education, impaired vision, and physical disabilities or for whom English is a second language, may require special assistance in completing some reports.

CONCLUSION

For many persons, health promotion for elders is an essential and viable alternative to the increasing physical and mental disease or disability, institutionalization, and the tremendous waste of human potential that occurs when people do not know how to take actions that promote healthy aging. At a time when the political and economic climate is stifling social and preventive health programs, it is especially important for advocates and providers of health promotion services to persevere in their efforts. A creative use of existing resources, efforts to influence legislation and to secure insurance coverage for preventive health services, conclusive and well-researched articles and proposals backed by documentation of program benefits, and the networking of all those interested and involved in health promotion for elders will help keep this important movement alive and growing.

Chapter 15

The Dartmouth Self-Care for Senior Citizens Program: Tools, Strategies, and Methods

Jeannette J. Simmons, D.Sc.
Ellen Roberts, M.P.H.
Eugene C. Nelson, D.Sc., M.P.H.

As Lowell and Levin states, self care is "a process whereby a lay person can function effectively on his or her own behalf in health promotion and decision-making, in disease prevention, detection, and treatment at the level of the primary health resource in the health care system."[1] Taking care of one's own health (self-care) has been a part of cultural traditions throughout recorded history, and in comtemporary American society, many groups encourage self-care. The drug industry uses all forms of mass media to promote the sale of nonprescription medications and vitamins for common ailments. Home medical tests for pregnancy, blood pressure, diabetes, and other conditions are widely advertised. Advice on how to maintain and improve health appears in books, popular magazines, and newspapers. Some television programs include a regular commentary by a physician. An ever-increasing number of self-help groups are being formed for specific health problems. The number of such groups in the United States was estimated by Katz and Bender to be several hundred thousand.[2] According to Butler, only a few self-care groups have been designed specifically for the elderly, although many of the other groups are appropriate for their needs.[3] Programs and studies on self-care for the older adult, which have been described in the professional literature from 1982–1985, range from information and skill training programs for a specific illness to problems expressed by patients trying to manage a chronic disease. There have been fewer descriptions of health promotion programs for older adults; most emphasize exercise and nutrition.

Although the number of community self-care programs is growing, only a few have been evaluated under controlled conditions to assess their effect.[4,5,6] The program described in this chapter is designed specifically for the elderly and was evaluated under controlled conditions to assess the effect of medical self-care education on health knowledge, self-care skills, life style, utilization of health and social services, functional health, and life quality of older persons.

The Self-Care for Senior Citizens Program (SCSC), developed and sponsored by the Dartmouth Institute for Better Health (DIBH), a nonprofit organization based at Dartmouth Medical School in Hanover, New Hampshire, is a comprehensive self-care program. Its overall aim is to promote intelligent self-reliance in health and social areas by helping the elderly help themselves to achieve better physical and mental health, to make judicious use of the health and social service system, and to maintain their capacity for independent living. Its specific objectives are to educate seniors in medical self-care, illness prevention, and appropriate use of health and human services.

HISTORY

The SCSC Program grew out of a series of community self-care courses that were first offered to the community at large and later tailored to the needs of older adults. To test whether the popular educational sessions had a positive effect on the participants' confidence and ability to apply self-care skills, a research and demonstration program was funded for three years by the Administration on Aging.

Two communities in New Hampshire—Manchester and Nashua—were selected as test and control communities, respectively. The communities provided DIBH two geographically close research sites and a good mix of health, social service, and aging networks to test the community program. The research and demonstration project began in July 1979 in Manchester and the surrounding rural area. In 1981, the SCSC project was transplanted to Miami, Florida, to test its adaptability to an urban area.

Participants for the study were self-selected. They had to meet the following criteria: be 60 years of age or older, consent to be interviewed three times during a 12-month period, be willing to participate in an educational experience, and be physically able to attend classes. The preenrollment interview provided baseline data about the seniors and gave them sufficient information about the program on which to base their decision to participate.

STRATEGIES

The key groups used in organizing the research and demonstration program were (1) senior citizens: persons who participated in the program; (2) community health and human services organizations and aging network: the co-sponsors of the program in all phases from planning to evaluation; and (3) Dartmouth and University of Miami Medical Schools: the professional experts who developed the course content, trained self-care educators, provided technical assistance in all aspects of the program, and conducted the study. The academic institutions served an essential role in the development and research phases of the SCSC program. However, after completion of the research and demonstration phases, the SCSC program continues to be conducted by some community groups who are not affiliated with an academic institution.

Recruitment of Seniors

A critical aspect of the process of adapting the SCSC program to a particular community is development of a recruitment plan that fits local conditions. Multiple approaches have been tried and found successful. Examples include:

- live "advertisements" at senior citizen centers, followed by (a) informational teas about self-care and (b) brochures hand-delivered or placed in key locations
- personal letters from the primary physician or hospital administrator, followed by phone calls to promote registration
- active recruitment of new participants by recent self-care course graduates
- newspaper, radio, and posters
- preprogram enrollment personal health assessment interviews that clarify the relevance of the course content for potential participants and alert course instructors to the needs of each group

Basic Steps

The following five steps in conducting an effective SCSC Program are recommended. First, an organization or an interested professional must take the leadership in working with the community's health and human services agencies and aging network to establish a consensus on the need for the program and to identify local organizations prepared to co-sponsor it. Second, self-care educators need to be selected from the co-sponsoring agencies and then be trained to teach the course by participating in an intensive, three-day workshop. Third, a recruitment plan must be developed to attract participation in the program. Fourth, the core SCSC Program is conducted, with all 13 two-hour sessions carried out on the basis of the learning process covered in the workshop. The fifth and last step involves followup of the core educational experience and a thorough evaluation. Both are undertaken with sponsoring organizations and senior participants to (1) facilitate specific actions that seniors wish to take (e.g., life-style change programs); (2) reinforce the core education program through group refresher/reunion sessions, publication of a self-care newsletter, and postcourse skills testing; and (3) measure the effect of the program on participants.

Tools

A package of educational materials has been developed into a curriculum to help the self-care educators lead a high-quality, systematic, semistructured learning experience with minimal training. Materials for the educators include:

- *SCSC Instructor Manual*
- SCSC course flipcharts
- *Give Yourself a Break: A Book on Exercise Breaks*
- pre- and postpersonal health assessment questionnaires

Materials designed for the seniors to tailor information, promote retention, and use as a tool for health decision making and self-directed change include the *Self-Care Planner* and *The Family Medical Handbook*. All these educational materials, with the exception of *The Family Medical Handbook* by Sehnert and Eisenberg,[7] were developed by Dartmouth.

To maintain a quality program, two ingredients are required: careful organization and effective education. The first ingredient, careful organization, is provided by a community coordinator who is trained to carry out the functions described in Exhibit 15–1.

Effective education requires two elements. First, a curriculum with an appealing set of learning tools and experiences designed to shape attitudes, increase self-confidence, build knowledge, and teach self-care skills is essential. Second, the course leaders must be prepared to orchestrate and fine tune the planned learning experiences to achieve maximum effect. To help meet this second objective, the SCSC Program has specified functions for members of an educational team and developed a workshop for training the team members.

Education Team: Facilitators and Core Instructors

The SCSC program curriculum is taught by a teaching team consisting of facilitator(s) and core instructor(s). Their functions are listed in Exhibit 15–1.

The facilitators are volunteers 60 years of age or older. They often are past SCSC program participants. Their only qualifications are (1) they feel comfortable appearing before the class and setting the stage for the instructor and/or the resource person, and (2) they are able to establish working relationships with class participants to help them learn self-care skills.

The core instructors, who are persons of various professional backgrounds, range from retired persons to young persons employed in community agencies. The number of instructors serving each course has fluctuated from one person being responsible for the entire program to three professionals serving this role in each of the content blocks: medical self-care, life style, and independent living. If

Exhibit 15–1 Functions of Community Coordinator, Facilitators, and Core Instructors

---

Community Coordinator

1. Recruit and select instructors and facilitators.
2. Recruit program participants.
3. Select the classroom site.
4. Acquire the education resources necessary for program implementation.
5. Design program schedule.
6. Monitor and/or supervise the program instructors and facilitators.

Facilitators

1. Attend a facilitator training workshop.
2. Assist in the recruitment of program participants.
3. Set up chairs, flip charts, and equipment at the start of each session, and put equipment away at the end of the session.
4. Take responsibility for the coordination and continuity of the self-care course:

   - Record participant attendance at each session.
   - Open and close each session.
   - Serve as a resource person to program participants.
   - Contact resource person.

Core Instructors

1. Attend an instructor training workshop.
2. Take responsibility for the instruction of assigned self-care program sessions:

   - Teach assigned subjects and skills.
   - Recruit and orient appropriate resource person(s) to co-instruct the session(s).
   - Obtain resource materials for session.
   - Serve as a resource person to program participants.

---

a core instructor does not feel comfortable with the content of a session, he or she often invites a resource person for this discussion. The medical block instruction has been taught by nurses, physical therapists, educators, and social workers. The independent living block instructor has usually been a social worker; however, nurses and educators have also served this function.

An effective system for training these self-care educators was developed. Both facilitators and core instructors are trained in an intensive, three-day workshop, which aims to:

- introduce the educators to self-care philosophy
- sharpen their group process and active learning education skills

- help them master the self-care skills and self-directed behavioral change techniques taught in the course
- introduce the health and social service information covered in the course

Course Content

Each SCSC course consists of 13 two-hour classes for 15 to 25 seniors. The classes are divided into three content blocks:

- medical self-care: acquiring access to the medical care system, learning medical self-care skills, and correctly utilizing the medical care system
- life style: assuming responsibility for one's own welfare (e.g., physical fitness, emotional well-being, dietary patterns)
- independent living: being aware of the social services available in the community and having the ability to use such agencies

Exhibits 15–2, 15–3, and 15–4 show the material covered in the three sections of the course.

A building-block approach has been used in planning the learning sequence for the course. This approach starts with the simplest, least threatening task, which can be readily mastered, before proceeding to more difficult tasks. Educational

---

Exhibit 15–2 Self-Care Program Outline: Medical Section (Sessions 1–5)

SESSION 1
   HEALTH CARE: Whose Responsibility
   SKILL: Reading a Thermometer

SESSION 2
   COMMON ILLNESSES: Symbols and Treatment
   SKILL: Throat and Neck Examination

SESSION 3
   MEDICATIONS: Facts and Fallacies
   SKILL: None

SESSION 4
   EMERGENCIES: How to Help
   SKILL: The Heimlich Method

SESSION 5
   CHRONIC CONDITIONS: Making the Best of Them
   SKILL: Taking Blood Pressure

Exhibit 15–3 Self-Care Program Outline: Lifestyle Section (Sessions 6–9)

SESSION 6
 LIFESTYLE: Taking Action to Promote Health
 SKILL: Blood Pressure Review

SESSION 7
 EXERCISE: Getting Fit and Feeling Fine
 SKILL: Taking a Resting and Exercise Pulse

SESSION 8
 NUTRITION: Eating to Stay Healthy
 SKILL: Nutritious Meal Planning

SESSION 9
 EMOTIONAL WELL-BEING: It's Your World
 SKILL: Relaxation Technique

---

objectives for each session are provided in the *SCSC Instructor Manual*. The educators use this resource to plan and evaluate their teaching efforts. Each session presents new information, provides an opportunity for practicing skills, allows participants to discuss feelings and reactions, and sets the stage for the following session.

Exhibit 15–4 Self-Care Program Outline: Independent Living Section (Sessions 10–13)

SESSION 10
 SOCIAL SERVICES: How They Can Help
 SKILL: Using the Local Directory of Human and Social Services Agencies

SESSION 11
 SOCIAL SERVICES: Discovering the Benefits
 SKILL: Review Using the Local Directory of Human and Social Services Agencies

SUMMARY
SESSION 12
 OPEN SESSION FOR REVIEW AND SPECIAL TOPICS

SESSION 13
 SELF-CARE CONTRACT: Planning a Better Tomorrow
 SKILL: Designing a Self-Care Contract

Methods

Each class session uses a variety of teaching and learning strategies that support the theme of learning through participation, which runs throughout the entire program. Some of the techniques that are used to foster active learning are group discussion, role playing, skills training, self-directed change, and record-keeping and self-observation. These learning strategies are designed to (1) engage the senior actively in the learning process; (2) provide the learner with an opportunity to gradually increase knowledge, skills, and confidence; (3) allow the individual to tailor the general material covered in the session to him- or herself; and (4) enable the participant to record self-observations and to record personal plans in a permanent place, i.e., the *Self-Care Planner*. This workbook is a ready reference for refreshing the participant's memory about what was learned in the course.

The program uses educational methods and techniques that correlate with Whitbourne's fundamentals of the learning process as they apply to the elderly.[8] For example, the instructor needs to consider adjusting the rate of presenting new materials to older adults through informal experimentation of how they respond to it; to adapt educational materials to the sensory limitations of vision and hearing; and to observe carefully verbal and nonverbal clues for mental fatigue, rather than expecting an open admission by the elderly. In addition, the instructor must clearly separate the presentation of items that have semantic or auditory similarities; for example, cardiac fibrillation versus flutter and ingestion versus digestion.

Whitbourne suggests four teaching strategies to use with the older adult learner. It is important to relate new information and skills to prior experience and knowledge and to differentiate where changes in practices contradict previous methods. Problem-solving skills should be developed through several varied and concretely different structured learning tasks that demonstrate the effectiveness of alternate strategies. To overcome cognitive difficulties, the learning experience should be based on actions, rather than verbalization, and should include concrete demonstrations before presenting abstract symbolization in the form of general principles. Finally, the learning situation must try to reduce the learner's anxieties by being sensitive to his or her background knowledge and feelings so these can be capitalized on to build success in learning new tasks and gaining self-confidence.

Throughout the 13 sessions, the SCSC material is tailored to the participants' knowledge. When they perceive the knowledge and skills as relevant to their own lives, they develop a greater retention and application.

EVALUATION

To measure the level of success attained, the Dartmouth SCSC Program developed a methodology for monitoring participant behavior as an outcome of the program effort. A controlled study was conducted to evaluate the effect of medical self-care education on health knowledge, self-care skills, use of health and social services, functional health, and the life quality of older persons. Data were collected on 330 elderly participants with an average age of 71 and chronic conditions as follows: 46 percent had hypertension, 33 percent had learning impairments, 33 percent had permanent stiffness, 24 percent had angina, 15 percent had diabetes, 8 percent had myocardial infarction, and 7 percent had a stroke. The test group—which consisted of 204 elderly persons—participated in a 13-session educational intervention. The control group—made up of 126 elderly persons—received a two-hour lecture demonstration. Both groups were assessed pre- and postintervention and one year after entry.

Major Findings

The results from the controlled trial demonstrated that it is possible to educate the elderly about self-care and that the skills and knowledge thereby acquired do not deteriorate substantially within the year following training. The results showed the intervention group health knowledge index (10 = excellent) was a mean score of 6.4 at three months posttest, as compared to 5.8 for the control group. At one-year follow-up, the scores were 7.1 for the intervention group and 5.8 for the control group.

The participants also demonstrated better performance in their ability to perform self-care skills (5.6 vs. 4.5, p < .0001) and confidence in skills performance (8.3 vs. 7.3, p < .001). They expressed the belief that they could communicate more effectively with their personal physician (84 percent as compared to 41 percent).

The course taught medical problem-solving behavior by promoting the use of a reputable home treatment book that could enable participants to decide when home care is safe and when physician contact is needed. At posttest, 93 percent of the participants owned a self-care book, and 35 percent reported using it initially to solve a medical problem.

The course stimulated a greater number of attempts to change health habits related to physical fitness, nutrition, weight control, and stress management. The average number of change attempts for the intervention group was 2.3, compared to only 1.3 for the control. The facets of life style that were most often the subject of short-run change attempts were, in rank order, weight loss (56 percent of test versus 32 percent of comparison group, p < .001), nutrition (55 percent versus 31 percent, p < .001), physical fitness (51 percent versus 31 percent, p < .001), and tension reduction (45 percent versus 21 percent, p < .001). There was no significant difference in self-reported success between groups; a substantial proportion of both groups rated their life-style change attempts as "very successful."

In addition, the self-care intervention had a favorable effect on two measures of life quality. First, quality and quantity of social activities were significantly higher for test subjects at follow-up (social interaction scale: 1.5 versus 1.6, $p < .05$). This increase was mostly due to gains registered among persons who had lower levels at pretest ($p < .001$). There were no overall differences between groups on the second global measure of life quality; however, when subgroups on pretest level were examined, it was found that test group participants who had lower baseline values scored significantly better one year later than their counterparts in the comparison group; life quality ratings at follow-up among persons with low values at pretest were 7.6 versus 6.4, $p < .05$.

Despite these favorable outcomes, there were no changes in two bottom line measures of effect—medical care utilization and health status. The number of physician visits was not influenced by the program; both cases and controls averaged slightly over five visits per person per year. However, the patterns of utilization did change among the participants in the course. Their report of decision making for medical care utilization suggests more selectivity and appropriate use of other community resources. All the health status measures had high values at pretest and did not improve or decline.

The evaluation concluded that medical self-care education can increase the capacity of the elderly to take an active role in managing their health.

Participants' Response

Participants expressed great enthusiasm for the self-care program; many requested "postgraduate" courses. In addition, the program proved to be an initiator of more active functioning for the participants. For example, they joined other health promotion programs (exercise, nutrition, etc.), developed new support systems through alliances with other participants, and returned for more training to become facilitators and instructors of the SCSC Program and also served as recruiters for new program participants.

Community Response

The communities that served as experimental sites went through three evolutionary stages: pilot, research and demonstration, and ongoing services. At the research and services phases, the medical school's involvement diminished and the communities' role increased. To date, the ongoing service stage is still underway, with courses being held regularly. The control community was provided with an initial training workshop, and this community has gone on to establishing SCSC Programs every six months.

COST OF PROGRAM

Ongoing costs for the program include those associated with marketing the program, teaching, education materials, managing and evaluating it, and space. Fortunately, many of these costs can be covered through in-kind donations or contributed services. The cost depends mostly on the extent of the use of volunteers as instructors, facilitators, and/or community coordinators and the availability of space. The program fees have ranged from $10 to $50 per person for a 13-session, 26-hour group education program for a group of 10 to 25 older persons. A modest charge for tuition or requesting a donation should be considered for course participants. The majority of communities using the Dartmouth SCSC Program have collected $8 to $15 from participants.

CONCLUSION

Although the Dartmouth SCSC Program is built on the ground-breaking work of such persons as Levin[9] and Sehnert,[10] it is unique to the self-care field. The content and education methods have been tailored to senior citizens who function independently in the community. Moreover, it provides for coordination and collaboration among health, social service and aging networks. When the educational teams have been trained to use appropriately the Dartmouth SCSC program strategies in the organization of the program, recruitment of seniors, and presentation of course content, the program has been equally successful with urban and rural groups.

NOTES

1. L.S. Levin, "The Layperson as the Primary Care Practitioner," *Public Health Reports,* 91 (1976): 206–210.

2. A. Katz and E. Bender, eds. *The Strength in US: Self-Help Groups in the Modern World* (New York: Franklin Watts, 1976).

3. R.N. Butler, et al., "Self-Care, Self-Help, and the Elderly," *International Health Aging and Human Development,* 10, no. 1 (1979–80): 95–119.

4. S.H. Moore, J. LoGerfo, and T.S. Innui, "Effect of a Self-Care Book on Physician Visits," *Journal of the American Medical Association* 243 (1980): 2317–2320.

5. D.W. Kemper, "Self-Care Education: Impact on HMO Costs," *Med Care* 20 (1982): 710–718.

6. J. Zapka and B.W. Averill, "Self-Care for Colds: A Cost-Effective Alternative to Upper Respiratory Infection Management," *American Journal of Public Health,* 69, no. 8 (1979): 814–816.

7. K.W. Sehnert and H. Eisenberg, *The Family Medical Handbook* (New York: Grosset and Dunlop, 1978).

8. S.K. Whitbourne and O.J. Sperbeck, "Health Care Maintenance for the Elderly," *Family and Community Health*, 3, no. 4 (1981): 11–27.

9. L.S. Levin, et al., *Self-Care Lay Initiatives in Health* (New York: Prodist, 1976).

10. K.W. Sehnert, "A Course for Activated Patients," *Social Policy*, 8 (1976).

Chapter 16

The Wisdom Project of the American Red Cross in Greater New York: A Blueprint for a Community-Based Health Care and Health Education Program

Stephanie Lederman, E.dM.
Mary Farrar, M.A.

The Wisdom Project of the American Red Cross in Greater New York is a program for older persons that focuses on preventive medicine and health education. Through services delivered at 30 senior centers in the southeastern section of Queens and in the South Bronx, the Wisdom Project provides affordable health care and education aimed at enhancing individual self-reliance and improving the life style of older adults. The program benefits area residents with a range of services offered within their own communities, including:

- total medical care for persons over 65 years of age with health disorders
- assistance to patients who receive referrals by way of "escort through the system" of cooperating hospitals
- transportation of medical supplies, laboratory specimens, and prescriptions to and from hospitals involved in the program
- individual counseling and group education sessions that enable patients to make informed decisions and maintain their optimal health

The American Red Cross is a community service organization that historically has developed and implemented programs based on community need. Recently, its thrust has been in the area of health services, particularly in the development of replicable programs that not only benefit the community but have a measurable degree of success. In planning the Wisdom Project in Queens and later in the Bronx, New York, an ad hoc committee was formed to assist the Red Cross in developing a model that would facilitate the delivery of preventive health care services to the elderly. Representatives from the New York City Departments of Health and Aging, the Municipal Hospital Corporation, and other key community agencies comprised the committee. The committee studied the community and its needs and found that the geriatric population frequently cited four major barriers to their acquisition of health care: impersonal attitudes of providers, inaccessibility of care, high cost, and extensive waiting time.

The committee also found that, because of the steady decline in the number of private physicians in the inner city, more older people were forced to turn to the hospital and, in some cases, the emergency room for outpatient care. Consequently, there was inappropriate utilization of health care,[1] which affected patient satisfaction, staff efficiency, cost, and the quality of personal care.[2] The committee concluded that early diagnosis and treatment of many diseases and the reduction of risk factors by changing certain health habits or the general life style represented the greatest hopes for reducing morbidity and mortality among the elderly.[3] A cost-effective program was needed that would provide accessible, affordable, personalized health care, utilize volunteers, and be replicable in other community settings.

Once the ad hoc committee set the goals and philosophy of the program, an agreement was made with a hospital to serve as the cooperating back-up facility. The Queens Hospital Center, in affiliation with The Long Island Jewish Hillside Medical Center, offered its services.

This chapter discusses the six components of the Wisdom Project:

1. assessment of need
2. visibility in the community—promotion/marketing
3. screening and treatment
4. health education of patients
5. training and recruitment of staff and volunteers
6. evaluation and follow-up

ASSESSMENT OF NEED

Review of the Literature

A review of the literature was conducted to ascertain the types of preventive health care programs that exist for the elderly, using a computer search of the following topic areas: community-based primary care programs, health education methodology, materials specifically developed for older people, disease incidence in inner-city elderly, the elderly as community health educators, and evaluation of elder health programs. This review indicated that, although many programs addressed the problem of health maintenance for the elderly, few had a comprehensive approach of health maintenance, follow-up, and health education.

Surveys

In order to implement a health care program effectively, the project needed information on the needs of the elderly in the target community. A telephone survey was developed to ascertain whether the older respondents (1) knew which services were offered at senior centers, (2) knew if a center was located in their own community, (3) attended the center, and most important, (4) would utilize health services if they were provided without cost at senior centers. A total of 167 calls placed randomly in the catchment area using a reverse phone directory yielded 60 completed surveys. Ninety-five percent of those over 65 years of age who responded to the survey were unaware that there was a senior center in their community. Thirty-five percent indicated that they would utilize free health services if offered at a nearby center. The majority of the respondents felt that senior centers were primarily for social events, not for health-related activities.

These results indicated the need for education about the availability of health services offered through the Wisdom Project at selected senior centers. The findings also indicated that most older people are averse to accepting charity. Therefore, a free program would not be acceptable to them. Although there are no out-of-pocket expenses, participants' health insurance is billed for medical service rendered through the Wisdom Project. For those participants who are not covered by Medicare/Medicaid or other insurance, services are provided at no cost.

Needs Assessments

Three needs assessments were conducted in the first year of the program to senior center members selected at random in six senior centers. Senior centers were chosen in cooperation with the New York City Department for the Aging, the Archdiocese of New York, and the Jamaica Service Program for older adults. The first needs assessment sought information from potential participants on how they received health care, how they paid for it, how often they saw a physician, how they traveled to receive health care, and what their main problems were in obtaining health care. The survey also provided information on the kind of medical advice in which this population was interested. The results of this survey indicated that most members of the target population had a primary care provider, but considered medical care a financial burden. This population—normally not recognized as in need—could readily be described as "falling between the cracks." Many were on fixed incomes, but were not eligible for Medicaid and may have had to pay an exorbitant amount for health care. The Red Cross has always provided services to this group.

In order to promote the program, the Wisdom Project conducted several blood pressure screenings. A letter was sent to those individuals identified as having high blood pressure inviting them to join the program. Because a considerable number of those who were invited to participate did not, a second needs assessment was conducted to determine why the program was underutilized by this population. Results indicated that these hypertensive individuals were under the care of a physician and were not interested in making a change.

The third needs assessment survey was conducted with potential participants to determine whether they would utilize the program. Eligibility requirements were modified to include all persons 65 and over with any chronic condition. Of those who responded, 77 percent said that they were interested in receiving medical services at their senior center because medical costs are too high and they often have too far to travel to receive health services. In addition, 51 percent assessed their health as only fair.

These needs assessments provided the necessary information on the target population to enable the program to modify its eligibility requirements to best meet their needs. Eligibility requirements evolved in three stages during the first three years of the project:

1. treatment for people 65 and over with high blood pressure
2. total treatment for people 65 and over with high blood pressure
3. treatment for any chronic condition

In the Bronx, these eligibility requirements were changed when the program was able to accommodate additional numbers and types of conditions served, and after approval from the cooperating hospital.

Health History Form

A health history form was distributed to a screened population, those who had their blood pressure taken by the Wisdom Project. The form consisted of a list of diseases that participants could check off indicating whether they or their mother or father had suffered from any of these conditions. Results of this survey provided information indicating the medical problems extant in the subject population.

VISIBILITY IN THE COMMUNITY: PROMOTION/MARKETING

In order to stimulate the target population to join the Wisdom Project, the concept of self-responsibility for health had to be promoted in the target community. First, the name of the program had to be conceived. A logo, depicting a large tree surrounded by the slogan, "Keep Healthy, Enjoy Aging," was created. This logo, along with the title of the Wisdom Project and the emblem of the American Red Cross, which was usually placed below, was used on brochures, flyers, posters, and other promotional material. (See Figure 16–1.)

Brochures were mailed to religious groups, community boards, community groups, local politicians, health-related agencies, and randomly selected elderly persons residing in the catchment area. Posters were placed on community bulletin boards and in libraries, Social Security offices, supermarkets, and post offices. Articles were placed in local and neighborhood newspapers describing the program and soliciting volunteers. An "Open House" for political representatives, the aged themselves, and key community people was held at the local chapter of the Red Cross, during which a ribbon-cutting ceremony was held to launch the program. Staff were invited to participate on a health-oriented television talk show that was arranged for by the public relations department of the American Red Cross. A slide presentation was developed to be shown at senior centers, golden age groups, and other locations where the elderly population congregated.

These promotional strategies are ongoing to allow for maximum exposure. However, as important as these methods are, the two most effective promotional techniques continue to be blood pressure screenings and word-of-mouth. Blood pressure screening or any health screening allows for a personalized intimate approach and an opportunity for volunteers and staff to meet elderly participants face-to-face and explain the benefits of the program. In addition, trust is developed through an accurate blood pressure reading, distribution of timely health information, and a personalized blood pressure card. Once in the program, satisfied participants relate their positive experiences to their peers.

SCREENING AND TREATMENT

Initially, the program adhered to a nationally accepted hypertension protocol developed by Cornell Medical Center. Because systolic blood pressure may fluctuate widely in elderly patients, this protocol calls for 3 blood pressure screenings before labeling any patient as hypertensive or deciding on treatment.

The first screening was open to all senior center participants. Second and third screenings were conducted by appointment for those who were identified as having a high reading. To those participants whose blood pressure was deemed high after three blood pressure screenings, a letter was sent to their home inviting them to participate in the Wisdom Project. Treatment for high blood pressure could be obtained at the senior center; however any other medical conditions were brought to the attention of the participant's primary care physician. On agreement by the participant and the Wisdom Project, a letter was sent to the physician that provided a medical update on the patient and a description of the program.

These eligibility requirements restricting treatment to hypertensive patients were in place for six months. However, because most hypertensive elderly in the

Figure 16–1

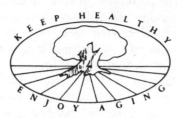

THE WISDOM PROJECT

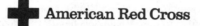 **American Red Cross**

GOOD HEALTH CARE BEGINS IN YOUR COMMUNITY SENIOR CENTER WITH THE WISDOM PROJECT

Get involved in your own health care!
The American Red Cross "Wisdom Project"
provides quality Health Services
at neighborhood senior centers.
Older adults have special health needs,
and we know what they are.
These Health Services include:

• Physical examination, treatment and
follow-up care by our geriatric health
care team
• Diagnostic tests
• Medications, when prescribed
• No out-of-pocket costs
• Medicare / Medicaid or other insurance
accepted
• Individual and group health education

For more information or an appointment
Please call: 870-8806

THE WISDOM PROJECT

THE AMERICAN RED CROSS IN GREATER NEW YORK

Source: Courtesy of the American Red Cross in Greater New York.

catchment area were already under the care of a physician, the eligible population was very limited. Moreover, participants felt uncomfortable using the Wisdom Project for treatment of hypertension and a different health care source for other conditions, so many did not take advantage of the program. Therefore, the eligibility criteria were changed from treatment of hypertension only to the Wisdom Project acting as the primary care provider for the hypertensive. This change increased enrollment.

One of the most important purposes of the program is to provide health services to those who have a chronic health complaint, but do not have a primary care provider. Often, when there are no restrictions on program admittance, the elderly shop around for second and third opinions and may become confused and over-medicated. To avoid having to turn away the "shoppers" and to ensure that the target population is reached, enrollment in Queens is limited to individuals with chronic conditions who are willing to make the Wisdom Project their primary care provider. Of course, some participants still shop around.

Currently, in the Bronx, participants in need of a primary care provider are served, regardless of whether or not they have a chronic complaint. This broad eligibility criterion was set because of the desire of the cooperating hospital and the nature of the population, which is much more difficult to reach. Because this target area is not as geographically concentrated as in Queens, there is less chance of long waiting lists of participants.

In Queens, the target population is made up of persons 65 years and older with a middle to low income level. Sixty percent of the population are black, and 40 percent are white. In the Bronx, the population is comprised of an indigenous Jewish population and a relatively recent Spanish-speaking population that has yet to be served. Although the income levels are similar in both areas, the diversified ethnic backgrounds provide interesting research data.

In summary, patients are admitted to the program who lack medical care and who meet the eligibility criteria set for each site. If prospective clients are satisfied with their present medical services, they are encouraged to remain with that source of care. Before gaining admittance to the program, the interested participant is given a short questionnaire to ensure that the program meets his or her expectations and needs. It is made clear to the applicant that the Wisdom Project is specifically designed for those who are in need of primary care services.

On admission to the program, the participant completes a detailed medical history form, which is brought to the first appointment. The medical history form includes five areas: past history, personal history, social history, family history, and a review of systems. The geriatric nurse practitioner assists the participant in completing any unfinished portions of the form. In addition, participants are provided with instructions for the first visit and are asked to bring in all medications, including over-the-counter drugs.

Each participant then undergoes a complete physical examination conducted by the geriatric nurse practitioner. Routine lab work includes a urinalysis, electrocardiogram, and hemoccult stool. The participant's second visit to the program includes a meeting with a health educator and a vist with the physician. The physician examines the patient, checks positive findings and all lab work, and dispenses any necessary medications. The medical team confers regarding the treatment plan and prescribes visits to the health educator as part of the treatment plan. All relevant findings are relayed to the participant.

The meeting with the health educator includes time for questions to allow the patient to understand completely the prescribed treatment. Once the health educator is confident that the participant is satisfied with the proposed treatment, a plan is jointly devised by the health educator and participant to help the patient follow the prescribed regimen. At this time, several goals may be set by the participant, or goal setting may be postponed until the participant is willing to make changes in health behavior.

The discussion between the health educator and the participant focuses on how to make the necessary changes in current life style, dietary habits, recreation plans, home environment, and mental health. Individuals may be seen on a one-to-one basis or encouraged to attend peer groups designed to address particular common needs. For example, small groups comprised of four to seven participants may meet to discuss diabetes management, weight control, or stress reduction. If the need arises, groups may be formed to address common issues concerning loneliness and depression, hypertension, medication management, smoking cessation, or exercise. The geriatric nurse practitioner may participate in the small groups along with the health educator. The health educator discusses and distributes appropriate educational material to the participant.

Follow-Up

The Wisdom Project is closely coordinated with the cooperating hospital's outpatient services, emergency department, and inpatient facilities so that necessary follow-up services can be provided in an integrated fashion. All medical equipment, laboratory services, medication, and physician services are provided by the hospital. Red Cross transportation volunteers deliver lab work, prescriptions, equipment and, in some instances, participants to the hospital. When participants need referral to the cooperating hospital for a procedure that cannot be provided at the center, all subsequent visits are conducted at the senior center by the geriatric nurse practitioner and/or physician. All the necessary information concerning the participant's visit is sent to the program site from the hospital to allow for continuing care of the individual. The geriatric nurse practitioner collaborates with colleagues in the department of nursing and other disciplines at the cooperating hospital to evaluate and meet the physical and psychosocial needs of all participants on an ongoing basis.

HEALTH EDUCATION: WHY IS THE WISDOM PROJECT DIFFERENT

The Wisdom Project is innovative in several respects, including the provision of primary care clinics in senior centers, the use of a geriatric nurse practitioner as the main provider of care, and the emphasis on health promotion through self-care education. However, what sets the Wisdom Project most clearly apart from traditional programs is the inclusion of the health educator as part of the medical team.

Health education can play a crucial role in the early detection of disease, minimizing the effects of existing problems and preventing further complications of the individual's health status. The elderly may in fact represent one of the most productive target groups for effective health education. As greater numbers of people live to age 65 or older, preventive health care can decrease the risks or morbidity and mortality, thereby improving their quality of life.

The Wisdom Project provides health education both to participants of the medical component of the program and to the general membership of the senior center. Participants in the medical component can be seen on a one-to-one basis or as part of a peer "Problem Group." How often patients are seen is determined by the entire medical team. A record of all health education encounters is kept in the patient's medical chart.

Group health education is available to all members of the senior center. Topics rated by preference in an earlier survey are presented to small groups. Each topic has an outline describing the overall goal for that particular subject, objectives of the presentation, content information, and methods and resources used for the presentation. Generally, the teaching plan is participant-oriented. By emphasizing the acquisition and improvement of knowledge and skill needed for everyday living, it helps the individual assume maximum self-responsibility for his or her overall well-being. Participants can use these tools for all aspects of their daily lives, not only those related to health. There are 23 topics, ranging from disease to a healthy life style.

The topics related to disease include:

- hypertension
- salt in the diet
- potassium and the hypertensive patient
- cholesterol

- arthritis
- diabetes
- cancer is curable
- hyperthermia
- alcoholism and the elderly
- constipation
- Alzheimer's disease
- foot care

The wellness-related topics include:

- using and abusing medication
- communicating with your doctor
- nutrition
- stress management
- exercise
- Medicare/what you should know
- food additives
- vitamins
- getting the most from your medical dollar
- safety and accident prevention
- loneliness and depression

The Wisdom Project bases its health education model on self-care education as it derives its goals from the learner's perceived needs and preferences. It is the learners who determine the desired outcomes in accordance with their decision as to which risks they choose to avoid or not to avoid.

Self-care education—with its diverse goals of promoting health and preventing, detecting, and treating disease at the primary care levels—not only emphasizes the individual as decision maker but also relies heavily on knowledge and skills that he or she already has. Self-care education avoids the victim-blaming orientation of some preventive health education efforts. Instead, it helps the learner identify those factors in society or the community that are complicit in disease production and for which solutions require sound action.[4]

The Wisdom Project's experiential learning groups use adult (andragogy) techniques. These are based on the principles of the ancient philosopher Confucius, who expressed his belief in the importance of learning from experience when he wrote, "I hear and I forget, I see and I remember, I do and I understand." Confucius related the acquisition of understanding and knowledge directly to living and experiencing: "I do and I understand."[5] Although an ancient method, this technique works well with the 23 topics in the Wisdom Project's repertoire. Older adults relay their own experiences as the group leader/facilitator follows a carefully planned teaching module. Two-way and multidirectional techniques, such as group discussion, simulation, role playing, case study, and question/answer, are utilized. In this way, the experiences of all learners are used as resources for learning.

Each module is a one-hour session, except for the exercise topic, which is more comprehensive and is presented in three, two-hour sessions. Each session includes an introduction, self-assessment, benefits, and demonstration. The average attendance for all Wisdom Project sessions is about 15 to 50 persons. A group size of 25 makes for the most informative workshop with considerable group interaction.

RECRUITMENT AND TRAINING OF VOLUNTEERS

All volunteers and students receive a manual as a guide to the program. It includes a detailed description of the Wisdom Project, a guide to education of older adults, an A.Q. (Aging Quotient) questionnaire adapted from Blue Cross and Blue Shield, sample discussion group outline, evaluation form, summary of the Wisdom Project services, a program brochure, current program statistics, information about the American Red Cross, and a policy and procedure manual describing the operation of the medical component.

Each volunteer position has a detailed job description that outlines the experience necessary for the job, day-to-day expectations, and how each specific job relates to the overall program. Volunteers are recruited from the community at large, the senior center, and local colleges and universities. Recruitment is done by letter, distribution and posting of flyers, personal appeals, ads in newspapers, and word-of-mouth through satisfied volunteers. Further, recruitment letters describing fieldwork opportunities are sent to all local colleges and universities with accredited programs in health education, nursing, and nurse practitioner certificate programs in gerontology. Students work on all aspects of the program under the supervision of the medical care team and the project director.

A peer volunteer program is the newest component of the program. This was designed to ensure the expansion of the health education services to older adults in community settings. When older adults work as peer educators, they successfully utilize their skills and talents, have the opportunity for continued development of their skills, and contribute to the community.

Peer educators have the advantage of having first-hand knowledge of the problems of older persons, which helps them develop a therapeutic bond of communication with older participants more quickly than could a younger professional.[6]

Peer educators are trained by volunteer instructors, many of whom are former peer educators, in three sessions. The first session covers the goals and objectives of the Wisdom Project, the purpose and value of the peer education system, the role of the peer educator, the training module, and the concept of adult learning using motivational learning techniques. The second session clarifies the role of the peer educator, acquaints the group with the support that the Wisdom Project could provide, and demonstrates teaching strategies. In session three, a typical teaching module is presented as it is taught to future participants, giving the trainees an opportunity to ask questions about the topics at hand and become familiar and comfortable with the proposed educational techniques. At the end of the three sessions, the trainee has the opportunity to evaluate the sessions and provide valuable input for future program development.

Peer educators are not expected to be experts in disease, nor are they expected to be able to answer all questions from participants. Rather, they are trained to guide participants to appropriate referrals if necessary, to assist participants in developing questions for their physicians, and to reinforce the importance of life-style management skills for maintaining optimum health.

The model of informational workshops and peer educators can be adapted successfully in settings as diverse as a university town, a rural community, a senior center, a nursing home, and a nutrition site in a low-income area.

EVALUATION

Evaluation of health promotion programs certifies their appropriateness and effectiveness and ensures that the practitioner is accountable for the patient (consumer), the community, and the administrators.[7] Evaluation mechanisms have been built into the Wisdom Project from the beginning. Surveys, questionnaires, and forms for patient status, patient enrollment, billing, medication review, and appointments kept are the instruments used to measure the success of the program. Each of these instruments are described below.

Numbers Served

In 1984, there were 247 participants enrolled in the medical component of the program, with 3,719 people screened for high blood pressure at 133 screenings in 30 locations throughout the Bronx and Queens. In addition, a total of 370 health education discussion groups were presented at 35 locations with some 11,500 people attending.

A monthly statistical report form is used to record all numbers served, as well as numbers of visits, appointments, clinic days, and any significant events. The health educator records numbers of participants attending each of the discussion groups on another form.

User Satisfaction

In February of 1984 an anonymous response questionnaire was sent to all participants enrolled in the medical component of the program, with a 45 percent return rate. Questions focused on participant satisfaction with the services in general and with the individual providers, money saved on health care, and whether waiting time was shorter than usual. In addition, participants were asked if they received satisfactory answers to their health questions. The overwhelming majority—98 percent—indicated that they were very satisfied with services; most were very pleased with the medical team, and 60 percent felt that waiting time was shorter than in the past. All the respondents said that they had saved a considerable amount of health care dollars since they had joined the program, that they had received satisfactory answers to their questions, and, most important, that their health status had greatly improved. This survey reported behavior quite satisfactory for program objectives.

Adaptability

The services of the Wisdom Project have been offered in senior centers, libraries, community centers, and churches. Programs can be implemented virtually wherever there is available space. Few changes are made as the program moves from site to site. Although no instruments measuring adaptability have been developed at present, the fact that the same program serves some 33 centers in four distinct communities is an impressive indication of its adaptability.

Replicability

In August of 1983, after 2½ years of operation, the Wisdom Project expanded its services to the Bronx. Another hospital was found that was willing to collaborate with the Red Cross to provide needed medical services to the community, and expansion occurred using the same staff without cutting services. In the near future, the program will continue to expand to other communities until it is offered on a city-wide basis.

Compliance

A quarterly review is done by the field coordinator to determine the number of nurse practitioner, physician, and health educator visits; number of appointments kept; participants' status on entering the program; and current medications. These results are recorded on a patient status review form. Current findings indicate that 65 percent of patients in the program are hypertensive, with 88 percent now under control using 160/90 mm Hg as the break-off point. In addition, 94 percent of participants who entered with a high cholesterol level are now within normal range, and 66 percent of those entering with a high glucose level are now stabilized. Periodic peer reviews of all charts are made to determine changes in such measures as lab reports, adherence to medications, or weight levels dropping. Ongoing meetings by the medical team ensure discussion of the problem participant. There is an 88 percent compliance rate for keeping appointments, a rate that is high for any age group. A health education checklist outlines important life-style information about the participant and indicates expectations for life-style change and future action. In addition, part of the form is used to record dialogue between the medical team. This checklist is part of the medical chart.

Health Education

In addition to the health education checklist, in June of 1984 a questionnaire was distributed to obtain additional information on the participants' attitudes and beliefs toward prescribed treatment. The questions centered around beliefs about certain health behaviors, such as weight control, exercise, keeping medical appointments, alcohol consumption, medication compliance, diet, smoking cessation, and safety. Although participants believed that their own actions influence their health, their answers to the questionnaire have not been compared as yet with their medical charts to see whether perceived belief is indicative of actual behavior.

Cost

Cost effectiveness can be analyzed in several ways. First, no out-of-pocket costs meant that the participants realized savings. Medicare payments are collected for medical visits, providing revenue for the hospital. In addition, costly physician time is replaced by the less expensive services of the nurse practitioner and health educator. In one year, 92.6 percent of patient revisits were conducted by the nurse practitioner, as opposed to only 7.4 percent by the physician, which is a considerable savings for Medicare.

The ultimate test of the value of outreach programs for the elderly, however, may be the degree to which, in a cost-effective manner, long-term disability and institutionalization are delayed in this population. In order to achieve this goal, programs should place special emphasis on health maintenance through early detection and early treatment of illness, which is achieved through self-help, including changes in life style. The Wisdom Project tries to remain a blueprint for reaching this goal.

CONCLUSION

The Wisdom Project of the American Red Cross in Greater New York is a cost-effective, replicable method for providing primary and preventive health care to older people. Red Cross volunteers help steer patients through the medical system to ensure adequate treatment for already existing conditions. Health education, making extensive use of volunteers and peer educators, helps prevent the onset of further health problems. Users report a high degree of satisfaction with this program.

NOTES

1. Marjorie H. Cantor and Mary Mayer, "Health of the Inter City Elderly" (Paper presented to Twenty-seventh Annual Meeting of Gerontological Society, Portland, Oregon, October 1975), published by the New York City Department of Aging.

2. Joel J. Alpert et al., "Attitudes and Satisfactions of Low-Income Families Receiving Comprehensive Care," *American Journal of Public Health* 60, no. 3 (1970): 499–506.

3. David Mechanic, "Sociology and Public Health: Perspectives for Application," *American Journal of Public Health* 62, no. 2 (1972): 146–151.

4. Lowell S. Levin, "Patient Education and Self-Care: How Do They Differ?" *Nursing Outlook*, March 1978, pp. 170–175.

5. U.S. Department of Health and Human Services, *Trainer's Guide To Andragogy: Its Concepts, Experience and Application* (Washington, D.C.: U.S. Government Printing Office, March 1972).

6. Francoise Becker and Steven H. Zarif, "Training Older Adults as Peer Counselors," *Educational Gerontology: An International Quarterly* 3 (1978): 241–250.

7. Larry Green, "How To Evaluate Health Promotion," *Hospitals*, October 1, 1979, pp. 106–108.

Chapter 17

The Healthwise Program: GROWING YOUNGER

Donald Kemper, M.S.I.E., M.P.H.

All people have two ages: a chronological age based on how long they have lived and a health age based on how much life they have left. No one can reduce his or her chronological age, nor should that be a desired goal. Yet, all of us can reduce our health age and, in a very real sense, grow younger.

Originating in Boise, Idaho, GROWING YOUNGER is a neighborhood-based health promotion program for people "sixty or better." It helps older adults celebrate their age and enjoy activities that will extend the years and enhance the quality of their lives. GROWING YOUNGER is positive, upbeat, and full of fun. It has given thousands of seniors an opportunity to laugh more, smile more, and feel better about themselves while, at the same time, improving their health. The program is symbolized by its butterfly logo. Just as the butterfly emerges beautiful and free at the end of its life cycle, so can older adults spread their wings in creating the most satisfying phase of their lives

BIRTH OF THE PROGRAM

The GROWING YOUNGER Program is the creation of Healthwise, a non-profit health promotion center developed in 1975 to promote self-responsibility for health. Earlier Healthwise efforts had developed nationally acclaimed health promotion programs for families, schoolchildren, and infants. Through the success of these efforts, a philosophy and approach to health promotion were developed that emphasized self-responsibility, the wellness approach, and direct efforts to develop a cultural environment supportive of good health.

As with many innovations, GROWING YOUNGER was created when two groups, with different concerns came together for a common purpose. In 1979, Healthwise was a small nonprofit health promotion center with a four-year history limited to working with young families to improve both their health and their

263

health care. The Healthwise staff had little experience with older adults. At an organizational planning session, several members of the Healthwise Board of Directors suggested that a practical community-wide, self-care program for seniors was long overdue.

That "rough cut" idea was taken to the Boise Council on Aging (BCA), a coalition of 30 or more senior citizen organizations devoted to serving the unmet needs of older adults in the Boise area. The BCA looked at the self-care concept as a means of accomplishing some of its own goals in providing social support for seniors. The two perspectives were then merged in a program that addressed both the health and social needs of the senior population.

The BCA was concerned that the program not simply preach to the older person. Rather, they wanted assurances that a broad and representative cross-section of elders would be brought into the program, and be involved in decision making, including those who did not normally participate in club and organizational functions. At the same time, the board of Healthwise was firm in insisting that the program focus primarily on *positive* health; it resisted suggestions to broaden that focus to include emphasis on understanding illnesses and direct screening for disease. It was agreed that an upbeat, positive approach would do more to meet the objectives of both groups.

In response to these concerns, the program was targeted to the average older person who was generally healthy and lived independently in the community. No socioeconomic group was specifically emphasized nor excluded, although special recruitment efforts were made to attract low-income seniors. The age limit was somewhat arbitrarily set at 60 and over. Funding for GROWING YOUNGER came from the Centers for Disease Control, the state of Idaho, numerous contributions from local employers and community organizations, and from modest fees paid by the participants themselves ($8 per person, $10 per couple). Funding totaled $384,000 over three years for development, implementation, and evaluation of the program.

GROWING YOUNGER was first implemented in Boise, Idaho, which has a predominately white population of 100,000, including 15,000 residents 60 or older. To ensure that the program would have meaningful impact on the community, a participation goal of 1,500 or 10 percent of all older adults was set. (That goal has since been exceeded.) The rationale for the goal was that, if 10 percent of the people went through the program, then most of the other senior adults would have at least indirect contact with it, and the opportunity for broad-based change would be present.

GROWING YOUNGER was developed and piloted at the Boise Senior Center, which serves as a focal point for 30 or more senior organizations. The open-ended concept of service that the center follows was key to the support and success GROWING YOUNGER has received.

GOALS AND OBJECTIVES

The overall goal of GROWING YOUNGER is simple: to improve the health of older people living in the Boise area. In support of the general goal, objectives were set in three areas: program participation, changed health risks, and cost containment.

1. Participation objective: Recruit 10 percent of Boise's 15,000 60 and over population into the GROWING YOUNGER program by October 1, 1983.
2. Health-risk objectives:
   a. Increase by 10 percent the percentage of seniors who exercise three or more times per week.
   b. Reduce age-specific resting heart rates by 5 percent.
   c. Increase by 10 percent the percentage of seniors who visit or are visited by others at least three times a week.
   d. Increase by 10 percent the percentage of seniors reporting to practice relaxation activities three or more times per week.
   e. Reduce by 10 percent the percentage of seniors who smoke.
   f. Reduce by 5 percent the age-specific mean diastolic blood pressure.
   g. Reduce by 10 percent the age-specific mean pounds overweight.
   h. Reduce by 10 percent the mean percent body fat of participants.
3. Cost-containment objective: Demonstrate a statistically significant positive effect on health care costs of participants during the 12-month period following participation.

In addition to these formal and measurable objectives, the program is guided by two additional informal goals. The first concerns the social quality of life for participants. Each aspect of the program is designed to improve friendships among participants and to encourage more smiles, hugs, and laughter in their daily routine. The final objective relates to broad community attitudes toward aging. GROWING YOUNGER strives to help people of all ages look to aging with positive anticipation. If the community raises its general expectations about aging, it will become much easier for older individuals to succeed at their own health promotion and self-promotion activities.

ENROLLMENT: A NEIGHBORHOOD MARKETING STRATEGY

GROWING YOUNGER's recruitment process enhances participant expectations and establishes a framework for continuing support through neighborhood-based recruitment plans. The target area is divided into neighborhood units estimated to contain 1,000 to 1,600 residents age 60 or over.

A "Tupperware" Approach

The actual program recruitment comes in home (Tupperware-like) parties held in each small neighborhood at the home of an older person or a neighbor. The home party atmosphere is informal, nonthreatening, and successful for encouraging the usual stay-at-home senior to become involved. The parties include health promotion activities of value by themselves and are designed to build or strengthen friendships within the neighborhood, whether or not enrollment follows.

An average of eight seniors attend each party, with about 60 percent agreeing to participate in the workshops. Each neighborhood is covered twice over a two- or three-year period to meet the 10 percent recruitment goal. Single floors in senior highrises or even church groups or clubs are often substituted for the neighborhood as the party focus.

Participant expectations are raised both through activities at the parties and public service announcements in the media. The image developed for the program is one of active seniors enjoying good health and good times. This image is created through high-quality television and radio messages in combination with a steady stream of news releases and media events. The media spots have been developed with grant funds and donations. All air time is free, with public service announcement time donated by the media.

The image is further developed in the neighborhood recruitment parties at which an introduction game, flexibility exercises, and the enjoyable style of the workshops are experienced. The introduction game asks neighbors to pair up with people they do not know well and to interview them about where they were raised, when they moved to the neighborhood, and what are their interests. Each person then introduces his or her partner to the group, highlighting what is learned in the interview. This process often helps the participants find new friends with similar interests and backgrounds. As a result, seniors enter the program looking both for a good time and for positive changes they can make to enjoy better health.

Finally, the individuals recruited at the parties are encouraged to be neighborly by sitting together at the workshop sessions and meeting once a week outside the workshop to take walks, share meals, or practice skills learned in the program. The creation of such a neighborhood group provides a continuing source of support for each person's efforts to improve his or her health.

WORKSHOPS ON FOUR INTEGRATED TOPICS

Four, two-hour workshops that cover physical fitness, nutrition, stress management, and medical self-care form the core of the program. The four main topics are integrated so that each is addressed in every session, as indicated in the session-by-session outline in Exhibit 17–1. A strong emphasis is placed on learn-by-doing activities that build knowledge, skills, and friendships among participants.

GROWING YOUNGER was limited to four sessions for both economic and logistical reasons. The initial program research uncovered enough content and activity ideas for 100 hours of workshops. However, realistic time and dollar requirements were needed if a significant proportion of the older population was to be recruited.

Four was an ideal number of sessions because participants found it easy to block out one morning a week for a month *and* because the program planners felt a significant impact could be made in that amount of time. The important decision was made to eliminate content before compromising approach, format, or style. Hence, the eight hours of program were the *best* activities, rather than a comprehensive digest of everything thought to be important. The four principal topics covered were "standouts" in an interest survey conducted early in the program design. The activities used to present them were those found to be the most enjoyable, the most likely to create behavioral change, and the most compatible with the socialization objectives of the program. The rest of the content was incorporated into the *Growing Younger Handbook*.

The workshops are coordinated by two presenters who lead the activities using a team approach. Laughter, exercise, role playing, and relaxation are built into each session to make them fun, positive, and successful. The participants begin to feel a part of a special, caring group of friends who are both interesting and interested in them.

To promote further enthusiasm for the program, participants receive useful health aids at each of the four sessions. The aids were selected first for use as focal points for opening activities in the workshops and then as aids for the continued development of self-care skills at home and in the small groups. They include a high-intensity penlight, a cryogel cold/hot pack, a fever thermometer, a magnifier for reading the thermometer, sunscreen, and an exercise stretchie band. Other aids considered but not used because of cost constraints included elastic bandages, first-aid kits, foot massagers, eye droppers, and medicine spoons. Each participant also receives a copy of the *Growing Younger Handbook* for both workshop and home use.

Activities are generally performed in pairs or in small groups representing each neighborhood. The groups then practice and discuss the skills and activities at informal weekly meetings in their neighborhood. The addition of four such informal sessions to the regular workshops, in effect, doubles the intensity of the program without adding to its cost. The practice also establishes a pattern for continued neighborhood group meetings after the workshops are completed.

Exhibit 17–1 Session-by-Session Description

Topics (Highlights Only)	*Format*
SESSION I.	
Definition of health and wellness	Dialogue
Shoulder and neck massage	Learn by doing
Seven key health habits	Dialogue
Target pulse rate for exercise	Learn by doing
Exercise: Flexibility and muscle tone to music	Learn by doing
Magic elixir presentation	Dramatics
Roll breathing	Learn by doing
Commitment and neighborhood group formation	Small group
SESSION II.	
Penlights as health tools	Learn by doing
Self-care—overview	Dialogue/human continuum*
Taking a temperature—fever	Learn by doing
Massage	Learn by doing
Doctor/patient relationships	Guided discussion
Exercise	Learn by doing
Eating changes/nutrient density/the ''80/20'' rule	Dialogue
Progressive muscle relaxation	Learn by doing
SESSION III.	
Use of hot/cold packs	Learn by doing
Back care	Dialogue and discussion
Arthritis	Dialogue and discussion
Massage and exercise	Learn by doing
Use of medications	Dialogue and discussion
Nutrition	Dialogue
Relaxation response	Learn by doing
SESSION IV.	
Foot rollers/foot massage	Learn by doing
Hospital costs	Dialogue and discussion
Walking	Dialogue and discussion
Fiber, protein, sugar	Dialogue and discussion
Roll breathing	Learn by doing
Personal plan for wellness	Individual and small group work
Neighborhood groups	Discussion
Graduation/diplomas	Celebration

*The human continuum allows people to express what percent of health problems they care for themselves by placing themselves along a wall with 0 percent on one end, 50 percent in the middle, and 100 percent on the other end.

SUPPORTING ACTIVITIES

The neighborhood groups provide the focus for continuing support to the GROWING YOUNGER graduates. Each group selects a volunteer leader or representative who facilitates each session and attends monthly Neighborhood Group Network meetings. The Network is set up to allow groups to share ideas for new activities and to coordinate multigroup events, such as fun walks, picnics, and the like.

Each active group leader receives a copy of the *Neighborhood Group Activity Guide*, which suggests fun and practical ways each group can develop new skills and interests in health. The Neighborhood Group Network is also used to find volunteers to help recruit for, present, or support the workshops.

Participants are brought back together for a formal "booster" session six weeks after the program is completed. The "booster" is presented as a class reunion, with reinforcement of key themes and an opportunity for participants to share both successes and barriers to success.

THE HAPPY HOOFERS AND OTHER SPIN-OFFS

In addition to the neighborhood group activities, the Network has initiated a number of spin-off activities important to the senior community. Most visible among these are the "Happy Hoofers," an informal group of seniors who walk three to eight miles, three times a week. The group size often exceeds 50 and, at times, has reached 100 persons. The success of the "Happy Hoofers" rests solely on the enthusiasm of its leaders, who make sure everyone has a good time and no one overdoes the exercise. The "Happy Hoofers" may soon split into two groups to reduce the numbers to manageable size, although combined events will still occur.

Other spin-offs include greatly expanded exercise and swim classes at the YMCA, an annual picnic, and official fun walks for seniors that are connected with the Great Potato Marathon, an annual marathon race in Boise.

STAFFING

GROWING YOUNGER has enjoyed a rich blend of talents and professions in its development and implementation. The core staff included people with backgrounds in health planning, health education, health systems engineering, nursing, and social work. In addition, volunteer help and consultation were received from physicians, dentists, physical therapists, nutritionists, advertising consultants, public relations executives, artists, and a rich mix of older adults of many diverse backgrounds. The integration of all these perspectives has added a great deal to GROWING YOUNGER's success.

Above all else, the staff of the GROWING YOUNGER Program has a positive view of aging and a respect for people of all ages. Following that, a good sense of humor and a basic understanding of health life styles are other important characteristics.

To boost the medical credibility of the program, it is helpful to include a nurse as one of the two instructors, particularly during the first six months of the program. A health educator (M.P.H.) or health promotion specialist complete the initial instruction team. The health educator should be experienced in drawing participants into discussions and activities. Experience has shown that two professional instructors are important in the early months of the program while refinements and style are being developed. Later, individuals with less formal education and experience can be substituted for either the nurse or educator. Because GROW-ING YOUNGER was developed by and for seniors, the authors recommend training GROWING YOUNGER graduates to be presenters (instructors) later on in the program.

Coordination of the overall effort should be the responsibility of a paid, full-time staff member. Although volunteers can be used effectively in many areas of promotion and recruitment, the task of coordinating and supporting recruitment efforts should not be underestimated.

MATERIALS

The *Growing Younger Handbook* is a large-print health guide for GROWING YOUNGER participants. It contains segments on fitness, nutrition, stress management, medical self-care, and personal health care management. The handbook serves both as a text during the workshops and as a reference guide for use at home.

Healthwise has also developed a complete replication kit, including a detailed *Presenter's Guide* with each of the four workshops scripted for reference by presenters. In addition, the kit includes complete documentation of the program in the *Growing Younger Organization & Promotion Guide*. Also available are high-quality television public service announcements that other communities can adapt to aid participant recruitment.

EVALUATION

GROWING YOUNGER is being evaluated on three levels. First, a six-month pre- and postquestionnaire has been used to monitor changes in self-reported health behaviors. Twenty-nine questions are divided into five groupings to obtain behavioral change index scores in exercise, nutrition, stress management/social, medical-care management, and dangerous behaviors (i.e., smoking, drinking, nonuse of seat belts).

A second level of evaluation involves observed changes in health measurements. Participants are asked to undergo an extensive health assessment during the first week of the program and again six months after graduation. The following biometrics are included: weight, flexibility, lung function (FEV–1/1), cholesterol (total and HDL), percent body fat (five-site caliper test), blood pressure, and resting pulse.

A third level of evaluation involves monitoring the Medicare costs of participants. A pre-/post-, experimental group/comparison group design is employed that controls for self-selection and general trend factors. Cost data are being obtained with cooperation from Blue Cross of Idaho, the Equitable Assurance Society of America, and the Health Care Financing Administration.

Although analysis of the data is not yet complete for any of the three levels of evaluation, preliminary data are available for health behavior changes and biometrics.

Health Behavioral Changes

Highly significant positive changes were found in four of the five behavioral change indices measured. Participants report exercising more, eating better foods, increasing stress management and social activities, and improving their management of health care problems. The only area in which significant improvements were not noted was in the dangerous behaviors index. The apparent lack of success in that area may be due to very low drinking (96 percent reported drinking seven or fewer drinks per week) and smoking (89 percent were nonsmokers) rates reported at the start of the program.

Biometrics

Preliminary data show significant, positive changes in weight, percent body fat, flexibility, cholesterol, and blood pressure.

Enrollment Success

Perhaps the best measure of the program's effectiveness is that over 1,800 Boise area seniors participated in its workshops over a 30-month period, a participation rate that exceeds 11 percent of Boise's entire senior population. Although seniors throughout the Boise area appear more active and visible now than at the start of the program, no formal evidence of broad community impact has been collected.

CONTINUATION AND REPLICATION

Grant support for the demonstration phase of GROWING YOUNGER ended in September of 1983. Since that time, the Boise program has been carried on under the co-sponsorship of the Boise Senior Center and two local hospitals.

Healthwise continues to refine and update GROWING YOUNGER and to make it available to other communities. The program has been described in a comprehensive replication package, which includes a detailed presenter's guide, an organization and promotion guide, a staff training program, and a large assortment of effective educational and promotional aids. A special low-cost package is available for rural areas. By April of 1984, the program had been purchased for replication by five clinics, four hospitals, three public health agencies, two senior centers, a university, a school district, and a rehabilitation center. GROWING YOUNGER programs are now starting in communities in Colorado, Florida, Idaho (4), Illinois, Kansas, Michigan, Missouri, New Mexico, Oregon, South Carolina, Texas (2), and Utah (2).

LEGACY AND LESSONS LEARNED

Although GROWING YOUNGER is so young and still alive in Boise and other replication communities, it has already begun to develop its legacy.

Graduates of the program are becoming increasingly involved in community activities, ranging from politics to poetry. In one particular effort, senior task forces are studying a large range of health issues affecting the older adult. One group developed, administered, and analyzed a questionnaire that asked seniors about the quality of their relationships with physicians. The results will be used in a continuing dialogue with physicians and hospitals. Other GROWING YOUNGER graduates joined other seniors in a creative writing project that culminated in publication of a book of their poetic writings, *Now My Soul Has Elbow Room*. Although GROWING YOUNGER can take no direct claim for these activities, its indirect effect on the interests and enthusiasm of its graduates appears obvious.

When the GROWING YOUNGER Program was being developed, the staff heard a number of theories relating to the folly of the plan: "Old people won't come," "Old people won't change their ways," "Old people can't learn new things," "And, anyway, if they did change, it's too late to do them any good." By mid-1984 after three years of experience with GROWING YOUNGER, each theory could be confidently dispelled as myth. Instead, for several reasons, health promotion for seniors is probably more fun, more rewarding and more cost-effective than for any other age group.

First, older adults have the freedom of time to make health a high-priority aspect of their lives. Time barriers are the greatest problems for programs focusing on younger persons. Second, older adults often appear more appreciative of the educational services, particularly if they are up beat and enjoyable. Their attendance is higher and their commitment more strong once they decide to make improvements. Third, older adults have three times the per capita health care expenditures of people under 65. A 10 percent reduction in costs for a senior is equivalent to a 30 percent reduction for the average nonsenior. If health promotion is to have any real effect on costs, it must certainly start with seniors. Finally, health promotion can make much more dramatic changes in the quality of life for seniors than for others. A 35-year-old person can suffer from poor nutrition, high stress, too little exercise, and a poor self-image without any dramatically obvious symptoms. For such a person, a health and wellness program often takes months to make a difference. With a large percentage of seniors, one can see the difference in a matter of a week or two.

A joyful, interesting, and stimulating wellness program can be the event that makes life worth living for many older people. For others, it can provide an opportunity for deepening friendships and reactivating interests in the community and themselves. For such people, the impact of health promotion is both obvious and lasting. GROWING YOUNGER has demonstrated that a large-scale health promotion program can make a real difference in a community: a difference in the quality of life and level of health of its seniors and in the attitudes all people have about aging.

Chapter 18

Hospitals and Health Promotion for Older Adults

Mary E. Longe, M.A.

Hospitals have been offering health promotion activities for many years, but the field has come of age since 1979. In August of that year, to encourage hospitals to expand their roles in promoting the health of the community, the American Hospital Association's House of Delegates approved the following statement:

> Hospitals have a responsibility to take a leadership role in helping ensure the good health of their communities. In addition to the primary mission of providing health care and related education to the sick and injured, the hospital has a responsibility to work with others in the community to assess the health status of the community, identify target areas and population groups for hospital-based and cooperative health promotion programs, develop programs to help upgrade the health in those target areas, ensure that persons who are apparently healthy have access to information about how to stay well and prevent disease, provide appropriate health education programs to aid those persons who choose to alter their personal health behavior to develop a more healthful lifestyle, and establish the hospital as an institution in the community that is concerned about good health in addition to one concerned about treating illness.[1]

Older adults are one of the populations that hospitals most frequently target for health promotion. In this chapter, program refers to the hospital's overall health promotion effort. Offerings and activities refer to the individual components within the hospital's health promotion program. Both are primarily developed to respond to the specific, immediate needs and desires of the elderly.

A 1981 survey of nearly 6,000 hospitals indicated that 43 percent of the respondents had health education programs for older patients and their families and 11 percent had special fitness programs for older adults.[2] In 1982 those hospitals reporting health education and fitness programs were surveyed again to learn more about their special health promotion programs for older adults.[3] In hospitals responding to the survey, it was apparent that most of the programming was loosely coordinated, with little conceptual focus and haphazard implementation. Since 1982, a review of the literature and informal surveys and interviews indicate that more hospitals are initiating health promotion efforts for the elderly. Those programs, which have written objectives and goals, seem to be better coordinated and developed, with more attention paid both to the older person and to the administrative needs of the hospital.

In general, hospitals organize promotion efforts in two ways:

1. Health promotion activities are frequently viewed as an integral part of hospital services that are designed especially for older persons, such as adult day care, home health care, and congregate meal programs. These activities are so integral, in fact, that they often are not specifically identified as health promotion.
2. Hospital staff identify older adults and other groups, such as children, employees, and the indigent, as target populations for the hospital's community program. Staff, depending on the hospital, community, and program topic, designate various segments of the older adult population for programming. Examples of various designated groups include those aged 55+, 60+, 65+, and 75+; the "old old"; and the homebound old.

This chapter provides an overview of all hospital-based community health promotion programs for older adults. It includes a rationale for hospital involvement in community health promotion, the administrative considerations in developing and managing a community health promotion program, a description of the kinds of activities and programs hospitals offer, and examples of hospital-based community health promotion programs for the elderly. Information used for describing administrative considerations is derived from hospital health promotion programs, rather than from older adult services. Specific examples of activities, however, are taken from both types of program organization.

RATIONALE

Hospitals provide health promotion programs for older adults in order to improve their health and quality of life. Moreover, each hospital identifies specific objectives to meet the needs of the particular population it serves. In addition, the aging of the population and changes in the economic and social environment of health institutions are encouraging hospitals to offer health promotion programs.

Frequently, hospitals initiate health promotion programs as a tool in their marketing activities. Hospitals have found that health promotion is a way to round out their image as a full-service institution. They are now providing prevention, wellness, and rehabilitation services, as well as the more traditional acute care services. Health promotion activities can be designed to bring people into the institution or be placed in the community to take the hospital to the people. Health promotion activities can also be viewed as a diversification option for the hospital or improve the hospital's image and relations with community organizations.

The Population

Eighty-three percent of persons 65 years and older have some type of chronic condition. Older adults have a higher incidence of most major serious diseases. Older people tend to be more vulnerable to infection, and they are in the hospital more frequently and for longer periods of time. Because of a high incidence of disease and the accumulation of chronic illnesses, older persons tend to have multiple illnesses, making diagnosis and treatment more complicated. Functional limitations frequently accompany chronic diseases. Nearly 20 percent of persons 65 and older have difficulty performing basic activities of daily living, and the degree of limitation increases with age. The compounding of all these factors with the changes brought about by the normal process of aging, such as weakening of sensory perceptions, is likely to affect all parts of an older person's life.[4]

Brody and Persily project that older persons will become the dominant users of the hospital over the course of the next 10 to 30 years.[5] They are already the largest health care market. In 1980, when they were 11.7 percent of the U.S. population, older persons accounted for almost 30 percent of all health care. They were responsible for $2,638 in health care spending per person, 29 percent of which was directly out-of-pocket. Although older adults are a major and increasing portion of the population hospitals serve, they have many unmet or inappropriately served needs. At the same time, it is projected that the income of the population will increase dramatically during the next 40 years,[6] and it is likely that an increasing portion of that income will be spent on health care. Because of these factors, hospital administrators are assessing and reorganizing their current lines of services in order to meet the increasing demand for services by older adults.

Social and Economic Environment

Hospitals are no longer being reimbursed under the same protocols as in the past. Federal and private third party payers are changing their financing policies and are paying prospectively, with limits on the total amount received for the diagnosis, rather than retrospectively, based on the cost of the hospitalization.

Administrators are taking a critical look at their institutions, eliminating programs that are no longer useful and adding programs that increase revenue.

Concurrently, the idea of marketing hospital services and of viewing patients and the community as consumers has dramatically influenced traditional hospital planning. At the same time, consumers are beginning to view health care as a product for which they can shop around, and they regard hospitals as only one of the many sources of that product.[7]

The complexity of health care needs of older persons requires that assessment be based on the individual's level of functioning, rather than on the absence or presence of disease alone. Many of the elderly and their families require an array of services to respond to these complex needs; for example, assistance in locating useful services, such as home care, adult day care, transportation, recreational opportunities, and low-cost, nutritious meals; information and skills in the management of disease or diseases; information on options for care and when and how to make choices; and information, strategies, and skills to protect and maximize health.

Hospital administrators view health promotion as one way to meet some of the needs of older adults and, at the same time, respond to the economic and social environment in which all health care institutions now find themselves. Health promotion programs and services can provide a link between the hospital and the community. Older persons and their families receive the services they need, and, in so doing, develop a relationship with an institution that they will likely turn to for other health needs. It seems safe to project that health promotion programs provided by hospitals will increase in number, variety, and scope of service as the older population increases.

PLANNING AND MANAGEMENT OF HOSPITAL-BASED OLDER ADULT HEALTH PROMOTION PROGRAMS

The mission and goals set by the trustees of the hospital provide a framework for the development and management of programs, products, and services in the hospital. Program planners need to be aware of the administration's operational objectives, such as more visibility in the community, and special problems or needs of the institution, such as the need to use underutilized laboratory or dietetic services. Most important, the program planner must set clear program objectives, such as increased mobility for program participants or decreased days of limited activity. The planning and management of health promotion programs for older adults include collecting information to assess needs and available resources, assembling appropriate staff, developing budget and financing mechanisms, providing services and activities to meet the needs of the community the hospital serves, and monitoring whether objectives have been met.

This section describes how hospitals plan and manage health promotion activities for older adults. For clarity, the discussion is confined only to activities for older adults conducted by hospital health promotion programs. However, examples of actual services and activities designed by other hospital program areas are provided.

Information Collection

To make administrative decisions about specific activities and services, location, and promotion and financing mechanisms, program planners collect information about the desires and preferences of older adults, the goals of the institution, and the resources available in the institution and the community. A variety of strategies that hospitals most often use to collect this information are listed below:

- *statistical documentation* to determine health problems and needs from such sources as hospital discharge records, state and local vital statistics, health departments, and health planning agencies
- *surveys* by phone, mail, or in person to determine the number of people interested in health promotion, the types of activities needed or desired, and the best times and places to offer the activities
- *literature reviews* of current publications for trends, environmental factors, and current state-of-the-art programs
- *internal audit* of the availability of the hospital resources, including personnel, facilities, finances, administrative support, and linkages with community agencies.

In addition, hospital staff often seek assistance from experts at local universities, health departments, and health planning agencies.

Staff

Staff arrangements for health promotion programs vary from hospital to hospital. Of 49 hospitals responding to questions prior to a 1983 invitational conference of hospitals with "innovative community health promotion programs," the number of full-time staff ranged from between 2 and 19 and the number of part-time staff from less than 5 to over 20.

Program staff usually consists of a director— who most likely holds at least a master's degree in health education, business, education, or nursing—and individuals responsible for the development and implementation of certain activities. Staff may have academic and professional experience in nursing, education, public relations, nutrition, physical therapy, or psychology. In some hospitals, one staff person is designated as coordinator of older adult programs; in other hospitals an individual responsible for a topic area, such as fitness or nutrition, develops activities appropriate to the various populations the hospital serves.

Often, the hospital sponsors activities, such as exercise or nutrition classes, with staff from other areas of the hospital, such as the social work or physical therapy departments. Individuals from other community organizations may also facilitate activities. For example, hospitals frequently work with voluntary organizations, such as the American Heart Association, American Lung Association, YM- or YWCA, and American Cancer Society; local and state government agencies, such as offices on aging, health departments, and park districts; churches; community colleges; and older adult residences.

Financing

Annual budgets for total health promotion programs range from less than $25,000 to over $1 million. These cover such items as salaries, program materials, audiovisual material development or rental, printing, supplies, promotion, travel, and capital expenditures, such as for furniture. Expenses for programs specifically geared to older adults include salary, program materials, supplies and equipment, space rental, and promotion.

Hospitals cover these expenses with income from several sources:

- *Hospital Contributions* cover all or part of most health promotions programs. Most hospitals contribute start-up costs; many cover indirect costs, such as a site, telephone, and electricity.
- *Grants* from federal, state, or local government agencies; local or national private foundations; the hospital's foundation; or local businesses are used to fund program start-up, research, and/or implementation costs.
- *Donations* of dollars, educational material, and of exercise or audiovisual equipment may come from participants, local businesses, retailers, or civic groups. These are used primarily to fund equipment and/or all or part of specific activities.
- *Fees* for health promotion activities for the general population are charged by most hospitals. For older persons, some hospitals use sliding scales to accommodate persons living on a fixed, limited, or no income. Other hospitals have developed tuition scholarships and special discounts for older persons.
- *Reimbursement* for health promotion activities differs from state to state and third party payer to third party payer. However, patient education integral to

care is generally reimbursable, whereas community health promotion generally is not.[8]

Unlike health promotion activities for the general public, programming for older persons is frequently viewed as a community service, and therefore services are often free or an individual donation is accepted. Hospitals are willing to provide services at little or no cost because they feel they are meeting an important community need and the hospital will gain a caring image and loyalty from individuals who participate in these activities.

HEALTH PROMOTION SERVICES AND ACTIVITIES

Because of the multiple problems and needs of older persons, it is nearly impossible to define and separate clearly the specific social and health services and activities that will assist the older person. It is also difficult to describe any one service or activity without mentioning others that it supplements or those that supplement it.

Hospital health promotion efforts for older persons vary as the older population served by different hospitals varies. No two hospital health promotion programs for older persons are exactly alike. However, they have some topics of concern in common, as well as a variety of unique strategies and mechanisms that can be used to deliver hospital health promotion activities for older persons. These topics are presented only to provide organization to a complex array of ways to promote the health of older persons. Examples are provided to illustrate, not to exclude, any possibilities.

Health Promotion Topics

From informed observations of hospitals across the country, six broad categories of health promotion topics can be identified:

1. *Patient education outreach* extends the health promotion activity begun when an individual was a patient to beyond the walls of the hospital. Examples include nutritional counseling, diabetes care and counseling, and stroke and ostomy clubs. This category also includes information and education for the well community about specific diseases and health conditions, such as "Living with Arthritis" or back care.
2. *Behavioral change* includes any activity that attempts to change an individual's unhealthy behaviors. Examples include smoking cessation, weight control, assertiveness training, and stress management.

3. *Wellness/life style* offerings integrate health practices into an individual's life style. Examples include survival skills for widows and widowers, cooking for one or two, sexuality and aging, "How to be an Effective Grandparent," tai chi, "Senior Pep," self-defense, and "Aging: A Family Affair."

4. *Medical self-care and utilizing the health care system* include skills and knowledge that prepare an individual to take a more active role in his or her own health care or in the care of another person. Examples from various hospitals include "Take as Directed: Understanding Medications," "How to Get What You Want from Your Doctor," "How to Care for the Homebound Ill and Disabled," and "Senior Citizen Orientation to the Hospital."

5. *Life savers,* which are some of the most common health promotion topics in hospitals, usually deal with health protection and safety. Examples include safety proofing the home, cardiopulmonary resuscitation, "Vial of Life," emergency communications systems, "Careline," first aid and automobile occupant protection.

6. *Preretirement planning* includes information and strategies for any age group on planning a physically, mentally, socially, and spiritually healthy retirement. Topics include health care benefits, planning a will, nutrition, coping with stress, and planning for leisure time.

Services and Strategies for Delivery of Health Promotion

At least 13 different strategies used by hospitals to deliver the various categories of health promotion topics have been identified. Most hospitals use a combination of these strategies described below:

1. *Classroom sessions* are usually single sessions or a series of sessions consisting of lectures, teaching and practicing skills, exercise, and other activities taught by a hospital staff member or an expert from the community. Classes vary in size and scope.

2. *Counseling* is any sort of individualized session to assist the participant to improve health and cope with change. Exercise, nutrition, grief, retirement, options for long-term care, arthritis, and diabetes are common topics for counseling efforts for older persons. Counselors may be specially trained health promotion staff, nurses, mental health professionals, chaplains, or peers.

3. *Screening and assessments* identify certain problems or determine the individual's level of health risk. Referral and follow-up are essential components. Often, hospitals offer screening for speech and hearing, blood pressure, hemoccult, and spirometry. Some hospitals assess aerobic capacity, body composition, endurance, strength, and health risks. One

hospital assesses the individual older person's home and makes recommendations for safe living environments for older persons. To date, few assessment tools are available that are tailored to the needs of the older person. Many hospitals adapt measurement instruments used for younger adults.

4. *Electronic media* disseminate health information to hospital patients and visitors through the hospital's closed circuit television system and to the community through commercial, cable, and public television. Hospitals have developed television series, 90-second and 2-minute spots, and "specials" for various television broadcasts.

5. *Support groups* offer education and a forum for mutual support and discussion on common concerns. Support groups are offered to individuals with certain diseases or conditions. Examples include ostomy or arthritis clubs, widows and widowers groups, and "Companionship and Support as We Age: What We Can Do for Ourselves."

6. *Telephone programs* provide the community with easy access to the hospital and health information. One hospital developed "Careline," an emergency response system. Another hospital developed "Telecare," in which a nurse contacts certain patients discharged the previous day. Other hospitals sponsor "Telemeds" and "Telhospitals" that serve as health information libraries, and still others have developed temporary and sometimes permanent hotlines for special community problems.

7. *Printed materials* are mainly used to supplement other strategies for disseminating information. Some hospitals offer cookbooks with healthy recipes, publish newsletters and periodic magazines on health topics, or provide handouts on certain topics. Materials are developed by hospital staff or experts in the subject area. Depending on the purpose and their role in the health promotion strategy, there may be no charge, the cost may be covered by a program fee, or the material may be used to generate a profit and the cost may include development and a profit margin.

8. *Libraries and resource centers* have been established to make books, tapes, films, pamphlets, and article reprints available to the community. Hospitals have located these resource centers in the hospital, as part of a community library, and in specially identified locations, such as senior centers. One hospital has developed a service to provide physician office waiting areas with health education materials.

9. *Fitness and other facilities* have been developed by hospitals to house their health promotion staff and to provide a guaranteed site for health promotion activities. Facilities frequently include a combination of indoor facilities, such as an aerobic exercise area, cooking facilities, racquetball or tennis courts, counseling and classroom space, a swimming pool, evaluation and exercise equipment, an indoor track, lockers and showers, and a stress

reduction/relaxation area, and outdoor facilities, including a running track, par course, and tennis courts. Mobile units are another strategy to reach the community; several hospitals use vans or trucks to carry materials and equipment to the community. To the author's knowledge, no hospital has facilities used exclusively by older persons; however, many facilities offer programming specifically for older adults.

10. *Health fairs* are frequently conducted with several departments of the hospital or in coordination with other community agencies. They are held on the hospital grounds, in shopping malls, at local libraries, or at a community facility. Hospitals frequently use the health fair as an opportunity to screen for certain health problems, such as cancer of the colon or hypertension. They may provide information on a variety of health topics, or they may focus on one theme, such as health in aging. Both types of health fair showcase the hospital's range of available and pertinent services.

11. *Live-in* smoking cessation or cardiac rehabilitation services have been developed by some hospitals. Most last from 5 to 30 days.

12. *Meals on Wheels and congregate meal programs* are offered on a daily or weekly basis.

13. *Vial of Life, Medic Alert* and similar programs monitor individual patients' medications, special conditions, and needs in an emergency. In some communities, individuals list all their medications, put the paper in a marked vial—the "Vial of Life"—and place it in a designated place in the house (the right side of the refrigerator). In the event of an emergency, emergency teams look there for the person's medication information. One hospital in a hurricane area in Florida developed an emergency evacuation system with local mail carriers. The mail carriers, because of their knowledge of individuals in the community, identify those who need assistance in evacuation and provide the list to the hospital's emergency department. In the event of an evacuation, the hospital knows which homes need assistance.

Hospital tours, equipment loan programs, fitness festivals, special walks, crafts, picnics, and vacation trips are also considered useful strategies to promote the health of older adults. These many strategies, in combination with the variety of topics that can be addressed, provide planners with an almost endless array of potential activities to offer.

EXAMPLES OF HEALTH PROMOTION PROGRAMS

Allentown Osteopathic Hospital

This hospital offers six, one-hour classroom sessions on prevention, promotion, and maintenance of health for seniors. The topics range from the appropriate use of health care services to hypertension, diet, exercises, and mental health and are taught by a nurse experienced in geriatrics and education. Teaching strategies include lectures, group discussion, audiovisual aids, handouts, and questionnaires.

In order to facilitate learning and encourage participation, classes are held in a friendly, supportive, and familiar environment; settings include older adult residences, community meeting places, and churches. Before the classes, hospital staff conduct an interview with each participant to assess his or her special needs and desires. With this information, classes are tailored to cover special interest areas, and actions are taken to compensate for any sensory deficits of the participants. For more information, contact Allentown Osteopathic Hospital, 1736 Hamilton St., Allentown, PA 18104, (215) 439–4000.

Augustana Hospital and Health Care Center

Through its Seniors' Health Program, this hospital offers information and activities on the aging process, nutrition, exercise, medication, disease management, stress, and coping with aging. Programs are conducted in older adult housing, senior centers, churches, libraries, and at the hospital. In 1982, in conjunction with two community churches, the Seniors' Health Program conducted "These Vintage Years, I'd Share with You," a one-day conference for older people and their families, friends, pastors, and community resource people. For more information, contact Seniors' Health Program, Augustana Hospital and Health Care Center, 2035 N. Lincoln Ave., Chicago, IL 60614, (312) 975–5000.

Mt. Zion Hospital and Medical Center

This hospital provides almost a dozen different geriatric services, several of which include health promotion. The Ruth Anne Rosenberg Adult Center is a medically oriented daytime program that enables participants to remain as independent as possible while living in the community. Among other services, the center provides a daily hot lunch, health and nutrition education, exercise classes, and recreational activities, such as field trips. The hospital's geriatric service also provides health screening and referral for individuals over 60 who have not seen a physician in more than a year. The screening includes a physical exam, a laboratory profile, and an assessment of dental needs and speech, language, and hearing abilities. A public health nurse conducts a follow-up report and makes referrals to a variety of medical and community services. For more information, contact Geriatric Service, Mt. Zion Hospital, 1600 Divisadero, San Francisco, CA 94115, (415) 567–2203.

Development of One Hospital's Older Adult Health Promotion Program

Walter O. Bosell Memorial Hospital (355 beds) was built by and serves the retirement community surrounding and including Sun City, Arizona. Sun City has a population of more than 50,000 people over the age of 55.

The hospital's Community Health Programs include: behavioral change and life enhancement activities, such as smoking cessation, breast self-examination, weight control, and microwave cooking; five separate support groups for individuals with Alzheimer's disease, Parkinson's disease, diabetes, multiple sclerosis, and ostomies; self-care, such as "How to Use Home Blood Pressure Equipment" and "How to Manage Medications"; and programs for family members, including "How to Live with an Ailing Spouse" and "How to Care for the Homebound Ill and Disabled." The latter program covers such topics as when to use a wheelchair, cane, or walker; how to give a bed bath; bowel and bladder problems; mouth care; and how to handle emergencies.

In 1983, over 17,000 persons 60 years of age and older from the Sun City area participated in the 200 activities offered by Community Health Progams. Staff attribute this large participation to the community's keen interest in education and health matters and to the staff's knowledge of the community. Every two years, a random sample of the community is surveyed to determine topics and preferable times and locations for activities. Activities are offered during the week from 9:00 A.M. to 4:00 P.M.; they therefore do not impinge on peak socializing times, such as late afternoon, evenings, and weekends.

The staff of the Community Health Programs consists of a part-time coordinator and a full-time secretary who organize the activities conducted by other hospital staff, such as pharmacists, social workers, physicians, and home care staff, and by individuals from other organizations, including the American Diabetes Association, American Cancer Society, and Jewish Family Services. Almost all the programs are free. For more information, contact Community Health Programs, Walter O. Boswell Memorial Hospital, P.O. Box 1690, Sun City, AZ 85372.

CONCLUSION

Hospitals have an important role in influencing the health of the community, and they are faced with an expanding role in caring for the older population. Community members look to the hospital as a health care institution; with the changing population and social and economic environment, the hospital is beginning to provide services and activities desired by community members to promote and protect their health.

NOTES

1. "The Hospital's Responsibility for Health Promotion" (Policy statement of the American Hospital Association House of Delegates, Chicago, 1979).

2. The 1981 survey was conducted by the Office on Aging and Long-Term Care of the Hospital Research and Educational Trust, research and development affiliate of the American Hospital Association. Unpublished, untitled.

3. 1982 follow-up survey was conducted by the Office on Aging and Long-Term Care and the Center for Health Promotion of the American Hospital Association. Unpublished, untitled.

4. *Hospital and Older Adults: Current Actions and Future Trends* (Chicago: The Hospital Research and Educational Trust, 1982), p. 1.

5. Stanley J. Brody and Nancy A. Persily, *Hospitals and the Aged* (Rockville, Md.: Aspen Systems Corporation, 1984), p. 9.

6. *Ibid.*, p. 15.

7. *Ibid.*, p. 4.

8. American Hospital Association, *Reimbursement Forum Proceeding* (Chicago: U.S. Department of Health, Education, and Welfare, 1979), p. 198.

Chapter 19

The Pharmacist's Role in Health Promotion and Wellness for the Elderly

Allen Frisk, R. Ph., M.S.

A careful and thoughtful approach to appropriate drug therapy and use for the elderly is essential for health promotion and wellness. Drugs become especially hazardous to elders due to age-related or altered physiology and pharmacokinetics, the higher incidence of drug interactions, inappropriate prescribing practices, inadequate monitoring of long-term medication, and inaccurate patient compliance. Choosing a safe, yet effective course of therapy, one that balances drug use between the benefits and risks, can aid in preventing illness and promoting health.

Promoting health and preventing illness are the primary missions of all health care professionals. Yet, pharmacists, as well as others in the health care delivery system, treat the sick primarily, rather than preventing illness. Certainly, pharmacists appear to spend much of their time dispensing drugs and related services to those who are ill. Although quality care for those who are ill is certainly desirable, the focus of many health services provided may be unbalanced.[1]

Pharmacist participation in health promotion and wellness therefore appears, at first glance, to be nearly nonexistent. Is this the case, or is there a role for pharmacists to become involved in preventive health care?

MODEL ROLE FOR PHARMACISTS

The pharmacist's position on the health care team is evolving from the traditional role of compounding and dispensing medication to involvement with direct patient care. The field of clinical pharmacy is growing; it involves total drug usage in a hospital, nursing home, or community; encourages specialization of pharmacists; deals with patients' attitudes toward drug therapy; and functions within the health care team concept.[2] Many of these functions related to the clinical pharmacy concept are now being performed by pharmacists.

The growth of clinical pharmacy is due in part to loss of the function of preparing medicines that formerly was a forte of all pharmacists. More important, however, is the *Megatrends* concept of "high-tech, high-touch."[3] Armed with sophisticated computers with programs to maintain and monitor patient's medication records, the pharmacist now has the time and desire to communicate with and counsel the patient. The pharmacist also has the time to participate in community education programs.

Pharmacies of the future will resemble those of the past. The old-time apothecary was operated by a well-trained professional who maintained personal contact with all his clients. Tomorrow's pharmacists will be educators and prescribers, guiding their clients away from questionable therapies, recommending self-medications that are safe and effective, and providing an environment for health promotion in the community.[4] The pharmacy facility itself will also change. Counseling areas for individual conferences will be utilized, and larger meeting rooms will be available for community events. Computers can assist in the educational process, as well as in recordkeeping.

RATIONALE FOR MONITORING DRUG THERAPY AMONG THE ELDERLY

An analysis of drug use patterns, problems, and diagnostic accuracy reveals that drugs are not used wisely by the elderly.[5] The elderly make up approximately 11.5 percent of the population of the United States, yet their use of medication accounts for 25 to 30 percent of the total U.S. drug expenditure.[6] It has been estimated that 84 to 87 percent of the elderly living outside institutions and 95 percent of the institutionalized elderly take prescription drugs.[7] The risk of adverse drug reaction in this group is almost double that in adults 30 to 40 years of age.[8] Elderly patients have a higher incidence of drug-related admissions to hospitals than younger patients.[9] Up to one-third of elders admitted to the hospital may have a drug-related problem that could have contributed to their admission.[10] These problems include misuse of medication, adverse drug reactions, and drug interactions.

The number of drugs prescribed for an individual also influences the rate of adverse drug reactions and compliance. Approximately one-third of elderly patients take five or more drugs.[11] Despite the great risks, overprescribing both in large numbers and dosages seems to occur often. Studies show that up to one-fourth of the drugs prescribed were found to be unnecessary and/or ineffective. Drugs are often prescribed for symptoms, rather than diagnoses, and compound drug problems are therefore overlooked.[12,13] Most of these drug reactions are direct extensions of the intended pharmacological action of the drug. Many others are due to unintentional misuse of the medication.

Clearly, 70 to 80 percent of these drug-related problems are predictable and preventable through appropriate drug therapy monitoring by pharmacists and other health care personnel.[14] Simple education and counseling could have prevented these problems. Other measures for monitoring drug therapy in the elderly, providing a means for predicting and thus preventing potential problems, are presented below.

PHARMACIST'S ROLE IN MONITORING DRUG THERAPY

Procuring Medication

The primary mission of the pharmacist is to provide appropriate medication to the patient. Yet, simply supplying a product is only one small phase of the entire dispensing process. For instance, with the prescribing physician's approval, most pharmacists are now allowed to select a generic equivalent, which may be a less expensive but an equally effective medication. Because certain properties of supposedly identical medications may vary between brands and result in therapeutic inequivalence, generic substitution is not risk-free. The pharmacist's knowledge of biopharmaceutics and pharmacokinetics must be the basis for deciding the appropriateness of generic substitution.[15]

One of the most valuable functions the pharmacist can provide the elderly is the procurement of nonprescription (over-the-counter) medication. The pharmacist's expertise can often save the patient a trip to the physician or encourage the elderly person to seek additional medical help when it is necessary.

Other examples of the pharmacist's assistance in procurement of medication include:

- determining the appropriate dosage form (liquid, tablet, capsule)
- locating difficult-to-find medication
- making home deliveries and checking on shut-ins
- seeking programs now available through pharmaceutical manufacturers to cover prescription costs for indigent clients

Documenting Previous Drug Therapy and Allergy

The pharmacist can often obtain a more accurate and complete drug history from patients than can physicians, nurses, and aides.[16] Drug histories are now taken by pharmacists whenever the patient seeks care from a different part of the health care system. They are conducted when the patient is admitted to the hospital, enters a nursing home, or returns home. During these drug counseling interviews, problems with drug consumption may surface and allow prevention of future problems. To take and maintain a good drug history, one needs an updated drug list, a good history technique, and frequent reevaluation of the patient's status.

This information should be documented and maintained in a patient medication profile and can then be used to make an intelligent assessment of the patient's status or perhaps help make a decision in the course of therapeutic management concerning medication. The profile becomes the common bond between the pharmacist and the patient.

Listed below are five commonly observed drug-related problems that health professionals should consider in discussing or monitoring drug therapy.

1. inappropriate drug therapy or dosage
2. lack of patient education on proper administration or precautions
3. misuse of medication or noncompliance (both overutilization and under-utilization)
4. interactions of medication with other drugs, diet, or disease states
5. adverse response to drug therapy

One-third of geriatric patients may have some problem with their medication that can be corrected, thereby preventing, potentially dangerous complications.

Determining if New Medication Is Contraindicated by Existing Therapy

Often, elderly patients are treated for more than one chronic disease simultaneously, but the medications may not all be compatible.[17] Each patient should be approached on an individual basis and a correct diagnosis be made for each problem. The drug therapy prescribed or recommended should have a definable end point and the risks weighed against the benefits. Reviewing this patient problem list each time a new drug is added can reduce unnecessary therapy. Some eminent geriatricians feel that the elder is best managed on *five* or fewer chronic-use drugs[18] because of cost and the fact that, as the number of medications grows, the likelihood of poor compliance and adverse reactions increases in geometric fashion. As many as 10 percent of geriatric patients receiving 6 to 10 different medications suffer adverse effects and require medical attention.[19]

Determining Contraindications to Other Preexisting Disease States

Aggravation of a preexisting disease by newly prescribed drug therapy can occur, especially when patients are being treated by more than one physician. Each doctor treating a separate disorder may be unaware of the patient's other conditions and medications. The pharmacist can help prevent this problem by maintaining patient medication profiles.

Providing Patient Education on Medication Therapy

Communication between the pharmacist or other health care personnel with the patient and family can often eliminate confusion about drug therapy, increase compliance, and help patients determine for themselves the effectiveness of drug therapy. Practitioners should be aware of their elderly patients' level of drug knowledge and information needs in order to promote more safe and effective drug therapy.[20,21]

In addition to traditional patient counseling, there are a number of systems and techniques for providing information on medication to patients. Listed in Exhibit 19–1 are a number of worthwhile references for aids in the educational process.

Pharmacists should use every means within their power to educate the elderly. Lectures, radio programs, videotapes, and various volunteer organizations are all tools that have been successfully utilized by pharmacists to reach this goal.

Documenting Medication Consumed

Through the maintenance of patient medication profiles, the pharmacist can detect overuse and underuse of medication by comparing the number of doses

---

Exhibit 19–1 Educational References on Geriatric Medication

ABOUT YOUR MEDICINES
  U.S. Pharmacopoeial Convention, Inc., Drug Information Division, 12601 Twinbrook Parkway, Rockville, MD 20852

CONSUMER DRUG DIGEST
  American Society of Hospital Pharmacists, 4630 Montgomery Avenue, Bethesda, MD 20814

ELDER-ED
  National Institute on Drug Abuse, Bethesda, MD 20205

MEDICATIONS AND THE ELDERLY
  William Simonson, Aspen Systems Corporation, Rockville, MD 20850

NATIONAL COUNCIL ON PATIENT INFORMATION AND EDUCATION
  Maloney, S.K., Office of Disease Prevention and Health Promotion, Room 2132, 320 C Street, S.W., Washington, DC 20201

PEOPLE'S PHARMACY—2
  Joe Graedon, Avon Books, 959 Eighth Avenue, New York, NY 10019

PRACTICAL GUIDE TO GERIATRIC MEDICINE
  Medical Economics Company, Cradell, New Jersey 07649

USP DISPENSING INFORMATION
  U.S. Pharmacopoeial Convention, Inc., Drug Information Division, 12601 Twinbrook Parkway, Rockville, MD 20852

dispensed and dates of refills. Records also should be kept of over-the-counter medications. Some nonprescription drugs, such as aspirin, antacids, and laxatives, can aggravate certain diseases, so the patient's use of these drugs should also be monitored.

Ensuring Proper Storage of Medication

Proper storage of medication ensures drug potency. Light, moisture, temperature, and age can all alter drug potency and effects. Such medication as nitroglycerin can begin to lose activity as soon as it is uncapped. Periodic checks of medication supplies and their storage can ensure that patients obtain the dose prescribed by the physician. Pharmacists can visit the homes of elderly and visually inspect medications and where they are stored.

Monitoring Proper Medication Compliance

Patient errors of commission and/or omission in the self-administration of drugs are common among the ambulatory elderly. Most studies indicate that over 50 percent of all drug takers do not comply with prescription directions.[22] The figure may be as high as 90 percent in elderly patients.[23] "The failure of an elderly patient to respond appropriately to an effective drug is nearly always due to the patient's failure to take the drug correctly rather than absorb it."[24]

Noncompliance may be due to a number of problems. The patient may fail to understand the importance of therapy, fail to understand instructions, lack appropriate supervision, feel too ill to take the medication, or have physical disabilities that prevent him or her from taking the medication. In addition, drug therapy may be too expensive, produce side effects or adverse drug reactions, be in unusual or difficult dosage form or in unusual or too frequent doses, or interfere with other concurrent medication or other activities. Finally, the health profession team may have a poor relationship with the elder, express doubt concerning therapy, or be unwilling to educate the elder.[25] Educating health care personnel about these causes of noncompliance can help them monitor drug therapy and prevent drug use problems.

The clinician should be willing to help ensure proper drug usage by continuously reinforcing instructions through both verbal and written communication. Various memory aids may also be of assistance; the most effective ones are daily calendars or diaries listing medication consumption. Also of value are medication pill boxes with exact times marked on the container that hold routinely prescribed medications set out in advance.

Monitoring Side Effects of Medications

In geriatric patients, side effects may be the first signs of acute drug toxicity. If anticipated and detected early, simple side effects, such as nausea, vomiting, or loss of appetite, can aid in preventing more dangerous reactions.

Anticipated side effects may contribute to noncompliance by geriatric patients; altering the time of administration or adding the drug to foods can improve compliance and drug effectiveness. Patients can be warned that certain side effects may occur with some medications, and they may continue taking the medication properly despite minor discomfort if they understand or expect the problems.

Government regulations require that the pharmacist warn the patient of certain side effects. This required responsibility has evolved with the support of most physicians and is an appropriate role for the pharmacist.

Monitoring Adverse Drug Reactions to Medication

Because response to medication is altered in geriatric patients, simple side effects can become adverse drug reactions that result in hospitalization and even death. Certain factors appear to put some patients more at risk than others. The list below describes those elderly who may be more prone to adverse drug reactions.[26]

- Patient is 75 years of age or older.
- Patient is of small physical stature.
- Patient is receiving more than five medications.
- Patient has some kidney or liver dysfunction.
- Patient has developed changes in overall condition.
- Patient is taking "high-risk" medication.

Once identified, elderly patients who have several of these risk factors can be educated through appropriate counseling and then monitored more closely than others.

Medications known to be of high risk in geriatric patients include digitalis preparations (Digoxin); aspirin and nonsteroidal antiinflammatory agents; prednisone and other steroids; antibiotics; warfarin (Coumadin); diuretics; central nervous system agents (tranquilizers, analgesics, sedative-hypnotic agents); and antihypertensive agents (beta-blockers and vasodilators).[27]

The altered effect of drugs may be unpredictable, although atypical responses are often anticipated. Lack of valid drug studies in the elderly contributes to the difficulty in predicting the response. Many of the differences are due to the aging process itself. These alterations, affecting the pharmacokinetic factors of the drug itself, are the major cause of adverse effects and drug toxicity in geriatric patients.[28,29]

Gastrointestinal changes may alter absorption of the drug, and decreased cardiac output and circulation affect its distribution. In addition, drug effects may be more harsh on cells stressed by age and lack of rejuvenation. Altered liver function inhibits metabolism, and decreased kidney function lessens elimination of the drug from the body. Because these factors usually prolong drug life, toxic levels build up as additional doses are consumed.

Because response to drugs is altered in the elderly, use of smaller doses should be considered. Some geriatricians suggest that, whenever medications are definitely needed in the elderly, their dosage should be reduced by 20 to 50 percent or more.[30] Close monitoring for untoward side effects and adverse reactions is also required. Pharmacists should reevaluate each medication and its dose every time another medication is added to the regimen. The medications of elderly patients in nursing homes should be reviewed monthly and those on maintenance medication at home should have their medications evaluated quarterly.

Monitoring for Drug Interactions

The susceptibility of geriatric patients to adverse drug interactions is influenced by a number of factors, some of which are patient-related and others are related to the disease or pathological state of the elder. When all factors are taken into account, there is an extraordinary incidence of drug interactions in this population. Epidemiologic studies demonstrate that the rate of adverse reactions to drugs increases from 4.2 percent when five or fewer drugs are given, to *45 percent* when 20 or more drugs are prescribed.[31,32] When "polypharmacy" is unavoidable, knowledge of the frequency of drug interaction and their mechanisms are essential.

The drugs most often associated with adverse reactions and interactions include: drugs affecting the central nervous system (central nervous system depressants, alcohol); cardiovascular agents (digitalis, beta-blocking agents); antibiotics (tetracycline, sulfonamides, aminoglycosides); diuretics (furosemide, thiazides); anticoagulant agents (Coumadin); and oral hypoglycemic agents (sulfonylureas).

Certainly, because so many drug interactions have been identified and documented, they should also be preventable. Prevention can be achieved by either avoiding certain combinations or by managing the potential interaction by considering such factors as proper dosage, time of administration, and condition of the patient. Sophisticated computer programs that monitor and/or warn health care personnel about the potential drug interaction and its severity are presently being put in place. Until they become commonplace, persons who work with the elderly should recognize that an alteration in the patient's behavior or an apparent deterioration in the individual's condition may be the result of a drug interaction.

The accessibility and proper utilization of the patient medication profile have proven the most successful means of preventing drug interactions.

Providing Educational Programs

Several leaders within the pharmacy profession have suggested the pharmacist can serve effectively as a drug information consultant and educator.[33,34,35] Descriptions of pharmacists' involvement in providing health education and information rarely distinguish between the two terms, even though they are fundamentally different. Health education refers to the provision of knowledge that results in a behavioral change, whereas information suggests simply the provision of facts.

The literature describes numerous examples of health education and information services with a community-wide focus that are provided by pharmacists. Often, pharmacists participate in formal, multidisciplinary educational programs. A number of pharmacists have used the media to promote preventive health issues, informing the public about health topics through newspapers, radios, and television. Public health messages addressing such issues as poison control or high blood pressure are made available during designated times of the year. Many pharmacies provide general health information centers. Informational pamphlets, brochures, and other handouts are readily available. In addition, pharmacists promote health education of the public by organizing and participating in health fairs.[36]

It is important to recognize that provision of health education or information services does not ensure the prevention of illness. Additional studies should be conducted to determine how patient education relates to preventive health care. Nevertheless, in many instances, health education should, and health information may, result in illness prevention.

CONCLUSION

Pharmacists can make a contribution to preventive health care in the elderly through their knowledge of drug therapy and position in the health care delivery system. They are generally well-trained in drug actions, reactions, and interactions—all problems in the geriatric patient.

In addition, pharmacists provide an important link between the prescribing physician and the patient. They may use this position to foster rational, safe, and effective drug therapy. The appropriate use of drugs in preventing illness and promoting wellness among the elderly is thus realized. Pharmacists have a real opportunity to achieve this objective.

NOTES

1. James M. McKenney, "The Pharmacist's Role in Community Preventive Health Care," *American Pharmacy* NS23 (August 1983): 16–22.
2. P. Allen Frisk, and William Simonson, "The Pharmacist's Expanding Role in Home Health Care of Geriatric Patients," *Geriatrics* 32 (December 1977): 80–85.
3. John Naisbitt, *Megatrends,* (New York: Warner Books, 1982), p. 35.
4. Joe Graedon, "The Pharmacy of the Future," *Medical Self-Care,* (Fall 1980): 16–17.
5. James W. Cooper, "Pharmacology: Drug-Related Problems of the Elderly," in *Eldercare: A Practical Guide to Clinical Geriatrics,* ed. M. O'Hara-Divereaux, L.H. Andrus, and C.D. Scott (New York: Grune and Stratton, 1981), p. 65.
6. William Simonson, *Medications and the Elderly,* (Rockville, Md.: Aspen Publications,1984), p. 7.
7. M.F. Laventurier and R.B. Talley, "The Incidence of Drug-Drug Interactions in a Medi-Cal Population, *California Pharmacist* 20 (1977): 18.
8. William Simonson, *op. cit.,* p. 125.
9. Kenneth L. Melmon, "Preventable Drug Reactions," *New England Journal of Medicine* 284 (1971): 1261–1270.
10. P. Allen Frisk, J.W. Cooper, and N.A. Campbell, "Community-Hospital Pharmacist Detection of Drug-Related Problems Upon Patient Admission to Small Hospitals," *American Journal of Hospital Pharmacists* 34 (1977): 738–742.
11. William Simonson, *op. cit.,* p. 65.
12. James W. Cooper, *op. cit.,* p. 66.
13. J.W. Cooper et al., "A Seven Nursing Home Study of Potential Drug Interactions," *Journal of American Pharmaceutical Association* NS15 (1975): 24.
14. K.L. Melmon and H.F. Morrelli, *Clinical Pharmacology,* 2nd ed. (New York: Macmillan Publishing Co., 1978), p. 967.
15. William M. Heller, "Drug Entity and Product Selection," in *The Practice of Pharmacy,* ed. Donald C. McLeod and William A. Miller (Cincinnati: Whitney Books, 1981), p. 16.
16. J.C. Craddock et al., "Postadmission Drug and Allergy History Recorded by a Pharmacist," *American Journal of Hospital Pharmacists* 29 (1972): 250–252.
17. William Simonson, *op. cit.,* p. 167.
18. James W. Cooper, *op. cit.,* p. 74.
19. K.L. Melmon and H.F. Morrelli, *op. cit.,* p. 972.
20. Steven R. Moore et al., "Receipt of Drug Information by the Elderly," *Drug Intelligence and Clinical Pharmacy* 17 (December 1983): 920–923.
21. Jack M. Rosenberg et al., "Elderly Ambulatory Care Patient's Knowledge about Drugs," *Hospital Pharmacy* 19 (April 1984): 280–301.
22. J.K. Cooper et al., "Intentional Prescription Nonadherence (Noncompliance by the Elderly)," *Journal of the American Geriatrics Society* 30 (1982): 329-333.
23. James W. Cooper, *op. cit.,* p. 80.
24. M.R.P. Hall, "Drug Therapy in the Elderly," *British Medical Journal* 3 (1973): 582–584.
25. William Simonson, *op. cit.,* p. 83.
26. William Simonson, *op. cit.,* p. 125.

27. P. Allen Frisk, J.W. Cooper, and N.A. Campbell, *op. cit.*

28. James W. Cooper, *op. cit.*, p. 67.

29. Gene A. Riley, "The Influence of Aging on Drug Therapy," *U.S. Pharmacist* 2 (November/ December 1977): 28–45.

30. James W. Cooper, *op. cit.*, p. 66.

31. Lawrence H. Block, "Drug Interactions and the Elderly," *U.S. Pharmacist* 2 (November/ December 1977): 46–55.

32. K.L. Melmon and H.F. Morrelli, *op. cit.*, p. 972.

33. James M. McKenney, *op. cit.*, p. 17.

34. James W. Cooper, *op. cit.*, p. 74.

35. William Simonson, *op. cit.*, p. 83.

36. James M. McKenney, *op. cit.*, p. 17.

Chapter 20

A Community-Oriented Approach to Health Promotion: The Tenderloin Senior Outreach Project

Robin Wechsler, M.P.H.
Meredith Minkler, Dr.P.H.

The Tenderloin area of San Francisco, California, has a long and widely publicized history as a high-crime, "red light district" with high rates of such health and social problems as heroin addiction, alcoholism, malnutrition, and suicide. The 45-block area houses large numbers of ex-offenders, prostitutes, and drug abusers, as well as former mental patients who were "mainstreamed" from state mental hospitals in the 1960s.

Less well known is the fact that the Tenderloin is one of the largest "gray ghettos" in the United States, with 8,000 elderly men and women or 40 percent of the total neighborhood population residing in its many single-room-occupancy (SRO)[1] hotels. A multiplicity of health problems are common among the Tenderloin's elderly residents, including alcoholism, depression, malnutrition, and hypertension. For many, the problems of social isolation and powerlessness are intimately connected with the health problems experienced.[2]

This chapter describes and analyzes a community-oriented health promotion program aimed at building supportive networks among elderly hotel residents and stimulating broader community action. Following an introductory look at the Tenderloin Senior Outreach Project that contrasts it with health promotion approaches that focus primarily on individual behavior change, the theoretical underpinnings of the project are explored. Two case examples then are used to demonstrate in more detail the usefulness of this alternative approach to health promotion for the low-income elderly of the inner city.

THE TENDERLOIN SENIOR OUTREACH PROJECT: AN OVERVIEW

The Tenderloin Senior Outreach Project (TSOP) provides a new way to approach health promotion from a community-oriented perspective. Programs typically designed for this population have involved (1) the provision of information about smoking, nutrition, exercise, and alcohol/drug abuse, and (2) screening and referral services for the early detection and treatment of disease.

Participants in these programs are encouraged to take simple steps to improve their health, including exercising, eating well-balanced and nutritious meals, and reducing alcohol use. Yet, integrating these seemingly simple behaviors into daily life in the Tenderloin is very difficult. Many residents are limited in their access to resources required to make the desired health behavior changes. For residents who have little access to sources of nutritious, affordable foods, for example, improving their diet may be difficult. Similarly, taking walks around the neighborhood for exercise is a frightening proposition for many elderly residents who have been mugged—some several times—when they ventured outside on an errand. Reducing alcohol use may take more than determination in a neighborhood where bars are more prevalent than any other type of business and where alcohol is more readily available than fresh fruits and vegetables. The Tenderloin environment, in short, neither provides support nor reinforcement for behavioral change and, in many ways, reinforces unhealthy life styles and behaviors.

TSOP is a community-oriented health promotion program in that it defines health problems within the context of the larger environment and seeks to address the role of the social, economic, and political determinants of health. Using relevant principles and methods of community organization, TSOP attempts to bring together elderly neighborhood residents to determine their own health priorities and to develop a base of power around their immediate health needs and interests. The elderly themselves thus play key roles in (1) identifying a health problem, (2) analyzing its root causes, (3) designing appropriate interventions and programs, (4) implementing the programs, and (5) evaluating program effectiveness. Indeed, a major aim of TSOP has been to help elderly residents move from the position of change *targets* to that of change *agents,* acting on their own behalf in collectively devising strategies and garnering resources to help alleviate shared social problems.

TSOP was established as a university-sponsored project in 1979 to address the interrelated problems of social isolation, poor health, and powerlessness common among elderly residents of the Tenderloin's low-income SRO hotels. The Project's two major goals were:

1. to improve the physical, mental, and emotional health of elderly residents by increasing social support and providing relevant health education
2. to facilitate individual and community empowerment by helping residents identify common problems or needs and to seek solutions to these problems collectively

The basic mechanism of action through which TSOP works to achieve these goals is the support group, held on a weekly basis in each of eight Tenderloin hotels. The support groups are facilitated by students in public health education and related disciplines who help elderly tenants identify common problems and develop action plans for addressing them.[3] An average of 20 students work with TSOP at any given time, spending a minimum of four to six hours per week in the community for periods ranging from three months to two years. Under the guidance of the full-time project director, the student volunteers are helped to use relevant educational and community organizing approaches in the hotel-based discussion groups that they coordinate.

Five of the eight TSOP groups have been meeting regularly for over four years. Since the project's inception, three additional hotel groups have been initiated. Hotels are recruited to sponsor TSOP groups based on several criteria:

- Does the hotel have a large percentage of elderly residents?
- Is the hotel manager supportive of the concept and willing to work with the group?
- Is there a lobby or adequate space in which to hold the meeting?
- Are trained TSOP volunteers available to facilitate the groups?

As the TSOP groups develop, a core membership of elderly residents forms in each of the hotels. Between 10 and 25 percent of the residents attend the meetings on a regular weekly basis, with another 25 percent attending sporadically. Special TSOP events, such as community speakers and meetings with the mayor or city officials, attract even larger numbers of participants.

TSOP volunteers are recruited from four local universities. Two student volunteers are trained and assigned to facilitate each of the eight groups. Once elderly group leaders emerge, they too receive training and eventually co-facilitate the groups with the students. As the older residents gain experience and self-confidence in their group skills, they ideally begin to facilitate the groups on their own, drawing on student volunteers primarily for back-up support.

As levels of trust and rapport increase, residents begin to discuss in more depth their shared health problems, their root causes, and plans of action for promoting health, both on individual and community levels. Many residents move beyond the confines of their own hotel support groups to attend meetings in other hotels and in the larger Tenderloin community. These interhotel and community-based meetings in turn generate broader social action approaches to problem solving, two of which are described in this chapter. To understand the success of the Tenderloin project in facilitating both increased social support and community health promotion efforts, it is necessary to examine its theoretical base.

THEORETICAL BASE

Two major theoretical frameworks have informed and guided this project since its inception. The first—social support theory—is based on the growing body of theoretical and empirical data demonstrating the important interrelationship among social support, sense of control, and health status.[4,5,6,7,8] The second theoretical underpinning is the educational philosophy and methodology eluci-dated by Paulo Freire as "education for critical consciousness."[9]

Social support may be conceptualized as "the resources provided by one's interpersonal relationships."[10] Social networks, in turn, are often defined as "that set of personal contacts through which the individual maintains his (or her) social identity and receives emotional support, material aid, services information and new social contacts."[11] Although this definition is useful in specifying some of the affective and other qualitative aspects of the supportive network, it should be amended to include a focus on the reciprocity of relationships; that is, the individual, through his or her network, both gives and *receives* a variety of types of support.

The basic tenet of social support theory was summarized by social epi-demiologist John Cassel when he noted that decreased social support affects the body's defense system, rendering the individual more susceptible to disease.[12] Although the precise mechanism by which social support influences health status remains unclear, several promising hypotheses have been set forth. One hypoth-esis, with particular relevance to the elderly in environments similar to the SRO hotel, suggests that social support influences health by increasing the individual's sense of control, which in turn may lead to positive health outcomes. Langer and others have demonstrated the influence of an enhanced sense of responsibility and control on the health status of the institutionalized elderly and have examined the implications of their findings for other elderly population groups.[13,14] As Langer has noted, many of the so-called aging problems in this country may in fact result from an environmentally induced loss of control. Decreased opportunity for interaction with others and for participation in decision making may be among the factors that contribute to this diminished sense of control, which in turn adversely affects morbidity and mortality. TSOP attempted to increase social support among tenants in the belief that such support may positively affect the physical and mental health status of residents.

A shortcoming of social support theory lies in its tendency to focus on the individual and his or her supportive network as the sole unit of analysis. Such an approach often overlooks the macrolevel changes that may take place as indi-viduals and communities, empowered by increased social support, work collec-tively to attack those shared problems that have contributed to their oppression.[15] In applying social support theory to the isolated elderly in the Tenderloin, TSOP staff have attempted to look beyond individual-level outcomes of increased social support to focus attention on institutional or community-level changes. This perspective is in keeping with the philosophy of Paulo Freire, whose concern with the development of "critical consciousness" also implies a focus on macro-, as well as microlevel, empowerment and change.[16]

Freire's use of "liberating dialogue" as a means of helping oppressed peasants critically examine their world and take action to transform it played an important role in shaping the development of the Tenderloin project. In an adaptation of the Freire method, TSOP student facilitators employ a process of posing questions at the weekly group meetings through which residents are helped to view the Tenderloin not as a fixed, immutable reality, but as a situation that can be transformed through collective effort.

As an initial stage in this problem-posing process, members of each hotel support group are encouraged by the student volunteers to describe the day-to-day situations that shape their lives. Expressions of helplessness and fatalism are common at this stage, with residents arguing that "nothing will ever change" and that the problems they face are too large and complex to challenge.

Through the group discussion, however, common themes begin to emerge, such as fear of crime; inability to obtain affordable, nutritious food; and the difficulties inherent in living on a small, fixed income. For each theme discussed, volunteer facilitators pose questions designed to help participants examine the root causes of the problems they face. As the residents begin to understand and talk about why these conditions exist, they move on to discuss what collective action they might take as a group to deal with the problem or issue being examined.

This type of dialogue is liberating for several reasons. First, it underscores the importance of the seniors' own perspective on the problem and of their proposed interventions. Such an emphasis differs markedly from the often disabling conviction that it is the outside professional or expert who "knows best" what the problem is and who in turn should be the one to intervene on behalf of the elderly. The concepts of community ownership and control implicit in the Freire approach thus help ensure the success and acceptance of proposed new projects or activities. A second liberating aspect of the dialogical method lies, as noted earlier, in its ability to help elders view their world as a situation that can indeed be transformed through collective effort. An outcome of this view is the serious commitment to developing community health promotion programs, which may result in environmental and social changes conducive to improved health and quality of life.

In summary, Freire's educational theory, as applied in TSOP, provides a framework for countering the learned passivity that is endemic among the Tenderloin's elderly. His technique helps older residents take an analytical look at the conditions of their lives. Residents begin to reflect critically on the substandard buildings in which they live, the lack of nutritious foods in their neighborhood, and the barriers to improving their own health status. As group members work together to plan their own health-promoting interventions, they experience an increased sense of control and self-determination. Two TSOP projects, the Safehouse Crime Program and the Nutrition Project, illustrate this process.

BUILDING INTERHOTEL COALITIONS: THE SAFEHOUSE PROJECT

Of the many health and related issues raised and discussed by elderly tenants, none was so frequently or fervently addressed as the issue of crime. Following the health education principle of "starting where the people are," the facilitators used the issue of crime and victimization of the elderly as a key focus of Freire education and organizing within individual hotels. The emergence of the crime project and the subsequent development by the elderly of their own interhotel coalition around this issue well illustrates the gradual empowerment of the elderly as individuals and as a community through TSOP.

In the fall of 1981, residents from six individual hotel groups viewed a police department film entitled "Senior Power," which focused on crime and safety for elders in the streets. The film advised elderly persons that they must be responsible for ensuring their own safety by carrying fake wallets and engaging in other individual-level crime deterrent measures. The residents reacted to the film with anger, arguing that it ignored the broader social and environmental root causes of crime and that its underlying message implied blame and guilt. Residents who had seen the film in one hotel were encouraged by group facilitators to visit other hotel support groups to discuss their feelings. As a consequence of these intergroup meetings, residents decided to hold a community meeting on the problem of crime in the Tenderloin. Representatives of local agencies were invited to attend, as were other nonelderly segments of the concerned community. Recognizing the power of the media in American society, tenants of several hotels successfully convinced local TV stations and newspapers to cover the meeting. The more than 50 residents who attended developed a proposal containing recommendations for dealing with crime in a nonvictim-blaming manner and requested appointments with district police captains, the chief of police, and the mayor of San Francisco to discuss their concerns.

Soon after the highly publicized community meeting, the elderly residents were granted a meeting with the mayor and chief of police. To increase their visibility and cohesion, the residents organized themselves into a formal interhotel coalition—Tenderloin Tenants for Safer Streets (TT–SS)—before this meeting.

The creation of Tenderloin Tenants for Safer Streets marked a turning point in the history of TSOP, with seniors beginning to meet among themselves, discussing shared problems, and developing action plans with far less reliance on the health education facilitators. In Freire's words, they began to see themselves as subjects capable of reflecting on and potentially changing the objective conditions of their reality.[17]

Tangible and immediate outcomes of the residents' organizing included a highly successful meeting with city officials, increased beat patrols in the Tenderloin neighborhood, and police cooperation in regularly visiting the SRO hotels and getting to know the elderly residents.

Of even greater consequence, however, was the "Safehouse Project" planned and implemented by elderly residents. This project evolved when the residents had the idea of approaching local businesses, agencies, bars, and restaurants and asking them if they would be a place of refuge where community residents could go in time of danger or medical emergency. The businesses and agencies were asked to put a decal in their window depicting a bird in the safety of its birdhouse, which would serve as a community message telling the person on the street that this was a Safehouse where emergency aid could be received.

In the first two weeks, the seniors managed to recruit 14 different stores and other community agencies that agreed to serve as Safehouses. The mayor was invited to open the first Safehouse, in November 1981. Over the subsequent two months, crime in the Tenderloin dropped 18 percent, and by the end of one year, with 48 Safehouses in operation, a 26 percent decline had occurred. Although other factors—for example, an unusually heavy rainy season—helped account for this dramatic decline, police in the area have attributed part of the decrease to this highly successful program. The Safehouse project has received widespread publicity on the *Today Show* and in national newspapers and magazines,[18] and efforts at replication are being considered in several other parts of California.[19]

THE TSOP NUTRITION PROJECT

Many critical facts of life for elders in the Tenderloin work against healthy nutrition practices. The problem of food access is complicated by the flight of major food chains from this and other inner-city areas for wealthier residential neighborhoods. Heavy reliance on "Mom and Pop" grocery stores and on neighborhood restaurants often translates into a diet heavy in processed and highly salted foods, and low in protein, whole grains, fresh fruits, and vegetables. Those foods that are available through corner stores, moreover, can cost up to twice as much as the same items in a major grocery store chain and thus may severely tax the already limited financial resources of the elderly on small fixed incomes. The problem of food access is worsened by the fire code regulations that prohibit Tenderloin residents from cooking in their rooms. Although many residents ignore the rules and regularly use hot plates, many others do not, and meals frequently consist of cold spaghetti, soup, or pork and beans eaten from the can.

The traditional approaches utilized by health and social service providers to meet the nutritional needs of this population are congregate dining for the ambulatory elderly and home-delivered meals for persons who are temporarily unable to attend the meal site. Despite the importance of these programs, however, neither has effectively dealt with the problem of malnutrition on a broad scale. Congregate meals and home-delivered meal programs combined reach only about 10 percent of the Tenderloin senior population in need.

In discussing the problem of malnutrition among the Tenderloin elderly, TSOP group members concluded that poor eating habits were less a result of inadequate nutrition education than of lack of access to food. In the summer of 1983, they responded by developing a multipronged nutrition project that deemphasized the delivery of nutrition education and information and focused instead on removing barriers to food access. Elderly TSOP members worked with another nonprofit community organization, the Food Advisory Service, which agreed to help them establish mobile minimarkets within SRO hotels. A pilot minimarket was subsequently established in one hotel, where fresh fruits and vegetables were sold at cost. Approximately 40 persons or 30 percent of the hotel residents regularly attend the market, buying produce and participating in biweekly food preparation demonstrations.

In addition to improving access to fresh and inexpensive foods, the minimarket affords elderly residents the opportunity to operate their own small business. Senior volunteers are responsible for setting up the market, selling the produce, maintaining market records, and taking inventory. Control of the market rests with the elders themselves, rather than with an outside professional or agency, and this senior control and involvement helps ensure the project's continued success. Perhaps most important, however, is the fact that the elders who manage the market experience an enhanced sense of responsibility and control in their lives, as well as increased opportunities for social interaction. The market thus serves multiple purposes of increasing access to foods, facilitating the development of social support networks, and helping the Tenderloin elderly develop more control over a critical aspect of their environment.

As a consequence of their success with the market, elderly TSOP members also have begun to consider other possible means of improving food access in the inner-city hotel environment. In one hotel, for example, residents are working to establish a "community kitchen," where supervised cooking on a regular basis could take place, and a rooftop garden is being discussed. In other support groups, cooperative food purchasing clubs are being planned, and residents are discussing effective means for advocating that buildings be brought up to code, so that cooking in one's room would become both safe and legal.

Although unconventional in form and content, these approaches to nutritional health promotion well illustrate the kinds of broad-based analysis and action that may take place when elderly participants are enabled to set their own agenda and when environmental change is seen by these elders as a clear prerequisite to effective individual-level behavioral change.

ORGANIZATIONAL DEVELOPMENT & PROJECT INCORPORATION

As TSOP has grown and taken on more projects, its structure has also evolved. In 1982 it became incorporated as a nonprofit agency. The project staff include a full-time director, a full-time nutritionist/assistant administrator, part-time clerical and accounting staff, and about 15 volunteers.

The organization's board maintains a delicate balance between community residents and outside professionals who are committed to the project's goals of empowerment, increased social support, and social action. It takes major responsibility for setting policy and direction. Subcommittees have been established in such areas as budget and finance, fund raising, personnel, and community action.

Although informal leadership development, particularly within hotel support groups, has been a part of TSOP since its inception, a new, more formal leadership training approach was developed in the teaching of group process skills to interested residents, the pairing of elderly residents with student facilitators to co-lead groups, the transferring of responsibility for running group meetings from outside facilitators to the elderly themselves, and intensive day-long leadership workshops. Residents in one group have written and submitted their own grant proposal, utilizing student facilitators and TSOP's project director as resource persons, rather than as primary sources of assistance. The grant was awarded in 1985.

TSOP has been fortunate to have attracted the interest and the financial support of several private nonprofit foundations. At the same time, heavy reliance on this source of funding has been problematic, in part because of the short—usually one year—duration of these grants and the fact that they generally do not provide core project funding. TSOP's 1984 annual operating budget of $89,000 consists of approximately $70,000 from private foundations and $10,000 from private donations and other sources.

With the addition of a half-time administrator, the development of a strong working board, and clear long-range planning mechanisms, TSOP is now in a position to develop a sound and diversified funding strategy. In particular, the generating of ongoing core support through private donations and local government agencies is seen as critical to its continued viability and growth. Finally, a three-year federal grant to support extensive evaluation of TSOP is being sought. Adequate funding for evaluation is particularly critical, because TSOP's effectiveness in the long run depends in part on whether this approach to community-oriented health promotion can be replicated in other areas.

In fact, a major objective of TSOP has been to provide a model of university-community cooperation through which this kind of project could be replicated to the advantage both of student volunteers and of the isolated low-income elderly in their communities. Development and dissemination of a detailed project replication manual and presentations at relevant professional and educational society meetings are a means of providing assistance and encouragement to other individuals and communities interested in developing similar programs in their areas. In this way, it is hoped that the benefits of the TSOP project may reach well beyond the 45-block Tenderloin area of San Francisco.

CONCLUSION

Practicing health promotion in the community differs significantly from practicing health promotion in the workplace or in a medical care setting, and the guiding principles for practicing health promotion in impoverished communities are different from those one would apply to affluent communities. The conditions of poverty itself bring new meaning to health promotion activities. It makes little sense, for example, to advocate life-style behaviors that delay death, prevent the onset of disability, or promote wellness when the barriers to adopting healthful practices are numerous. A more meaningful approach to promoting health in low-income inner-city areas involves empowering elderly residents to reduce and eliminate those barriers so that individual choices are possible. As demonstrated in this case study, such an approach may involve creative outreach to and work with other segments of the community—for example, local stores, the police, and the media—that may work effectively with elders in implementing change.

Although quantitative and qualitative analyses of the TSOP's effects on the health, morale, and sociability of residents have not yet been completed, informal assessments by student facilitators and the elderly themselves indicate impressive changes, particularly in the areas of mental health, perceived sense of control, and sense of community. Moreover, as noted earlier, an outgrowth of the elders' increased sense of control and commonality has been their willingness to tackle major problems in the community—high crime rates and malnutrition—and their effectiveness in working together for change.

Long-term evaluations of TSOP and other community health promotion approaches therefore must include a careful look at the effects these efforts may be having not only on individual health and well-being but also on the larger community. It is this dual focus of concern and action that characterizes community-oriented health promotion and makes it an important alternative approach to meeting the health and social needs of the low-income elderly.

NOTES

1. The U.S. Housing and Urban Development Office (HUD) defines SROs as one-room, one-person per room establishments in which occupants lack private access to plumbing and/or kitchen facilities.

2. Meredith Minkler, S. Frantz, and R. Wechsler, "Social Support and Social Action Organizing in a 'Grey Ghetto': The Tenderloin Senior Outreach Project," *International Quarterly of Community Health Education* 3, no. 1 (1982–83): 3–15.

3. For an expanded discussion of the history and metamorphosis of this project, see M. Minkler, S. Frantz, and R. Wechsler, *op. cit.*, pp. 3–15.

4. J. Cassel, "An Epidemiological Perspective on Psychosocial Factors in Disease Etiology," *American Journal of Public Health* 64 (1974): 1040–1043.

5. S. Cobb, "Social Support as a Moderator of Life Stress," *Psychosomatic Medicine* 38 (1976): 300–313.

6. E.J. Langer, "Old Age: An Artifact?" in *Aging: Biology and Behavior,* ed. J. McGaugh and S.B. Keisler (New York: Academic Press, 1981), pp. 255–281.

7. W.A. Satariano and S.L. Syme, "Life Change and Disease in Elderly Populations: Coping with Change, in *Aging: Biology and Behavior,* ed. J. McGaugh and S.B. Keisler (New York: Academic Press, 1981), pp. 311–327.

8. Meredith Minkler, "Applications of Social Support Theory to Health Education: Implications for Work with the Elderly," *Health Education Quarterly* 8, no. 2 (1981): 147–165.

9. P. Freire, *Education for Critical Consciousness* (New York: Seabury Press, 1973), p. 164.

10. S. Cohen and S.L. Syme, eds., *Social Support and Health* (New York: Academic Press, 1985), p. 390.

11. K.N. Walker *et al.,* "Social Support Networks and the Crisis of Bereavement," *Social Science and Medicine* 11 (1977): 35–41.

12. J. Cassel, *op. cit.,* pp. 1040–1043.

13. E.J. Langer and J. Rodin, "The Effects of Choice and Enhanced Personal Responsibility for the Aged: A Field Experiment in an Institutional Setting, *Journal of Personality and Social Psychology* 34 (1976):191–198.

14. E.J. Langer and J. Avorn, "The Psychosocial Environment of the Elderly: Some Behavioral and Health Implications," in *Congregate Housing for Older People,* ed. J. Seagle and R. Chellis (Lexington, Ma.: Lexington Books, 1981).

15. Meredith Minkler, S. Frantz, and R. Wechsler, *op. cit.,* pp. 3–15.

16. P. Freire, *op. cit.,* p. 164.

17. P. Freire, *op. cit.*

18. See "Safehouses Now Easing Fears of Elderly Residents," *Los Angeles Times,* 21 November 1982, p. 1, and "San Francisco's 'Safehouse' Area: Hopeful Signs in a Crime District," *Philadelphia Inquirer,* 11 June 1983, p. 1A and 6A.

19. For a fuller discussion of the Safehouse Project, see S. Frantz and R. Wechsler, "Tenderloin Tenants for Safer Streets: Inner City Elders Working Together to Fight Crime," *Aging* (in press).

Chapter 21

Research Issues in Health Promotion Programs for the Elderly

William Rakowski, Ph.D.

How effective is health promotion for the elderly? Which programs and policies result in the greatest benefits? Which health promotion strategies seem to be the most promising? In order to answer such questions as these with the greatest amount of certainty, research is clearly necessary. Policy makers, advocates, program directors, and elderly consumers all have a large stake in the results of this research. This chapter discusses several considerations that underlie and accompany the development of an empirical literature on health promotion and health promotion programs in later life. Areas to be covered in the chapter include different criteria by which health promotion evidence is evaluated, what we can *not* expect research data to tell us, and concerns for research design and the subsequent interpretation of results. This chapter is written on the assumption that material and financial support for health promotion and wellness programs (including research components) are desired from the highest levels of government, business, and the nonprofit sectors. To begin with any less expectation for necessary rigor and thoroughness will restrict our full use of research and virtually guarantee that the potential effect of its findings would be limited from the start.

A CONTEXT FOR RESEARCH

Research and program efforts guided by objectives of health promotion for older adults require as much conceptual and methodological rigor as do any other pursuits in gerontology. Health promotion in this way is similar to any concept or theoretical proposition that is the subject of research (e.g., the multiple jeopardy of certain groups of elderly, "relocation stress" following institutional placement). Data pertinent to health promotion will be given credence in major arenas of policy making and resource allocation only if basic criteria of sound empirical study are met.[1,2,3,4] At a very minimum such criteria include specification of clear short-range and long-range objectives to permit thorough evaluation; presence of a conceptual framework or clear rationale to underlie program activities; statements of testable hypotheses; representative and generalizable samples; a health promotion protocol that is sufficiently developed to permit replication and evaluation across several samples and settings; a representative and well-operationalized set of independent and dependent variables; measurement indices with satisfactory reliability and validity; data collection methods that minimize the risk of bias; statistical techniques that are appropriate for the research questions, for the number of variables being employed, and for the sample size; and, recognition of the limits to any particular study.

The traditional experimental/control research model, with random assignment of a target unit—individuals, families, communities—to different programs, will almost certainly continue to be the standard of quality against which the design of health promotion research and the credibility of its outcome data are judged. The appeal of this paradigm lies in its straightforward rationale. Comparisons can be made among intervention groups or strategies that are known to vary in specific ways, when all else is held equal and errors are randomly distributed through initial random assignment. Evidence for the long-term maintenance of program benefits is also likely to be required to provide a fully complete picture of the impact of health promotion programs. Realistically, research with any less rigor is not likely to command serious attention at the highest levels of policy formation and resource allocation.

When conducting research and interpreting its data, we must recognize that research is best able to identify health promotion strategies that have the *relatively* highest likelihood of reaching the *relatively* greatest number of persons for the *relatively* longest time. Literature on personal health behavior suggests that almost any well-reasoned health promotion strategy will work for someone. There is no single formula for success. Personality characteristics—for example, perceived control over health, future outlook—prior life-style health habits, skill level in dealing with health matters, and strength of informal social supports all need to be investigated as they interact with characteristics of health promotion programs (e.g., uses of media, level of responsibility placed on the participant, individual *vs.* group presentation). Such a task is undeniably a massive undertaking.

Eventually, research data and accumulated experience will indicate what most persons already accept as true—that the best results are obtained when participants are approached as individuals and the need for program flexibility is recognized. What we are in fact moving toward, however slowly, is the capability to build sufficient options for flexibility into health promotion packages in order to be most responsive to each person's unique situation. This responsiveness may be the most realistic, yet also the most demanding, expectation to hold for the outcomes of research guided by health promotion.

Finally, health promotion is certainly not an objective unique to programs planned for older adults. Unless a significant amount of support is directed toward other segments of the population—for example, school nutrition, environmental safety for younger adult workers—our society will simply be a revolving door of successive cohorts of older adults who show little evidence of gains made in morbidity, mortality, behavioral change, or quality of life. Research can provide estimates of the years of life that might be gained through efforts to reduce recognized risk factors at various points throughout the life span. Research on correlates of the health-related behaviors of older adults is also likely to show the desirability of directing attention to their life-style habits earlier in life. In a context of limited resources, however, the extent to which advocates for the elderly are willing to limit their requests for age-categorical support might become a delicate issue and one discussed quite separately from the results of any research showing the need for a life-span perspective.

THE "COURTS" OF EVALUATION

Perhaps the most basic question at issue for policy makers, advocates, and elderly consumers is whether health promotion and wellness programs for older adults are "worth it." Stated more subtly, how do such programs *pay* for themselves? Building a research literature to answer such questions is a time-consuming process, in which evidence usually accumulates only gradually, is sometimes contradictory, and is characterized by ever-present gaps. However, although there will always be gaps in our knowledge, policy and resource allocation decisions must be made based on the best information that is available at any given time.

In an already complex context of politics and searches for funding support, advocates for health promotion and wellness programs should be aware of several different areas in which evidence for the benefits of health promotion efforts can be obtained, presented to others, and judged. All types of benefits or outcomes may not carry equal weight in the eyes of political decision makers, planners, or funding sources. Because a judgment to provide or *not* to provide support for a proposed program is so final, it is useful to think about several possible "courts of evaluation" for organizing and presenting health promotion data.[5]

The Court of Cost Containment

The objective of cost containment is certainly predominant in current discussions of health care.[6] The attractiveness of using cost containment as a criterion for evaluating program success lies in its bottom-line "dollars-and-cents" logic and its ready presentation in monetary terms that most people understand. A central question, although deceptively complex, is whether health promotion and wellness programs can reduce the rate of growth in health care expenditures, if not actually decrease them. Even more important, can such savings be demonstrated for services that are primarily reimbursed by third party payers, as opposed to areas of health care usually covered by self-payment? Fewer hospital and physician visits, decreased demands on staff time, and lower volume of services per person should all have bottom-line cost-savings implications. However, it is possible that per person costs can decrease while overall costs increase due to greater numbers of persons being served.

For now, the hope of achieving cost containment has resulted in some research support for demonstration projects. Support for social/health maintenance organizations (S/HMOs), for example, is based on the hope that a comprehensive package of social and personal health-related care, delivered through the auspices of a preventively oriented service setting, can achieve cost control.[7] For any such initiative supported by outside funds, however, results of benefits will need to be evident in a short time for the "soft money" support to be continued.

The Court of Survivorship and Lowered Mortality

In certain cases—exercise training, stress management, postheart attack, or diabetes self-care—the outcomes or payoff from health promotion may include the prevention of unnecessary or premature death. Many issues and events of late life often studied by gerontologists have been seen as important because of concern over a risk of mortality that may accompany them. Relocation stress, widowhood, and even mandatory retirement have been among the areas investigated in regard to subsequent death rates.[8,9,10] The finality of death and the preservation of life provide a stark contrast, with powerful value implications, making lower death rates an especially attractive piece of evaluation evidence to employ. However, documenting an increased rate of survivorship may not be sufficient by itself, due to other considerations involving the quality of life that these persons have. Does living longer necessarily mean living better?

The Court of Illness Reduction and Improved Quality of Life

Reductions in levels of impairment, reduced presence of symptomatology and rates of illness, and the improvement in overall qualitative status of one's life are other measures for evaluating program impact. In fact, the significance of achieving gains in survivorship is enhanced when accompanied by data showing a high probability of improvement in the day-to-day health status of an intended target group. To be most convincing, these indices of lowered illness rates should be objective in nature (e.g., days of activity limitation, average length of an illness episode, hospital utilization rates). Verification should be possible through medical examination or other standard assessment procedures.

Because quality of life often denotes changes in social and psychological domains, it is a less easily measured indicator of reduced illness or dysfunction. The achievement and maintenance of an improved quality of life are probably the most important challenges to health and social policy for older adults and perhaps also the most frustrating to pursue. Increased life satisfaction, becoming a more informed consumer, participation in a meaningful social role, improved self-concept, gains in morale, enhanced capacity for self-care, better knowledge about aging, improved family communication, and social integration are among the outcomes often sought from health promotion programs. Results in such areas are currently more susceptible to challenge due to such issues as instrument reliability, validity, and the existence (or absence) of associations with observed changes in behavior. For example, what does a four-point shift on a scale of life satisfaction really mean? At the same time, an improved quality of life however generally it is defined, has the advantage of representing a goal that most people desire for themselves and can therefore readily identify for others.

The Court of Behavioral Change

Programs of health promotion may be evaluated simply by the presence or absence of observable changes in a specific behavior, relative to a predetermined level or objective. Weight loss, physical endurance, smoking cessation, knowledgeable selection of specific food groups, and control of alcohol intake are some specific practices that are often targeted for change. In such cases, broader effects on improved quality of life may not be a prime concern. Risk-factor reduction may be a sufficient and satisfactory objective in a limited but crucial area of life.

Similarly, programs of health promotion may make arguments for their effectiveness and the viability of receiving support based on the relative ease with which particular health-related activities can be changed. As literature develops on the elderly, certain health-related practices may be found to be easier to modify than others. If potential benefits of interventions in diverse areas are comparable, then resources may be easier to obtain for those behaviors that are most amenable to influence, especially when changes can be maintained over the long run. Objective evidence of behavioral change has the advantage of being translatable into cost-containment projections, if dollar figures can be attached to the consequences of behavior.

The Court of Productivity and Functional Independence

Reductions in mortality and rates of illness, and change in health-related behaviors are important outcomes of health promotion efforts, but they may not provide a complete set of evidence for their effectiveness. Not only should we focus on the *elimination* of problem situations and risk factors through health promotion initiatives, but we should also emphasize positive actions. When an undesirable situation, such as smoking cessation or dietary control, is modified, what *desirable* actions replace those that were given up? Is health promotion simply a matter of *not* doing something? Practically speaking, therefore, research investigations should attempt to identify and then monitor indicators that *clearly* reflect an *active* outcome of health promotion programs. An increased productivity (actual or potential) and greater capacity for functional independence are two areas in which such evidence can be gathered. This type of data possesses the attractive feature of implying what the individual may contribute *to* society. Costs of a program may therefore be recovered by some combination of actual savings and returns to society's reservoir of human, material, and monetary resources. The work setting, for persons still employed, is an important context for research to investigate such gains.

Priorities Among Courts of Evaluation

There is no *a priori* best or most appropriate court of evaluation as a basis for resource allocation decisions. Governmental policy, interest-group advocacy, and prevailing political philosophies may be the most important determining factors. Cost-containment is currently the most heavily emphasized measure and the one best able to stand alone, with the more direct bottom-line evidence of such types of benefits, the better. An ability to document reductions in illness (with evidence for health care cost-saving estimates), combined with either observed changes in a health-related behavior (with estimates for reduced morbidity risk), or with improved productivity (which might offset program costs to society) would appear to be a workable second strategy. Unless extremely dramatic effects could be demonstrated, arguments for long-term support of health promotion and wellness programs based *solely* on reduced mortality or improved psychological/social quality of life criteria would seem to face an uphill battle. To succeed, arguments using these two types of evidence will require political pressure, creative funding strategies, shifts in basic governmental health policy, or employer initiatives for sustaining employee morale.

Third party reimbursement sources and government health economists, for example, may place highest priority on evidence for cost containment. Reimbursement policies under Medicare are, in fact, routinely criticized for not covering services that are preventive or health-enhancing using broader quality-of-life dimensions. There is little reason to expect this coverage to broaden unless anticipated cost savings can be demonstrated through rigorous empirical study.

In contrast, state health planners or health systems agency staff might be especially concerned in their annual planning documents with outlining objectives tied to desired rates of reduction in illness and mortality (e.g., blood pressure control through self-care education) and to behavioral change (e.g., smoking cessation, physical exercise, self-examination). Even here, however, planning objectives may not be implemented state-wide or even regionally unless benefits are expected to exceed the cost of implementation. In turn, advocates for the elderly often try to marshal support around broader themes of improved quality of life, with less emphasis on the courts of cost-containment or lower mortality (e.g., "adding life to years, not just years to life"). Evidence of *cost containment* and lower mortality is a pleasant bonus, of course, but not a determining factor for viewing health promotion as a valuable societal endeavor.

Obviously, there is considerable potential for disagreement across the courts of evaluation. Each has its own attractive feature, and therefore each can be drawn on in selected circumstances to support selected lines of debate. Each type of evidence can therefore also serve the purposes of any proponent's or opponent's hidden agenda. Demonstration of cost-containment, for example, is a rigorous criterion because of the detail and scope of costs that must be monitored. Results, however, might be seen in a relatively short time. In contrast, death rates may be easier to monitor and count, yet take longer to accumulate as evidence, especially if *length* of survivorship is measured. Adamant positions for (or against) the value of any one court of evidence undoubtedly say more about the person or group taking that position than about the form of evidence on which they place the greatest (or least) value.

Any research study must take into account its intended audience, which helps determine an essential core of information that must be gathered and the sample that should be used to allow subsequent translation to the major issues at hand. Advocates for health promotion and wellness programs would therefore be well advised to determine with a bluntly critical perspective the court(s) in which the bulk of their existing evidence lies. Strategies for advocacy can then be determined more realistically and effectively, and an appropriate case can be presented. If research is in the planning stage, it is also essential to determine the type of data that will eventually be collected. Into which court(s) are your data going to fall? The initial selection of outcome measures sets boundaries for what can be discussed, inferred, or generalized when results are presented to others.

WHAT NOT TO EXPECT FROM RESEARCH

At its most basic level, research is a process of collecting information to answer specific questions, which are phrased as straightforwardly as possible. Research is designed to answer those specific questions with the greatest degree of certainty by providing data that carry the least risk of ambiguity. It is possible, of course, to overinterpret data, such as the now classic errors of inferring facts about aging from cross-sectional data, using a single score to represent a multidimensional concept, or implying that a health promotion program was a success in the absence of even short-term follow-up data. It is also possible to expect too much from research. In many instances, research data are at best only a necessary but not a sufficient component of a much larger picture.

Providing Supportive Data

Research plays no favorites. There are no guarantees that empirical investigations will document that benefits occur uniformly to participants from health promotion programs. Realistically, we should expect to see a patchwork quilt of favorable, ambiguous, and neutral outcomes. Moreover, even when considerations in research design and intrepretation are made to accommodate the imperfect control that exists in applied settings,[11,12] the need to establish a standard program protocol that will permit replication and the making of accurate inferences about program effectiveness may seem counterproductive. Program directors may see research as interfacing with a program's evolution toward greater effectiveness. In such cases, research data from a changing program will be as temporary and nonreplicable as the program itself.

It is clearly a professional judgment to decide when a program has achieved sufficient consistency and quality of presentation to merit investigation and evaluation. Once that decision is made, however, the requirements and risks of conducting quality research must also be accepted. Research *is* a risk, because the best we can do is to create an environment for the optimally valid collection of data, however those data turn out. The demands made by research and the potential consequences of research findings should in fact be an effective stimulus for thorough conceptual grounding of program efforts and a careful definition and evaluation of intended outcomes.

Establishing Goals and Priorities

Research data in and of themselves are not sufficient to establish federal, state, or community goals and priorities. Wellness and health promotion for older adults are competing against other attractive programs.

Within the area of health promotion itself, the list of potentially desirable health promoting behaviors and attitudes that we might hope to encourage is indeed lengthy and promises to grow even longer. Which one(s) do we wish to support? Are smoking cessation and nutrition education more important than physical self-examination skills and self-management of hypertension? Even advocates for the elderly may find themselves debating in the various courts of evaluation for their favored priorities. It is not likely that everyone will win. However, it is also possible that health promotion and wellness objectives can be stated in terms of reduction in the incidence and prevalence of major disabilities. Momentum to pursue the positive or active side of wellness—the maximization of personal potential—may need to be generated through broad-based political efforts of which research data are only a part.

Achievement of "Optimum Health"

Research can provide evidence to indicate whether clearly defined health objectives, such as those often found in health systems agency planning documents, state comprehensive health plans, and statements of national objectives, have been achieved. It is not possible, however, to specify when we have "done enough" to promote the health status of older adults, nor can research define when an abstract objective, such as the optimum health of the elderly population, has been achieved. In an absolute sense, there can be no predetermined ceiling on the objectives of good health status for a population. It is difficult to imagine any community of scientists, advocates, or citizens who would be satisfied for very long with any level of progress. Arguments to take the next step beyond are inevitable, creating pressure to promote health in new ways, toward more ambitious objectives. Research data, regardless of their complexity and the elegance of statistical analysis, are often nothing more or less than cannon fodder for assaults in the arenas of policy planning and resource allocation.

Maintaining a Successful Outcome

Health promotion and wellness programs are attractive largely due to the promise of their long-term benefits, whatever court of evaluation is being considered. Follow-up of program participants is obviously necessary, and research data can certainly document trends over time across outcome measures. There are few absolute criteria, however, for specifying *how long* a favorable outcome should be maintained before we claim success, unless we are discussing remission rates for disease processes in which cure is not recognized until a certain time period has passed.

Often, we focus on indicators that reflect changes in morbidity, changes in overt behavior, mortality, and quality of life. Is behavioral change for three months an appropriate time frame? Should morbidity reductions occur for six months, nine months, or a full year? We may need to use the experiences of earlier, similar efforts by others to serve as a guide. The general rule of thumb—"the longer the better"—for the maintenance of benefits will, of course, always hold true when viewed in combination with the program's cost/benefit ratio. The criteria that are established to define the minimum but still acceptable outcomes are the key issue, however, and research data will be only one element in the decisions that are made.

CONSIDERATIONS FOR RESEARCH

Limited Program Size

Health promotion and wellness programs with the elderly have traditionally been modest in size, primarily because of limitations on local resources that often support them. There have only been a few large-scale programs with hundreds or even thousands of participants. Research *can* be conducted with small samples. The flexibility for splitting participants into multiple groups to compare different interventions is limited, however, leaving less opportunity for research on a wide range of creative and theoretically based initiatives. Similarly, statistical methods often require a moderately large sample size to permit multivariate analyses. Although it is true in large samples that statistical significance is often achieved with seemingly small differences among groups, it is also the case that, with relatively small-sized groups, even notable differences may not achieve significance due to the greater possibility of error variance.

There is also the practical question of whether the evaluation of individual small programs, even with good research design, can have much effect on policy circles. Locally based political and funding sources may favorably evaluate the outcomes of relatively small programs, perhaps conducted with their own local constituency, although little attention would be given to the same data by state, regional, or national sources. The fiscal, bureaucratic, and political stakes that accompany decisions related to health promotion can be high. As a result, research planning in health promotion programs for the elderly must be sensitive to the arenas of desired policy impact. The size and generalizability of one's sample are prime considerations insofar as they enhance the certainty of policy makers that a given decision is correct. Similarly, the type of input and outcome variables that have been or are to be employed is also important to the degree that extensiveness of program/policy effect can be estimated.

The Replicability of Programs

To some extent, research is a process that requires replication of prior studies and the introduction of systematic variations, with all else held constant. No single study can answer all possible questions or sample all relevant groups of the older population. Programs therefore need to be repeated and evaluated more than once. The criteria used to determine that a program has been accurately repeated deserve some attention.

It is hard to imagine that any health promotion program could be or should be fully standardized across all leaders, all settings, and all groups of participants. The ideal of laboratory science replicability is unrealistic for health promotion programs. Direct service professionals must have the prerogative to exercise their best judgment when implementing a program plan. At the same time, if program modules, training packages, or standard guides are not available and based on clearly stated conceptual rationales, research is difficult. Programs that deserve to be considered as models need to *earn* such a status through empirically demonstrating their effects. To the degree that comprehensive data do exist to support claims of success, judgments to depart from the established protocol and consequent responsibility either for above-average success or failure to achieve objectives will fall more directly on the professional.

Built-in Bias

Although the experimental/control, random assignment paradigm sets an admirable standard, it is admittedly difficult to achieve. Our research often recruits convenience samples and participants who have made at least some commitment to health promotion, if only through attendance at a seminar or health fair. We can, of course, still randomly assign our sample and use statistical controls to check for possible bias. From the strictest research perspective, however, which is one readily taken by informed critics and political adversaries, the question of built-in bias can still be raised. If results are anything other than clear and dramatic, doubts about success to be expected from broader implementation of pilot projects might be voiced.

There is no simple resolution to this problem, especially when the samples on which arguments are based do not meet the ideal of experimental/control random assignment. Answers to questions raised may need to be crafted from some combination of a comparison to the results of any existing experimental/control research, a logical (if not empirical) rationale to argue that the sample was not unduly biased even though self-selected, reference to the magnitude of program effects (if sizable), and/or comparison of the sample to a larger population to suggest its representativeness. Anticipating such questions suggests foresight and awareness of one's intended audience and possible critics and not defensiveness.

Interdisciplinary Effort

Particularly in the area of health promotion, it should be clear that research must be interdisciplinary from its planning stage through interpretation of its results. General objectives to achieve optimum health are operationalized by indicators that include physiology, nutritional status, functional activities of daily living, biological integrity of particular organ systems, oral health, and psychological status, with each in turn having further specificity. Selection of appropriate indicators and subsequent translation of research data to practice can be achieved only through cooperative efforts. Our research is likely to become more comprehensive and wholistic in its application at the same time that indicators of health status become increasingly specialized and scientific. The challenge lies in effectively forming the pieces of many studies into a coordinated picture—a task of synergy that only interdisciplinary effort can accomplish.

Multiple Variables

Finally, studies on health promotion programs need to recognize the importance of multivariate statistics and longitudinal—or repeated measures—research methodology. To some extent, the new methodology is a double-edged sword. On the positive side, which the author considers to be more important, research efforts are able to incorporate much larger numbers of variables, in more detailed conceptual frameworks, which more closely capture the logic underlying our program efforts. Methodological and conceptual sophistication can only make health promotion appear to be an endeavor willing to achieve scientific and scholarly credibility. On the other hand, an increased number of variables also produces the opportunity for ambiguity of interpretation and even contradiction. For example, does the achievement of three out of six program objectives constitute "success," even though a control group program showed improvement in none of the target areas? What if the path-analytic models for the three successfully achieved objectives exhibit marked differences in structure? The use of several outcome and predictor variables also permits greater opportunity for apparent contradiction among studies and therefore extra leeway for value judgments and biases by policy makers in setting health promotion priorities and in their subsequent process of resource allocation.

CONCLUSION

Rigorous and sound research studies must be conducted to help answer the question of whether or not health promotion efforts with older adults deserve extensive commitment of time and resources. The experimental/control group model of research will probably continue to be the standard against which health promotion data are judged. However, the considerations that are involved in interpreting and implementing data often go far beyond research design itself. This chapter has discussed several of these additional factors.

One factor is the different "courts" of evaluation, including those of cost-containment, survivorship and mortality reduction, lowered rates of illness and an improved quality of life, behavior change, and productivity/functional independence. It is crucial for health promotion advocates to evaluate critically the weight that their particular type of evidence will carry.

A second factor is the inability of research to answer certain key questions by itself. There is no guarantee that data will confirm the benefits of health promotion programs for the elderly. Similarly, we need to be careful about extending data based on *group* results to what given *individuals* can expect to achieve. Research data can not tell us when we have achieved optimum health for older persons, nor can it tell us what our goals and priorities for health promotion ought to be. In addition, the time that must elapse before one can say a program has been successful is also difficult to define.

Other factors include the small size of many programs, the difficulty of developing a standard or replicable program, the complexities of multiple variables, and possible biases from self-selection.

Because of the highly analytical nature of hypotheses testing, theory, development, and statistical methods, research on health promotion and wellness in later life carries a risk of taking a fragmented approach toward an objective that has usually been viewed as wholistic. It is certainly true that research may employ excruciating detail and procedures, reaching the seemingly too common conclusions that we still need more research and can make few firm statements at the present time. Frustration in such cases is fully understandable. Unfortunately, this author knows no easy resolution to this problem. There is no guarantee that data will provide convincing evidence of benefits in any court of evaluation; but, in the absence of a dramatic change in fundamental governmental health policy, however, research is among the few factors supporting health promotion.

NOTES

1. Karl E. Bauman, *Research Methods for Community Health and Welfare* (New York: Oxford University Press, 1980).

2. Michael Q. Patton, *Utilization-Focused Evaluation* (Beverly Hills, Ca.: Sage Publications, 1978).

3. Claire Sellitz, Lawrence S. Wrightman, and Stuart W. Cook, *Research Methods in Social Relations*, 3rd edition (New York: Holt, Rinehart, and Winston, 1976).

4. Carol H. Weiss, *Evaluation Research* (Englewood Cliffs, NJ: Prentice-Hall, 1972).

5. William Rakowski, "Research Issues in Health Promotion with Older Adults," (Paper presented at the Annual Meeting of the National Council on the Aging, Detroit, March 16, 1983).

6. S.E. Berki, ed., "Health Care Policy in America," *The Annals of the American Academy of Political and Social Sciences* 468 (July 1983): 9–246.

7. Dennis L. Kodner, "Who's a S/HMO? A Look at Metropolitan Jewish Geriatric Center and Its Plans to Develop a Social/Health Maintenance Organization," *Home Health Care Services Quarterly*, 2 (1981): 57.

8. Suzanne G. Haynes, Anthony J. McMichael, and H.A. Tyroler, "Survival after Early and Normal Retirement," in *Second Conference on the Epidemiology of Aging*, ed., Suzanne G. Haynes and Manning Feinleib (Bethesda, Md.: National Institutes of Health, July 1980, NIH Publication No. 80–969), p. 187.

9. Knud J. Helsing, Moyses Szklo, and George W. Comstock, "Factors Associated with Mortality after Widowhood," *American Journal of Public Health* 71 (1981): 802.

10. Richard Schulz and Gail Brenner, "Relocation of the Aged: A Review and Theoretical Analysis," *Journal of Gerontology* 32 (1977): 323.

326 WELLNESS AND HEALTH PROMOTION FOR THE ELDERLY

11. Donald T. Campbell and Julian C. Stanley, *Experimental and Quasi-Experimental Designs for Research* (Chicago: Rand McNally, 1963).
12. John W. Farquhar, "The Community-Based Model of Life Style Intervention Trials," *American Journal of Epidemiology* 108 (1981): 103.

Chapter 22

Health Promotion and the Elderly: Evaluating the Research

Sharon Arnold, M.S.P.H.
Robert L. Kane, M.D.
Rosalie A. Kane, D.S.W.

Although prevention measures taken early in life have always been an acceptable way to mitigate, defer, or prevent the chronic diseases and functional problems of later life, more recently our society has promoted interventions directed at persons who are already old. Older persons, particularly in their seventies and eighties, are likely to suffer from one or more diseases or functional disabilities. Unfortunately, little definitive knowledge exists about the causes of these conditions and the efficacy of interventions to prevent them or minimize their effects. In this chapter, the authors take a broad view of health promotion and disease prevention, including activities taken to alter a person's susceptibility to disease, to reduce the extent of the disease, and to minimize the dysfunction that may accompany it. The general difficulties inherent in evaluating health promotion activities directed at the elderly are discussed, as well as the state of research on the efficacy of specific interventions, such as the prevention of cardiovascular disease and osteoporosis, the treatment of hypertension, and general health promotion activities, including smoking cessation, exercise, and dietary modifications.

EVALUATING HEALTH PROMOTION ACTIVITIES

The term "risk factor" has been used in the literature to connote a characteristic that identifies an individual as having an increased likelihood of developing a given condition. Risk factors may be of two types: mutable (e.g., personal habits, body weight) and immutable (e.g., demographic and genetic characteristics, such as age, sex, family history). Unfortunately, it is easy to confuse the two types of risk factors. For example, weight may be mutable at any age, yet the effects of obesity on risk of disease may be immutable at some given point. Presently, we lack good information about the risk associated with various behaviors of the elderly and the effect of behavioral change in old age on that risk.

The traditional taxonomy of prevention is difficult to apply to the elderly. The distinctions between primary, secondary, and tertiary prevention fit poorly into the language of chronic disease. A condition may be simultaneously a preventable disease—and thus a problem in its own right—and a precursor (or risk factor) for another condition that could follow. For example, osteoporosis is a common geriatric problem and also a risk factor for hip fracture. Hypertension is a problem in itself and a risk factor for stroke and heart disease. Thus, one can attempt primary prevention of hypertension (e.g., through diet modification), whereas control of hypertension (tertiary prevention) becomes primary prevention for stroke.

Another poorly understood issue is the propensity of the elderly individual to change his or her behavior in order to reduce the risk factor. Modifying personal behavior is difficult at any age, and evidence of noncompliance with treatment regimens is well documented in the elderly. Furthermore, although motivation may be high to change risk factors after the manifestations of disease, the possibility of irreversible damage cannot be excluded. Epidemiologic studies provide evidence of associations, but few studies have demonstrated that, even when a characteristic is changeable, reducing that factor leads to reduced risk in the elderly. Moreover, few investigators have even asked the question in this age group.

Even though a risk factor can be altered, it does not follow that the alteration is effective in preventing the disease or problem of interest. At best, some risk factors are connected to the disease by secondary associations. In other cases, time of exposure may prove to be an important element in the value of preventive intervention, especially in the elderly. On the one hand, a risk factor may need to have been present for a minimal period before it is associated with increased risk of the disease; for example, obesity does not appear to have a substantial role in heart disease, unless it has been present for some time.[1] On the other hand, once a risk factor has existed for a substantial period, it may have produced its effect, and thus any subsequent efforts to alter it may be unproductive; some British geriatricians have taken this position with regard to treating established hypertension.[2]

Other difficulties exist in the evaluation of preventive interventions in the elderly. Discussions about health promotion and disease prevention tend to get bogged down around related issues of cost and efficacy. Efficacy is often difficult to demonstrate; once risk factors have been identified and a treatment plan determined, one must demonstrate that people do, in fact, follow the treatment and that the treatment makes a difference in risk. This effort often entails establishing the nonoccurrence of rare events, which usually require large-scale, expensive studies. In addition, the cost of health promotion includes more than the direct costs of the programs. A cost-effectiveness analysis must also consider inconvenience costs, indirect costs (such as the costs of evaluating false positive cases), and untoward consequences of interventions (such as drug side effects or the psychological consequences of being labeled as having a disease or at high risk of developing one).

Another issue concerns the distinction between the prevention of specific diseases and the promotion of a higher level of functioning. Although the focus of prevention has traditionally been on conditions or disease states, a more appropriate focus for the elderly may be on the level of functioning; in this case, an increase in the level of functioning would replace the absence of disease as evidence of success.

The long past-time horizon of the elderly poses difficult questions of when during the life course to apply interventions, especially when time of exposure to risk is a significant factor. It is also difficult to isolate any specific intervention in the life course of the individual as the definitive one that affected the outcome. On the other hand, the relatively short future-time horizon (and higher prevalence) makes certain preventive efforts, such as influenza vaccines, more cost-effective for older than younger age groups. These issues should be taken into account when estimating the effects of interventions on the elderly.

The benefits to be derived from applying interventions to prevent future disease or disability in someone who is already old is influenced by the narrow therapeutic window that characterizes the elderly person. The line between doing good and doing harm with an intervention is hard to distinguish. With drugs, for example, the range between dosage levels for benefit and side effects narrows for older patients. Aging does not imply inevitable decline, but it does intensify the risk of iatrogenic consequences of the best-intended actions.

EFFICACY OF INTERVENTIONS

Preventive strategies may be classified into two general groupings: strategies aimed at those *conditions or disease states* that may be addressed in traditional preventive terms and strategies focused on specific *behaviors* that are likely to produce beneficial or adverse effects on various conditions and thus on health states. These two approaches overlap a great deal. Both types of established preventive strategies being applied to the elderly are discussed below. The authors' intention is not to be exhaustive, but rather to use these concrete examples to illustrate the state of research on the efficacy of preventive interventions in the elderly.

However, in general, the elderly have been excluded from these studies of preventive strategies. Arguments for the application of findings to this age group are frequently based on extrapolation. Yet, the authors' knowledge of aging suggests that such an approach is sometimes very hazardous.

Cardiovascular Disease

Underlying host factors that predispose a person to cardiovascular disease have been well documented in several long-term studies, such as the Framingham study,[3] and include both genetic and behavioral factors. Such underlying conditions as hypertension, hypercholesterolemia, and impaired glucose tolerance are well-known risk factors for cardiovascular disease. Although a relatively large proportion of research has gone into identifying these risk factors, relatively little research has looked at the mutability of risk in the elderly.

Cigarette smoking plays a significant role in mortality and morbidity from cardiovascular disease.[4,5] Although few specific data are available on the effects of smoking on the elderly and the benefits to them from stopping, there is considerable evidence of benefit from smoking cessation for middle-aged men.[6,7] However, much more research is needed to examine the benefits of smoking cessation directly on the elderly.

The definitive link between physical exercise and reduction in risk of cardiovascular disease has not yet been found. Although the Paffenbarger study[8] of Harvard alumni did find a modest association, one cannot blithely extrapolate from data derived from studies on middle-aged men. Even though the results of some research demonstrated that exercise may have some positive physiological effects on elderly persons,[9] there are no studies that show a decrease in risk of cardiovascular disease specifically in elderly persons as a result of physical exercise.

Poor dietary habits have also been implicated as a causal factor in cardiovascular disease.[10] Obesity has been associated with an increased risk of hypertension and hypercholesterolemia, two other well-documented risk factors for cardiovascular disease; however, it is unclear whether current obesity or a history of obesity is the risk factor. If only a long-standing history of obesity correlates positively with cardiovascular disease, then it is questionable whether weight should be considered a modifiable risk factor in the elderly. Presently, no studies have examined the effect of weight reduction on decreased risk of cardiovascular disease in the elderly.

Diets low in sodium and saturated fats and high in vegetables and fiber have also been recommended for the prevention of cardiovascular disease. Although these dietary changes have been shown to reduce the average blood pressure of the subjects,[11,12,13] it is unclear whether they actually reduce the incidence of cardiovascular disease. Long-term compliance with exercise and dietary regimens, although clearly desirable, has not proven satisfactory in the past. In addition, it has not yet been proven that late-life behavioral change will erase a lifetime of damage.

High levels of stress have been associated with hypertension and cardiovascular disease. The type A personality, characterized by impatient, time-conscious behavior and high levels of stress, appears to correlate with an increased risk of cardiovascular disease in middle-aged men. However, recent evidence suggests that aggressive, competitive behavior may have a positive effect on morbidity in elderly persons.[14] Whether this is a case of Darwinian survival of the fittest or the adaptation of new, adaptive behavior patterns remains to be seen. In any event, persons characterized by nursing home staff as belligerent and/or cantankerous have shown a better ability to achieve functional rehabilitation goals than their more passive and better-liked counterparts.[15] This phenomenon has been found serendipitously and has not been studied systematically with respect to specific diagnosis; no studies have distinguished between type A and B personalities in the elderly.

These findings are especially significant in that they illustrate the dangers inherent in extrapolating data derived from studies of younger persons to the elderly. Unfortunately, elderly persons are frequently excluded from studies that examine preventive approaches, such as smoking cessation, diet control, exercise, and stress reduction; the usual reasons given are that underlying conditions and foreshortened life expectancy make it difficult to study the effects fully. However, such findings as these emphasize the potential differences in the roles of risk factors that exist between middle-aged and elderly persons and the importance of studying the effects of interventions directly on the elderly.

Hypertension

Because hypertension is asymptomatic and decreases in blood pressure are clearly associated with reductions in risk, substantial resources have been devoted to community screening programs. Recent studies show that the proportion of persons who are aware of their blood pressure is increasing and that elderly persons are more likely to know their blood pressure than are younger persons.[16] One substantial problem with past hypertension screening efforts is that, while they may detect many cases of hypertension, they do not usually offer a satisfactory treatment program and, in fact, may be repeatedly detecting the same cases of hypertension. The low proportion of untreated and previously undetected hypertensives identified in more recent programs[17] does not appear to justify the high costs involved in continuing these screening programs.

Isolated systolic hypertension has been correlated with an increased risk of stroke,[18,19] but there is conflicting data concerning the efficacy of treatment for isolated systolic hypertension.[20,21] The data on the benefits of treating mild hypertension are even less clear. The Joint National Committee on Detection, Evaluation, and Treatment of High Blood Pressure[22] cites the findings of the Hypertension Detection and Follow-up Program to argue the benefits of treating any level of hypertension in the elderly. Elevations in diastolic blood pressure are related to an increased risk of cardiovascular death and myocardial infarction;[23] however,

overall mortality does not appear substantially different between treated and untreated persons with mild hypertension.[24]

The adverse side effects of antihypertensive medications have been well documented and include impotence, gout, impaired glucose tolerance, and postural
hypotension.[25] Although the benefits of drug treatment of high-risk patients
appear to outweigh the dangers, the data are inconclusive regarding borderline
hypertensives. Many researchers have advocated the modification of poor dietary
habits and sedentary life styles as an alternative to drug treatment of hypertension;
however, the elderly may be uninformed about the risks of poor diets and lack of
exercise. Of persons aged 65 and older, only 18 percent believe that being
overweight causes hypertension, whereas 11 percent believe excess salt, 6 percent
believe smoking, and 3 percent believe lack of exercise cause hypertension.[26]
These knowledge deficits, in turn, may be partly blamed on professionals. It is
often stated that poor compliance with behavioral change has made drug treatment
for hypertension necessary, but the survey just cited also found that 61 perent of
the elderly had never been told to go on a weight-loss diet, and only 66 percent had
been told to eat less salt to control their blood pressure. It becomes obvious that
well-designed studies are needed to determine the potential for long-term control
of hypertension in the elderly through nondrug treatments. Not only is it necessary
to determine if the nondrug treatment will, in fact, reduce blood pressure over
sustained periods of time but also the potential for actually changing an elderly
person's behavior and maintaining these changes over sustained periods must be
assessed.

Diabetes

Impaired glucose tolerance has been implicated as a risk factor for cardiovascular disease because of the high incidence of vascular complications in
persons with diabetes mellitus. The efficacy of long-term management of diabetes
in the prevention of cardiovascular disease remains unclear;[27] however, the trends
suggest a favorable prognosis with sustained close control.

Cholesterol

The association between serum cholesterol levels and cardiovascular disease
appears to be a function of the atherosclerotic lesions that may develop on the
arterial walls. The National Heart, Lung, and Blood Institute Type II Coronary
Intervention study has provided evidence that, for persons with Type II hyper-
lipidemia, or extremely elevated levels of cholesterol, treatment with the drug
cholestyramine in addition to a diet low in fat and cholesterol will lower serum
cholesterol levels.[28] The same study provides suggestive evidence that reductions
in serum levels may correspond to reductions in the incidence of coronary artery
disease.[29,30] However, studies on persons with mildly elevated levels of serum
cholesterol have not provided similarly positive results.[31] In addition, the Fra-

mingham study found that the association between serum cholesterol levels and cardiovascular disease decreases with age, having little impact on the elderly.[32]

Osteoporosis

Fractures in the elderly cause enormous disability. Hui and his colleagues[33] have estimated that low bone mass, associated with osteoporosis in elderly women, is probably the greatest determinant of fracture. Decreased calcium and Vitamin D intake[34] and decreased physical activity have been associated with a positive risk ratio for osteoporosis.[35] Many researchers advocate calcium and Vitamin D supplements and exercise regimens to reduce the loss of bone mass, although there have been no large-scale studies to determine the long-term efficacy of modification of these risk factors. Administration of estrogen appears to be the best method of arresting loss of bone mass;[36] however, estrogen alone does not reverse the symptoms of osteoporosis and is usually given in combination with Vitamin D, calcium, and fluoride. The treatment of osteoporosis with estrogens, even in low doses, is not without its risks, and adverse side effects, such as an increase in vaginal bleeding and endometrial cancer, are significantly more frequent in women taking estrogens. A recent recommendation by the American Medical Association Council on Scientific Affairs indicates:

> There is general agreement that women who undergo *premature* meno-
> pause should receive estrogen replacement, at least up to the average age
> of menopause to retard the early onset of bone loss. The election of
> estrogen replacement for this purpose in the normal menopausal patient
> can be based only on assessment of the relative risks and benefits
> applicable to the individual patient. The duration of such treatment is
> also a matter of individual judgment.[37]

The efficacy of the preventive and treatment courses of therapy for osteoporosis has not been subjected to many prospective clinical trials because of the nature of the disease. Osteoporosis is characterized by long asymptomatic periods, and the clinical course of the disease is variable. Most patients who have diminished bone mass do not develop fractures, whereas many women treated for osteoporosis still develop fractures.[38] Unfortunately, much more must be known about the specific risk factors for osteoporosis and the risks and benefits for long-term therapy before a large-scale program of prevention can begin.

Infectious Diseases

The prevention of infectious diseases is an essential component of a health promotion program for the elderly. The decreased skin thickness and altered mucosal membranes brought on by aging make the older person more susceptible to infection, as does the decreased immune response. Malnutrition has been linked to immune deficiency,[39] possibly because of a reduction in body vitamin or zinc concentration.[40] However, not enough is known about the various roles of these nutrients to recommend a specific diet for the prevention of infectious diseases.

The Public Health Service has recommended influenza vaccination for populations at high risk, but only 20 percent of the elderly receive these vaccines.[41] Several studies have concluded that pneumococcal pneumonia vaccine is more cost-effective for the elderly.[42,43] At the same time, several questions have been raised about the efficacy of these vaccines in the elderly. The elderly show a poorer antibody response than do younger people and thus do not respond as well to vaccines.[44] Preliminary trials of the pneumococcal pneumonia vaccine showed a 75 to 95 percent efficacy in young, healthy adults. More recent evidence shows a mean efficacy closer to 36 percent in the elderly population.[45] More evidence is needed before vaccination can be recommended as a national program for the prevention of pneumonia in persons at high risk.

Rehabilitation

Stroke

Although modifying risk factors and treating diseases early in their course are obviously desirable, health promotion also includes the rehabilitation and subsequent reduction of disability throughout the course of the disease. Rehabilitation has become an accepted part of treatment following stroke. Because a randomized trial to determine the benefits of rehabilitation versus no rehabilitation would surely be ruled out on ethical grounds, studies must be confined to assessing the relative benefits of different intensities of rehabilitation given in different settings on different levels of impairment. It is generally accepted that intensive rehabilitation after stroke is not indicated for all patients.[46] Patients who are unconscious during acute stroke are likely to remain dependent, and patients who remain conscious and are able to walk unaided generally exhibit spontaneous functional recovery.[47] Consequently, the results of clinical studies that do not differentiate between the levels of initial impairment may be biased.

A recent, well-designed study[48] showed that patients receiving intensive rehabilitation in a specialized stroke unit experienced greater functional recovery in a shorter time than did patients given traditional rehabilitation on the medical wards. As representative of patients likely to survive but unlikely to experience spontaneous recovery, the investigators selected patients who remained conscious during acute stroke but who exhibited developed or established hemiplegia. Therefore, they could validly compare the two intensities of treatment. Another study found that age (under 80), sex, and presence of concurrent medical conditions did not affect functional outcomes after rehabilitation, suggesting that the degree of impairment is a valid criterion for patient grouping.[49]

Heart Disease

There is active interest in rehabilitation—usually in the form of exercise regimens but including drugs, stress reduction, and other techniques—after the episode of coronary heart disease has been resolved. The elderly have generally been excluded from such efforts or have not been examined as a specific subgroup.

Several classes of drugs may be used to prevent a recurrence of coronary heart disease. Medical treatment with antiarrhythmics has not proven successful in clinical trials. Although the results are not statistically significant, the outcome of the control groups, in terms of mortality, appeared better than the treated groups. The beta-blocker and platelet-active drugs appeared to exert an overall positive effect in several trials.[50] A small daily dose of aspirin has proven beneficial in the prevention of recurrent myocardial infarction.[51,52] Although the overall picture is mixed, exercise rehabilitation programs appeared to exert a positive effect by reducing mortality in several trials.[53] Coronary bypass surgery has proven successful in patients with more than one coronary artery affected.[54]

The benefit of intensive rehabilitation after the manifestation of coronary heart disease is not as well substantiated as is rehabilitation after stroke. The goals of cardiac rehabilitation include improved quality of life, enhanced risk-factors modification, and improved ability to perform such activities as recreational exercise, work, or sex.[55] A controlled study of the effect of an intensive exercise program showed improved ability. However, the improvement was apparent only in formal testing; it did not appear to reflect a significant difference in actual activity.[56] More evidence is needed before physical rehabilitation after coronary heart disease can be recommended for widespread use.

Fracture

Hip fracture is probably the most debilitating type of fracture suffered by the elderly. An important factor in recovery is a total rehabilitation program, which includes both physical and occupational therapy.[57] Early fixation of the fracture, early mobilization, and early weight bearing appear to be instrumental in successful rehabilitation and prevention of loss of independence. In a study comparing early (one day postoperatively) and late (two to three weeks postoperatively) weight bearing, length of stay was found to be considerably shorter (27 versus 44 days), and a greater proportion of patients were able to be discharged directly home with rehabilitation utilizing early weight bearing.[58]

After hip fractures, patients generally require more assistance with activities of daily living, even after receiving intensive rehabilitation. A greater proportion of patients are able to return home if they live with someone else; due to a combination of the physical assistance and psychological support provided.[59,60] In a study assessing hospital rehabilitation one year after fracture, the proportion of patients utilizing some form of home-help services increased from 29 percent before fracture to 62 percent.[61] Although specialized rehabilitation clinics provide a more intensive level of rehabilitation than do nursing homes, one study concluded that patients discharged from specialized rehabilitation clinics ultimately used more social services, such as Meals-on-Wheels and home help, than did patients discharged from nursing homes after rehabilitation for hip fractures,[62] implying that nursing homes may be more cost-effective than are the specialized rehabilitation clinics. However, simply determining the utilization of services is not an optimal way to determine the functional ability of elderly persons. Although the provision of social services may imply a loss of function, it may also signify the greater ability of rehabilitation clinics to return patients to the community with less functional ability. If the rehabilitation clinics are able to discharge patients to the community who would otherwise be institutionalized, even the increased use of social services would not negate the financial savings and increased quality of life of the elderly patient.

The sparse data on rehabilitation after hip fracture leave many unanswered questions. It is not clear what the differences are between patients who benefit greatly from rehabilitation and those who do not or whether those differences can be modified. Although the intensity and setting of rehabilitation may be important in aiding functional recovery, few studies have compared results by randomly allocating patients to different rehabilitation programs. Clearly, much more research is needed before we can determine the most effective way to prevent much of the disability and institutionalization resulting from hip fracture.

General Behaviors

Many health promotion programs focus on the modification of personal habits to effect a reduction in the risk of chronic diseases. In general, the evidence linking behavioral changes to reduced risk of disease is fragmentary at best. However, even those behaviors without any clear-cut evidence of benefit may be worthy of encouragement because they are more likely to do good than harm.[63] Some offer a direct benefit by increasing a sense of well-being or social participation; others involve some sacrifice of immediate gratification. All are potential vehicles for exploitation, especially economic exploitation of the economically marginal elderly. Various unnecessary or ineffective services may be sold to those least able to afford them.

Smoking

The evidence linking smoking behavior with increased risk of mortality and morbidity from cardiovascular disease, stroke, and a variety of cancers is perhaps the best substantiated of all the behavioral risk factors. In a study to determine the smoking habits and related mortality of a defined population, Scholl estimated that one-third of all deaths occurring in men aged 50 to 60 could have been avoided if all smokers had quit at age 50.[64] Although decreases in the incidence of lung cancer are not seen until several years after cessation, rates of coronary heart disease, chronic bronchitis, and emphysema exhibit a rapid turnaround with smoking cessation. Some evidence points to a decrease in mortality after quitting for one to four years in men aged 50 to 69.[65] Although the benefits of smoking cessation should not be extrapolated to the elderly from studies done on middle-aged men, the evidence suggests a reduction in risk with cessation in the elderly.

Diet

The evidence linking dietary modifications with reduction in risk of disease is not as well substantiated as that with smoking cessation. Dietary modifications include a wide variety of changes from caloric restriction to adding or deleting specific food components. The dangers of obesity have probably been exaggerated, and no compelling evidence is available to support active weight reduction in the elderly except those well above—50 percent or more—ideal body weight.[66] Reduced intake of specific constitutents usually means limiting salt and saturated fats. Sodium reduction has been shown to reduce hypertension: A 25 percent reduction in salt intake may be associated with a 5 to 10 mm Hg reduction in blood pressure.[67]

A reduction in saturated fat intake has been shown to reduce blood pressure in normotensive subjects,[68,69] but no studies have examined the effect on elderly subjects at high risk. There is presently no conclusive evidence establishing that reductions in saturated fat intake in persons with normal or mildly elevated serum cholesterol levels will decrease the risk of cardiovascular disease.

Dietary modification in the form of vitamin supplements raises special concerns. The recommended daily allowance of calcium and Vitamin D is likely too low, and inexpensive supplements are indicated to prevent osteoporosis. However, there is no good evidence to support the widespread use of general-purpose vitamins. The elderly seeking longevity and vitality may be especially vulnerable to the promises of those making unsubstantiated claims for large doses of these substances. Schneider and Nordlund[70] canvassed community-based elderly in Ohio and found that about half their sample were using some kind of vitamin or mineral supplement. Use was directly correlated with age and *inversely* correlated with income. In only half the instances was the supplement recommended by health care providers. The authors also discuss two common misconceptions: The value of the supplement increases with its price, and the larger the dose, the more beneficial the result.

Exercise

Although the role of exercise in preventing heart disease and controlling arthritis in elderly persons is unclear, several studies have shown positive physiological responses to exercise in elderly subjects.[71,72] The Paffenbarger study of

Harvard alumni found a modest association between lack of physical exercise and risk of stroke in middle-aged men; present nonparticipation in athletics was a much stronger risk factor than previous nonparticipation.[73] A growing body of reports suggests that exercise may play a positive role in delaying osteoporosis, but the results to date cannot permit a definitive recommendation.[74,75,76]

Social Isolation

The correlation between social isolation and subsequent risk of morbidity and mortality has prompted a number of innovative interventions targeted at the elderly. Although the anecdotal data from these activities are impressive, clear scientific evidence of reduced risk is not yet available. One reason for this lack of evidence may be that these interventions generally do not take into account the individual's lifetime history of socialization. There is no basis for anticipating benefit from socialization for individuals who have pursued an isolated life style throughout most of their adult life, but those recently isolated by bereavement or loss, where the isolation exacerbates other stresses facing them, may indeed be helped. Another reason is the lack of a good definition for social isolation. At present, it is unclear whether social isolation and subsequent risk of mortality are a result of the lack of interpersonal relationships or the lack of support—either emotional or instrumental—derived from those relationships.[77]

Functional Impairment

As they age, the elderly are more likely to suffer from chronic impairment and disability. An important part of any health promotion plan should examine the effects of interventions to prevent or minimize functional impairment from such conditions as hearing loss, visual impairment, dental problems, and incontinence. Unfortunately, little is known about the natural course of these conditions and the risk factors that, if modified, may prevent or delay impairment. Longitudinal studies following cohorts of elderly persons are rare, and such studies almost never include information on functional status. Reasons for the lack of data on functional impairments in the elderly include the commonly held belief that declines in functional status are inevitable and social taboos that militate against voluntary reporting of early manifestations. More research is needed to understand these conditions and enable the development of a health prevention strategy targeted at high-risk individuals.

Nursing Home Admission

Finally, an important goal for health promotion in the elderly is the prevention of unnecessary admissions to nursing homes. Studies that follow elderly community-based persons to determine the characteristics of those who enter residential care are rare and may be limited in the amount of medical data included.[78,79,80,81] Demonstration projects attempting to prevent nursing home admission in a cost-effective manner have produced mixed results. More research is needed to identify the risk factors associated with nursing home admission in order to target interventions at those with high risk.

CONCLUSION

The field of health promotion and disease prevention suffers from a general lack of attention to the elderly. Although clinicians and health professionals are beginning to recognize the need to include older persons in activities aimed at preventing future diseases and disability, there is a serious lack of scientific data to direct them in their attempts. At present, the majority of popular health promotion and disease prevention interventions directed at the elderly derive their expected benefit from data on middle-aged men or, worse yet, from secondary associations without clear-cut evidence of merit. Although some preliminary results may appear promising, many issues need to be resolved before health professionals can unconditionally call for these interventions to be encouraged for the elderly as part of a national emphasis on health promotion.

Although many studies have already discovered risk factors for heart disease, cancer, and stroke, data remain scarce on the relative importance of these risk factors in the elderly. The Framingham studies[82] and the Alameda County studies[83] are examples of existing longitudinal studies that can be used to address specific questions about risk factors in the elderly. These studies have long periods of follow-up that establish the relationship between the existence and persistence of risk factors and consequent morbidity. Other lines of research should begin to establish the incidence, prevalence, and risk factors for functional disabilities not usually followed, such as hearing and vision impairments and incontinence. Each of these conditions can dramatically impair the elderly person's functioning; however, not enough is known at present to recommend a plan for their prevention.

Elderly persons should also be included in studies that examine the effects of preventive approaches, such as diet control, weight control, stress reduction, hypertension control, and cancer screening. For example, the MRFIT study to modify risk factors for cardiovascular disease included only men aged 35 to 57[84] (MRFIT Research Group, 1982), and the North Karelia study in Finland included persons aged 25 to 59.[85] Older persons are inappropriately excluded with the best of intentions. Often-cited reasons are that multiple diagnoses cloud interpretation of the data, and foreshortened life expectancy may make it difficult to study effects fully. Yet, to explore interventions with the elderly, it is important to be able to study the relationships in just those situations with multiple diagnoses. Elderly persons included in intervention studies should be specifically stratified to include both those with long-standing and those with newly acquired risk factors.

Particular attention must be paid to teasing out the importance of various behaviors as risks for the elderly. Serious gaps exist in our knowledge about the mutability of such risks and, therefore, the pay-off in stopping or starting various behaviors at different ages and in the presence of specific conditions. Concerns about the elderly have focused on both the value and the feasibility of intervention, but more recent experience offers much optimism about the feasibility of behavior change. The goals of such research should include identifying factors that suggest an older person is likely to change his or her behavior.

Improving our understanding of intervention and treatments requires clinical research. More effective intervention techniques are needed, especially for the improvement of functioning and the minimizing of disability and handicap. Clinical trials including the elderly should be encouraged. As discussed previously, it is important to study the effects of interventions in elderly persons with multiple diagnoses to obtain a true indication of efficacy in that population.

Health professionals have made a positive step in their new interest in health promotion and disease prevention in the elderly. It is now necessary to evaluate existing interventions in terms of their efficacy in the elderly and encourage new research to increase knowledge in this field. Although it is easy to point out deficiencies in existing knowledge, it is much more difficult to contend with the practical issues of study design and stiff competition for funding. Indeed, it is impractical to restudy all established interventions for their efficacy in the elderly; however, new studies should certainly include a cross-section of elderly subjects representative of the groups targeted for the specific intervention. Health professionals should be aware of the limitations of existing research and avoid making unsubstantiated claims about the potential effects of prevention on elderly persons. For the moment, we must balance the need for optimism about prevention, to counter the stereotypes of aging with caution in the light of poorly established effectiveness. The enthusiasm for a preventive practice should be tempered by the same concerns about the ratio of benefits to risks that are applied to any intervention with the elderly.

NOTES

1. A.L. Stewart, R.H. Brook, and R.L. Kane, *Conceptualization and Measurement of Health Habits for Adults in the Health Insurance Study: Vol. II, Overweight* (R-2374/2-HEW) (Santa Monica, Ca.: The Rand Corporation, 1980).

2. J.G. Evans, "Stroke Predictors," in *Advanced Medicine–18*, ed. M. Sarner (London: Pitman Books, 1982), pp. 288–301.

3. W.B. Kannel, and T. Gordon, "Cardiovascular Risk Factors in the Aged: The Framingham Study," in *Second Conference on the Epidemiology of Aging*, ed. S.G. Haynes and M. Feinlieb (NIH Pub. No. 80–969).

4. L.M. Schuman, "Smoking as a Risk Factor in Longevity," in *Aging: A Challenge to Science and Society*, ed. D. Danon, N.W. Shock, and M. Marois (Oxford: Oxford University Press, 1981), pp. 204–218.

5. J.L. Izzo, "Hypertension in the Elderly: A Pathophysiologic Approach to Therapy," *Journal of the American Geriatric Society* 30 (1982): 352–359.

6. N. Scholl, "Smoking Habits in the Glostrub Population of Men and Women, Born in 1914," *Acta Med. Scand.* 208 (1980): 245–256.

7. L.M. Schuman, *op. cit.*, pp. 204–218.

8. R.S. Paffenbarger, Jr., "Early Predictors of Chronic Disease," in *Social Factors in Prevention*, ed. R.C. Jackson, J. Morton, and M. Sierra Franco (Berkeley, Ca.: University of California Public Health Social Work Program, 1979), pp. 111–119.

9. J.L. Hodgson and E.R. Buskirk, "Physical Fitness and Age, with Emphasis on Cardiovascular Function in the Elderly," *Journal of the American Geriatrics Society* 25, no. 9 (1977): 385–392.

10. A.L. Stewart, R.H. Brook, and R.L. Kane, *op. cit.*

11. P. Puska et al., "Controlled, Randomized Trial of the Effect of Dietary Fat on Blood Pressure," *Lancet* 1, no. 8314/5 (1983): 1–5.

12. I.L. Rouse et al., "Blood-Pressure-Lowering Effect of a Vegetarian Diet: Controlled Trial in Normotensive Subjects," *Lancet* 1, no. 8314/5 (1983): 5–10.

13. J.L. Izzo, *op. cit.*, pp. 352–59.

14. J. Sparacino, "The Type A (Coronary-Prone) Behavior Pattern, Aging, and Mortality," *Journal of the American Geriatrics Society* 27 (1979): 251–257.

15. E.M. Brody et al., "Excess Disabilities of Mentally Impaired Aged: Impact of Individualized Treatment," *Gerontologist* 11 (1971): 124–132.

16. R.H. Brook et al., *Conceptualization and Measurement of Physiologic Health for Adults: Hypertension* (R–2262/3 HHS) (Santa Monica, Ca.: The Rand Corporation, 1981).

17. A.R. Folsom et al., "Improvements in Hypertension Detection and Control from 1973–1974 to 1980–1981—The Minnesota Heart Survey Experience," *Journal of the American Medical Association* 250 (1983): 916–921.

18. M.R. Stegman and G.O. Williams, "The Elderly Hypertensive: A Neglected Patient?," *Journal of Family Practice* 16 (1983): 259–262.

19. W.B. Kannel et al., "Epidemiologic Features of Chronic Atrial Fibrillation," *New England Journal of Medicine* 306 (1981): 1018–1022.

20. Joint National Committee on Detection, Evaluation, and Treatment of High Blood Pressure, "The 1980 Report of the Joint National Committee on Detection, Evaluation, and Treatment of High Blood Pressure," *Archives of Internal Medicine* 140 (1980): 1280–1285.

21. J.L. Izzo, *op. cit.*, pp. 352–359.

22. Joint National Committee on Detection, Evaluation, and Treatment of High Blood Pressure, *op. cit.*, pp. 1280–1285.

23. M.R. Stegman and G. O. Williams, *op. cit.*, pp. 259–262.

24. E.D. Freis, "Should Mild Hypertension Be Treated?," *New England Journal of Medicine* 307 (1982): 306–309.

25. M.F. Oliver, "Risk of Correcting the Risks of Coronary Disease and Stroke with Drugs," *New England Journal of Medicine* 306 (1982): 297–298.

26. Urban Behavioral Research Associates, Inc., 1981. *The Public and High Blood Pressure: Six-Year Followup Survey of Public Knowledge and Reported Behavior* (NIH Pub. No. 81–2118).

27. R.H. Brook et al., *Conceptualization and Measurement of Physiologic Health for Adults: Diabetes Mellitus* (R-2262/7 HHS) (Santa Monica, Ca.: The Rand Corporation, 1981).

28. J.F. Brensike et al., "Effects of Therapy with Cholestyramine on Progression of Coronary Arteriosclerosis: Results of the NHLBI Type II Coronary Intervention Study," *Circulation* 2 (1984): 313–324.

29. R.I. Levy et al., "The Influence of Changes in Lipid Values Induced by Cholestyramine and Diet on Progression of Coronary Artery Disease: Results of the NHLBI Type II Coronary Intervention Study," *Circulation* 69 (1984): 325–337.

30. "The Lipid Research Clinics Coronary Primary Prevention Trial Results Part 1: Reduction in Incidence of Coronary Heart Disease; Part 2: Relationship of Reduction in Incidence of Coronary Heart Disease to Cholesterol Lowering," *Journal of the American Medical Association* 251 (1984): 351–374.

31. R.H. Brook et al., *Conceptualization and Measurement of Physiologic Health for Adults: Hypercholesterolemia* (R–2262/11 HHS) (Santa Monica, Ca.: The Rand Corporation, 1981).

32. W.B. Kannel and T. Gordon, *op. cit.*

33. S.L. Hui et al., "A Prospective Study of Change in Bone Mass with Age in Postmenopausal Women," *Journal of Chronic Diseases* 35 (1982): 715–725.

34. L.G. Raisz, "Osteoporosis," *Journal of the American Geriatrics Society* 30 (1982): 127–138.

35. J.F. Aloia, "Exercise and Skeletal Health," *Journal of the American Geriatrics Society* 29 (1981): 104–107.

36. J.C. Stevenson et al., "Calcitonin and the Calcium Regulating Hormone in Postmenopausal Women: Effects of Estrogens," *Lancet* 1 (1981): 693–695.

37. American Medical Association Council on Scientific Affairs, "Estrogen Replacement in the Menopause," *Journal of the American Medical Association* 249 (1983): 359.

38. L.G. Raisz, *op. cit.,* pp. 127–138.

39. R.K. Chandra, "Nutrition, Immunity, and Infection: Present Knowledge and Future Directions," *Lancet* 1, no. 8326 (1983): 688–691.

40. E.L. Schneider, "Infectious Diseases in the Elderly," *Annals of Internal Medicine* 98 (1983): 395–400.

41. F.L. Ruben, "Prevention of Influenza in the Elderly," *Journal of the American Geriatrics Society* 30 (1982): 577–580.

42. J.S. Willems et al., "Cost Effectiveness of Vaccination Against Pneumococcal Pneumonia," *New England Journal of Medicine* 303 (1980): 553–559.

43. K.M. Patrick and F.R. Wooley, "Cost-Benefit Analyses of Immunization for Pneumococcal Pneumonia," *Journal of the American Medical Association* 245 (1981): 473–477.

44. E.L. Schneider, *op. cit.,* pp. 395–400.

45. C.V. Broome, R.R. Facklam, and D.W. Fraser, "Pneumococcal Disease after Pneumococcal Vaccination: An Alternative Method to Estimate the Efficacy of Pneumococcal Vaccine," *New England Journal of Medicine* 303 (1980): 549–552.

46. K. Sheikh, "Evaluation of Stroke Rehabilitation," *Journal of Chronic Diseases* 36 (1983): 427.

47. W.M. Garroway et al., "The Triage of Stroke Rehabilitation," *Journal of Epidemiology and Community Health* 35 (1981): 39–44.

48. *Ibid.,* pp. 39–44.

49. J.S. Fergenson, "Stroke Rehabilitation: Effectiveness, Benefits, and Costs—Some Practical Considerations," *Stroke* 10 (1979): 1–3.

50. G.S. May et al., "Secondary Prevention after Myocardial Infarction: A Review of Long Term Trials," *Progress in Cardiovascular Disease* 24 (1982): 331–352.

51. M.G. Bousser et al., "AICLA: Controlled Trial of Aspirin and Dipyridamole in the Secondary Prevention of Athero-Thrombotic Cerebral Ischemia," *Stroke* 14 (1983): 5–14.

52. Enquete de Prevention Secondaire de l'Infarctus du Myocarde (EPSIM) Research Group "A Controlled Comparison of Aspirin and Oral Anticoagulants in Prevention of Death after Myocardial Infarction," *New England Journal of Medicine* 307 (1982): 701–708.

53. G.S. May, *op. cit.*, pp. 331–352.

54. European Coronary Surgery Study Group, "Long-Term Results of Prospective Randomised Study of Coronary Artery Bypass Surgery in Stable Angina Pectoris," *Lancet* 2, no. 8309 (1982): 1173–1180.

55. P. Greenland, "Cardiac Fitness and Rehabilitation in the Elderly," *Journal of the American Geriatrics Society* 30 (1982): 607–611.

56. R. Mayou et al., "Early Rehabilitation after Myocardial Infarction," *Lancet* 2, no. 8260/1 (1981): 1399–1401.

57. "Old Woman with a Broken Hip," *Lancet* 2, no. 8295 (1982): 419–420.

58. L. Ceder et al., "Rehabilitation after Hip Fracture in the Elderly," *Acta Orthop. Scand.* 50 (1979): 681–688.

59. *Ibid.*, pp. 681–688.

60. H.W. Nickens, "A Review of Factors Affecting the Occurrence and Outcome of Hip Fracture, with Special References to Psychosocial Issues," *Journal of the American Geriatrics Society* 31 (1983): 166–170.

61. L. Ceder, *op. cit.*, pp. 681–688.

62. J.S. Jensen, E. Tondevald, and P.H. Sorensen, "Social Rehabilitation following Hip Fracture," *Acta Orthop. Scand.* 50 (1979): 777–785.

63. A. Warner-Reitz, *A Health Lifestyle for Seniors: An Interdisciplinary Approach to Healthy Aging* (New York: Meals for Millions/Freedom from Hunger Foundation, 1981).

64. M. Scholl, *op. cit.*, pp. 254–256.

65. L.M. Schuman, *op. cit.*, pp. 204–218.

66. A.L. Stewart, R.H. Brook, and R.L. Kane, *op. cit.*

67. J.L. Izzo, *op cit.*, pp. 359–362.

68. P. Puska et al., *op cit.*, pp. 1173–1178.

69. I.L. Rouse et al., *op. cit.*, pp. 5–10.

70. C.L. Schneider and D.J. Nordlund, "Prevalence of Vitamin and Mineral Supplement Use in the Elderly," *Journal of Family Practice* 17 (1983): 243–247.

71. J.L. Hodgson and E.R. Buskirk, "Effects of Environmental Factors and Life Patterns on Life Span," in *Aging: A Challenge to Science and Society*, ed. D. Danon, N.W. Schock, and M. Marois (Oxford: Oxford University Press, 1981), pp. 189–196.

72. P. Franks, P.R. Lee, and J.E. Fullarton, *Lifetime Fitness and Exercise for Older People* (San Francisco: Aging Health Policy Center, 1983).

73. R.S. Paffenbarger, Jr., *op. cit.*, pp. 111–119.

74. J.F. Aloia, *op. cit.*, pp. 104–107.

75. E.L. Smith, W. Reddan, and P.E. Smith, "Physical Activity and Calcium Modality for Bone Mineral Increase in Aged Women," *Medicine and Science in Sports* 13 (1981): 60–64.

76. E.L. Smith and W. Reddan, "Physical Activity—A Modality for Bone Accretion in the Aged," *American Journal of Roentgenology* 126 (1976): 1297.

77. L.F. Berkman, "The Assessment of Social Networks and Social Support in the Elderly," *Journal of the American Geriatrics Society* 31 (1983): 743–749.

78. B. Havens, "A Longitudinal Study of Manitobans," *Essence* 3 (1980): 125–142.

79. A.J. Stark, G.M. Gutman, and B. McCashin, "Acute Care Hospitalizations and Long Term Care," *Journal of the American Geriatrics Society* 30 (1982): 509–515.

80. A.J. Stark et al., "Placement Changes in Long-Term Care: Three Years' Experience," *American Journal of Public Health* 74 (1984): 459–463.

81. J.M. Mossey and E. Shapiro, "Self Rated Health: A Predictor of Mortality among the Elderly," *American Journal of Public Health* 72 (1982): 800–808.

82. W.B. Kannel et al., *op. cit.*, 1918–1022.

83. L. Berkman and L. Breslow, *Health and Ways of Living* (Oxford: Oxford University Press, 1983).

84. Multiple Risk Factor Intervention Trial (MRFIT) Research Group, "Multiple Risk Factor Intervention Trial: Risk Factor Changes and Mortality Results," *Journal of the American Medical Association* 248 (1982): 1465–1477.

85. P. Puska et al., "Changes in Coronary Risk Factors during Comprehensive Five-Year Community Programme to Control Cardiovascular Diseases (North Karelia Project)," *British Medical Journal* 2 (1979): 473–477.

Index

A

Congregate housing , 119
Congregate meals, 284, 307
Constancy of behavior, 122
Consultation in community, 142, 143
Consumer role
  of community, 278
  of nursing home residents, 129
  of patients, 278
Continuation of program, 272
Continuing education (CE), 81
  grants for, 78
Continuum of care, 120-129
Contraindications
  for drugs, 292
  for exercise, 171, 172
Control, 304
Control Data Corporation, 158
  STAYWELL program of, 159-160
Cookbooks, 283
Cooperative food purchasing clubs,
  41
Cooperative Health Education Project
  (CHEP), 76
Coordinating Council for Senior
  Citzens, Durham, North Carolina,
  113
Coors Industries, 155
Coping skills, 40, 138
Copper, 188
Core instructors, 238-240
Cornell Medical Center, 251
Coronary artery disease (CAD), 170,
  171, 209
  in centenarians, 204
  and exercise, 167
  symptoms of, 171
Coronary bypass surgery, 335
Coronary heart disease. *See* Coronary
  artery disease (CAD)
Corporate contributions committees, 95
Corporate culture, 147
Corporations
  See also specific companies
  funding from, 91-96, 98
  in-kind donations by, 98
  medical departments of, 150

Costs
  containment of, 315-316, 319
  health care. *See* Health care costs
  hospital care, 120
  medical care, 92
  program, 245, 260, 318
  psychoanalytic service, 139
Coumadin, 295, 296
Council on Aging, 15
  See also Office of Aging
Council of Financial Aid to Education, 93
Council of Foundations, 93
Council on Scientific Affairs, AMA,
  333
Counseling, 142-143, 145, 282
  drug, 291
  life-style change, 76
  one-to-one medical, 67
  patient, 79
County Senior Councils, 141
Couple-oriented society, 135
Crapo, Lawrence, 19, 62, 63
Credibility of program, 270
Cremmins, James C., 102
Crime, 136, 305, 306
  reduction in, 41
"Critical consciousness" education,
  304, 305, 306
Cross-sectional studies, 49
Curriculum, 229-230, 238, 240-241
Cutler, Neal, 15
Cycling, 166, 170

D

Dairy products, 181, 182, 186, 206
  See also specific products
  nonfat, 184
Dartmouth Institute for Better Health
  (DIBH), 235, 236
Dartmouth Medical School, Hanover,
  New Hampshire, 236, 238
Dartmouth Self-Care for Senior
  Citizens Program, 235-245
Davies, David, 207, 208

H

Hammond, E. Cuyler, 204
"Happy Hoofers," 269
Hardening of arteries, 190
Harnes, Curtis, 209
Hartford Foundation, 76
Harvard University, 201, 330
 Medical School of, 81
 School of Public Health of, 154
Hawaiian "Iron Man Competition," 11
HCFA. *See* Health Care Financing
 Administration
HDL-C. *See* High-density lipoprotein
 cholesterol
Health
 biomedical definitions of, 56, 57, 61
 defined, 51-52, 55, 56, 57, 58, 61, 65, 80
 environmental determinants of, 66
 individual self-responsibility for,
  250, 263
 information on, 72
 knowledge on, 243
 measurement of, 271
 monitoring of, 40
 optimum, 321
 social determinants of, 66
Health age, 263
Health agency networks, 90
Health aids, 267
Health care
 See also Medical care
 access to, 63
 continuum of, 120-129
 goals of, 73-74
 home. *See* Home care
 inappropriate utilization of, 248
 institutional. *See* Institutionalization
 organization of, 71
 preventive. *See* Prevention
 quality of, 63, 289
 self-responsibility in, 105
 in senior centers, 110-111
 and social policy, 55-67
 team for, 77
 utilization of, 282

Health care costs, 60
 individual responsibility for, 61
Health Care Financing Administration
 (HCFA), 76, 89, 271
Health care insurance, 57
Health care personnel
 See also specific occupations
 education of, 46, 71-84, 143-144, 294
 roles of, 45-46
 training of, 71-84
Health education, 62, 67, 247, 255-257,
 260, 270, 275, 276, 297, 306
Health fairs, 152, 153, 284
Health Guard, 150
Health habits, 243
Health history forms, 250
Health insurance, 76
Health maintenance, 45, 76, 80
Health maintenance organizations
 (HMO), 76, 316
 senior center link with, 115
Health Professions Education
 Assistance Act, 78
Health promotion, defined, 52
Health Promotion with Elders project,
 New Mexico, 219, 220, 221, 223, 225
Health Promotion with the Elderly
 Project, School of Social Work,
 University of Washington, 80
Health promotion specialists, 270
Health Resources and Services
 Administration, DHHS, 81
Health status, 56, 304
 individual responsibility for, 65
Health systems agencies (HSA), 318
Health and welfare insurance, 232
Health and Welfare Trust, Storeworkers
 Union, New York City, 148
Healthwise Program, 263-273
Healthy Lifestyles for Seniors (HLS)
 program, New York, 230
Healthy Lifestyles for Seniors (HLS)
 program, Santa Monica, 221-232
*Healthy People: The Surgeon General's
 Report on Health Promotion and
 Disease Prevention*, 21, 64, 71, 88

Medical care
See also Health care
costs of, 92
seperation of wellness from, 84
Medical care model, 39, 120
vs. social care model, 130
Medical counseling, 67
Medical credibility of program, 270
"Medic Alert," 284
Medical establishment dominance, 65
Medical evaluation before exercise,
170-172
Medical insurance, 67
Medical professions
See also Physicians; specific
occupations
education of in aging, 78-79
Medical schools, 78
teaching hospital affiliation with, 79
Medical screening programs, 149
Medical self-care, 240, 243, 244, 266,
282
Medical/social model of chronic care,
120
Medicare, 15, 45, 48, 56, 57, 60, 65,
67, 76, 87, 88, 89, 92, 100, 120,
129, 130, 134, 140, 249, 271
Medications. *See* Drugs
Megatrends, 290
Memberships, 99
Memorandum of Understanding, Office
of the Surgeon General, 89
Memory, 137
aids to, 294
loss of, 12
Mental faculties, 190
Mental health services, 136, 139-145
for employees, 152
escorts to, 144
funding of, 140
institutionalization stigma of, 141
negative attitudes of elderly toward,
140-141, 142
sliding fee scale for, 143
stigmatization of, 141
youth-orientation of, 139-140

Mental Health Systems Act, 140
Mental illness, 12
See also specific types
worker's compensation awards for, 157
Mental stimulation, 213
Mercy Medical Center, Denver, 47
Metabolism
abnormalities in, 184, 187
carbohydrate, 182, 187, 190
drug, 296
rate of, 180
vitamin D, 191
Mettler, Molly H., 219
MFMFFH. *See* Meals for Millions/
Freedom from Hunger Foundation
Miami, Florida, 236
Michaelangelo, 13
Microlevel empowerment, 304
Middlescence (young old), 14, 15
Milio, N., 51
Milk, 189, 206
Mineral oil, 191
Minerals, 184
See also specific minerals
Minimarkets, 308
Minkler, Meredith, 39, 63
Mixtures of drugs. *See* Interactions
of drugs
Mobile minimarkets, 308
Moderate aortic stenosis, 172
Modernization, 214
Monitoring
of compliance, 294
of drug interactions, 295-297
of drug side effects, 295
of drug therapy, 290-297
of health, 40
Monoamine oxidase inhibitors, 191
Monroe Senior Citizens Center, Monroe
County, Michigan, 111
Mood changes, 170
Morale, 317
Morbidity, 76
See also Disease
compression of, 34-37, 76-77
premature, 63